Pharmacology Clear & Simple

A Drug Classifications & Dosage Calculations Approach

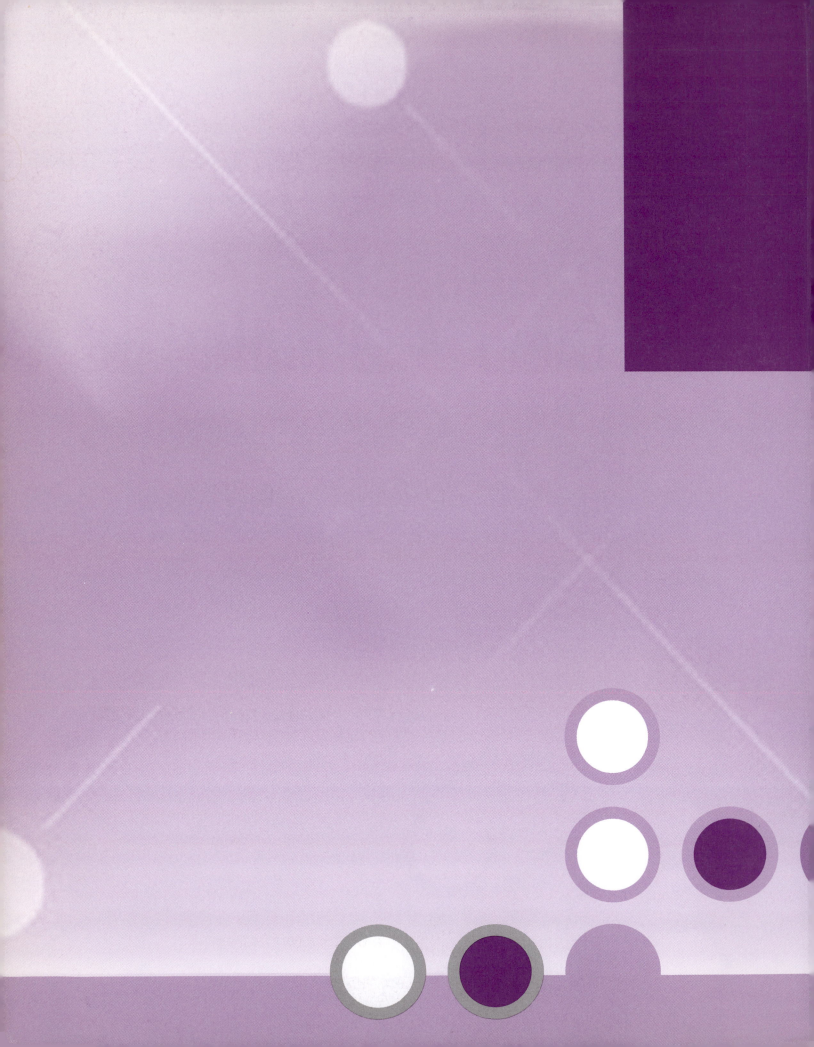

Pharmacology Clear & Simple

A Drug Classifications & Dosage Calculations Approach

NINA BEAMAN, MS, RN,C, CMA(AAMA)
Allied Health (Medical Assisting) Subject Area Coordinator
Bryant & Stratton College
Richmond Campus
Richmond, Virginia

F. A. DAVIS COMPANY • Philadelphia

F. A. Davis Company
1915 Arch Street
Philadelphia, PA 19103
www.fadavis.com

Printed in the United States of America

Last digit indicates print number: 10 9 8 7 6 5 4 3

Publisher: Margaret M. Biblis
Acquisitions Editor: Andy McPhee
Developmental Editors: Jennifer A. Pine, Yvonne N. Gillam
Manager of Content Development: Deborah J. Thorp
Art and Design Manager: Carolyn O'Brien
Illustrator: Laurie O'Keefe

As new scientific information becomes available through basic and clinical research, recommended treatments and drug therapies undergo changes. The author(s) and publisher have done everything possible to make this book accurate, up to date, and in accord with accepted standards at the time of publication. The author(s), editors, and publisher are not responsible for errors or omissions or for consequences from application of the book, and make no warranty, expressed or implied, in regard to the contents of the book. Any practice described in this book should be applied by the reader in accordance with professional standards of care used in regard to the unique circumstances that may apply in each situation. The reader is advised always to check product information (package inserts) for changes and new information regarding dose and contraindications before administering any drug. Caution is especially urged when using new or infrequently ordered drugs.

Library of Congress Cataloging-in-Publication Data

Beaman, Nina.
  Pharmacology clear & simple : a drug classifications & dosage calculations approach / Nina Beaman.
      p. ; cm.
  Includes bibliographical references and index.
  ISBN-13: 978-0-8036-1239-6
  ISBN-10: 0-8036-1239-7
  1. Pharmacology. 2. Allied health personnel. 3. Drugs—Dosage. 4. Drugs—Classification.
  I. Title. II. Title: Pharmacology clear and simple.
  [DNLM: 1. Pharmaceutical Preparations—administration & dosage—Problems and Exercises.
  2. Allied Health Personnel—Problems and Exercises. 3. Dosage Forms—Problems and Exercises.
  4. Drug Administration Routes—Problems and Exercises. 5. Medication Errors—prevention & control—Problems and Exercises. QV 18.2 B366p 2008]
  RM300.B33 2008
  615′.1—dc22   2007037440

Dedication

Certainly, I wish to thank my parents, Chester and Mary Beaman, for encouraging me to always strive for the best at everything I do. I could not have written this book without the support of my family: Kayla and David Christianson, Bonny and Troy Glidewell, Mary Ruth and Adam Schuknecht, Belle Blodgett and Emily Blodgett and my best friends, Marty Shapiro and Walt Roberts.

Preface

Having taught medical assisting for more than 15 years, I know the challenges students face as they study pharmacology. They know it's a pivotal class and that the safety of the patient depends on their mastering this course.

This book was conceived as an answer to numerous complaints from students about the futility of memorizing drugs and the overwhelming fear they have when doing math. I tried to design the book to alleviate their fears by providing enough information to arrive at the correct answer but not so much that they feel helpless. The book starts by covering the basics of pharmacology, then moves into math and dosage calculations, and finally delves into drug classifications.

● UNIT BREAKDOWN

Unit 1 seeks to acclimate the student to the role of the allied health professional in pharmacology. The student is introduced to patient safety principles; governmental regulations regarding the development, testing, and administration of medications; sources and actions of drugs including how they affect specific populations of patients; formulations of drugs and how they're administered; prescriptions and labels; and useful resources for learning more about the drugs being given.

Unit 2 covers techniques for administering medications by all common routes, including oral, ophthalmic, otic, nasal, inhalation, transdermal, vaginal, rectal, parenteral, and even intravenous (IV). Medical assisting students are being asked more and more to provide some level of care to patients receiving IV therapy. This unit will help students better understand this important therapy and ultimately provide better care to their patients.

Unit 3 introduces mathematics and dosage calculations. I've tried to introduce math gently but completely. Addition, subtraction, multiplication, and division are explained clearly and simply, not once but several times throughout the unit, depending on the calculation being described. The unit builds from the most basic mathematical concepts to the more difficult ones, one clear and simple step at a time. The student is also introduced to the various measurement systems, including avoirdupois and apothecary, household measurement, equivalents, and the metric system.

The pinnacle of this unit, Chapter 10, outlines several methods of calculating dosages that all yield the same results. These methods include dimensional analysis, ratio and proportion, word problems, and two formula methods. Why discuss all these ways of arriving at the correct answer? Because each student learns differently and not all methods fit everyone. One student may like the more visual ratio and proportion (means and extremes) method, while another may like the more sequential dimensional analysis method. Allowing students to select the method that best fits them relieves much of the "math anxiety" that many students experience.

The final unit, Unit 4, covers all major drug classifications in a clear, systematic way. Individual drugs are mentioned but each chapter focuses on key attributes of that particular classification. This focus on classifications allows students to understand how a particular set of drugs work and then know that all the individual drugs within that class function the same way. For instance, students learn that anyone who takes an ACE inhibitor—whether the specific drug is lisinopril, benazapril, or fosinophil—is at risk of a sudden drop in blood pressure.

All classifications are based on the classification structure used in the best-selling *Davis's Drug Guide for Nurses,* 10th edition, by Judith Hopfer Deglin, PharmD, and April Hazard Vallerand, PhD,

RN, FAAN. Throughout the book, key terms are highlighted in bold, and drug classifications are italicized.

The book also offers several useful appendices, including:

- Drug classification index organized by generic name, to easily determine to which classification a particular drug belongs
- Routine pediatric and adult immunization guidelines, a must-have for any MA working in a medical office
- Medication administration in children, a highly descriptive tool for giving drugs to a special population
- Pediatric dosage calculations, for figuring out children's dosages based on weight

KEY FEATURES

This book is filled with great features to help students learn. Here's a quick rundown:

- Plenty of practice exercises throughout the book, especially at the end of each chapter to help students commit what they've learned to long-term memory
- Critical thinking activities to engage students and enhance their understanding of pharmacology
- Checkup questions sprinkled throughout each chapter to let students gauge their progress as they move through the chapters
- Drug classification review tables to reinforce need-to-know information in each class
- *Master the Essentials* tables, which cover side effects, precautions, contraindications, and interactions for each classification in a view-and-go format—again, keeping pharmacology content clear and simple!
- "Fast Tip" boxes that provide quick-read pieces of key information
- "Virtual Field Trips" to foster each student's use of the many online resources available
- "A Closer Look" boxes to examine important information in greater detail

INTERACTIVE CD-ROM

To aid the student even more, an interactive CD-ROM has been included. This powerful tool teaches all major methods of calculating dosages, and every method can be used for every problem. Students can work at their own pace through the entire program or focus on areas of weakness.

In addition, section quizzes allow students to check their progress and see where they need further review. Students can also print their test scores so they can show their teachers how far they've come in understanding this critical content.

The software is divided into eight modules, each containing:

- Learning objectives
- Tutorials
- Interactive exercises
- Section quizzes
- Module review
- Two tests per module with more than 320 questions on all eight modules.

A High Alert Drugs button on each module screen leads to detailed information on the safe administration of medications identified by the Institute for Safe Medication Practices as having a greater potential for harm than others.

WEB RESOURCES

Students are further helped through several valuable online resources, available on DavisPlus (davisplus.fadavis.com). Check out these great resources:

- Online review questions

- Syringe-pull activities in which students can practice pulling back on a lifelike syringe plunger to specific marks on the syringe–a great practice tool for administering parenteral medications
- Preventing medication errors tutorial
- Illustrative animations that show drug absorption, distribution, metabolism, and excretion

● FOR TEACHERS

A teacher's manual accompanies this book and offers hundreds of multiple-choice questions to help prepare students for national certification examinations, as well as a PowerPoint presentation in lecture-note format for every chapter.

Nina Beaman

About the Author

Nina Beaman, MS, RN,C, CMA is the Allied Health Coordinator for Bryant and Stratton College in Richmond, Virginia. She holds dual credentials as a registered nurse certified (RN,C) in ambulatory women's health and as a certified medical assistant (CMA) through the American Association of Medical Assistants (AAMA). Miss Beaman was the recipient of the AAMA's 2004 Golden Apple Award. In addition to coordinating the Allied Health Department and teaching courses, she practices nursing working with patients with disabilities, brain injury, and developmental delays at the Arc of the Piedmont in Charlottesville, Virginia. She is currently a doctoral student at Walden University. Previous education includes studies at Capella University (MS), Randolph-Macon College (BA with Honors), University of Nice, France (Diplome d'etudes francaises), John Tyler Community College (AAS in Nursing), and Luther Rice College (AA in Business). She is also a health psychologist and the author of numerous books and articles on current behavioral health issues, such as obesity reduction and workplace violence.

Acknowledgments

I wish to express my sincere appreciation to Campus Director Beth Murphy of the Richmond Campus of Bryant and Stratton College for her support of my continuing education, and to the students of Bryant and Stratton College for teaching me more about the field of education than courses ever could.

Additionally, I would like to thank Andy McPhee for embracing the concept of this book and encouraging me to write it. Thanks also go to Cindy Saver, RN, MS; Lisa Bonsall, RN, MSN, CRNP; and Jennifer Pine for developing the book to publication.

Reviewers

Carol A. Alexander, MSN, RN
Associate Professor
Nursing Department
Palm Beach Community College
Lake Worth, Florida

Kathleen Brassea-Atencio, RN, BSN, CGC, CGRN
Nursing
Southern Colorado Clinic
Pueblo, Colorado

Brenda K. Frerichs, MSM, BSM, CMA
Manager
Medical Assisting Program
Colorado Technical University
Sioux Falls, South Dakota

Dori Y. Gilman, RN, BSN
Instructor
Nursing
North Country Community College
Saranac Lake, New York

Cheryl Gilton, MEd, BSN, RN
Coordinator
Special Health Initiatives
Allegany College of Maryland
Cumberland, Maryland

Kris A. Hardy, CMA, RHE, CDF
Director
Medical Assistant Program
Brevard Community College
Cocoa, Florida

Glenda Hatcher, BSN, RN, CMA
Director
Medical Assisting Program
Southwest Georgia Technical College
Thomasville, Georgia

Marsha Hemby, RN, CMA, BA
Chair
Medical Assisting Program
Pitt Community College
Greenville, North Carolina

Geraldine Kale-Smith, MS, CMA

Coordinator & Associate Professor

Medical Office Administration Programs

Harper College

Palatine, Illinois

Nancy Kuncl

Assistant Professor

Nursing Program

Weber State University/Davis Applied Technology College

Kaysville, Utah

Gayle Mazzocco, BSN, RN, CMA

Adjunct Faculty

Medical Assisting Program

Oakland Community College

Waterford, Michigan

Kay A. Nave, CMA

Former Director

Medical Assistant Program

Hagerstown Business College

Hagerstown, Maryland

Karen Rhonda Snipe, CPhT, AS, BA, MAEd

Coordinator

Pharmacy Technician Program

Trident Technical College

Charleston, South Carolina

Bennita W. Vaughans, RN, MSN

Coordinator

Performance Improvement

Central Alabama Veterans Health Care Center

Tuskegee, Alabama

Brief Contents

APPENDICES

Contents

UNIT 3 Calculations

CHAPTER 8
Basic Review of Mathematics   131

CHAPTER 9
Measurement Systems   163

CHAPTER 10
Dosage Calculations   179

UNIT 4 Classifications of Drugs

Pharmacology Clear & Simple

A Drug Classifications &
Dosage Calculations
Approach

Safe and Legal Dispensing of Medications

Patient Safety

This chapter discusses the basics of how to administer medications safely. Safely administering medications includes identifying the right patient, obtaining the right medication, measuring the right dosage, administering the medication at the right time, using the right route, and documenting the procedure in the right manner. In addition, you need to memorize some abbreviations used in prescribers' orders and learn how to respond to allergic reactions and poisoning incidents.

OBJECTIVES

At the end of this chapter, the student will be able to:

- Define all key terms.
- Discuss the responsibility of allied health professionals in administering medications.
- List the six rights of medication administration.
- Discuss the ethics of medication administration.
- State circumstances when you would call a poison control center.
- Describe how to respond to patients' allergic reactions.

KEY TERMS

a.c	ID	Pharmacology
a.d.	IM	prn
Anaphylaxis	IV	qid
a.s.	npo	PO
a.u.	o.d.	s̄
bid	o.s.	SC
c̄	o.u.	tid
HIPAA	p.c.	Urticaria

● PATIENTS' RIGHTS

Allied health professionals play a pivotal role in ensuring that the patient safely receives a medication. What makes this task more challenging is that patients often feel vulnerable when they come to a medical facility. They may be in pain, overcome with grief, depressed, frightened, or not fully functioning at the top of their mental or physical capabilities. Therefore, you must take care when explaining and administering medication to patients.

To help you safely administer drugs, follow the 6 *Rights* of medication administration:

• Give the drug to the right *patient*.
• Give the right *drug*.
• Give the drug in the right *dose*.
• Give the drug at the right *time*.
• Give the drug by the right *route*.
• Chart the drug using the right *documentation*.

Right Patient

You must give the ordered drug to the correct patient. In a medical office or clinic setting, patients do not have identification bands. Even in the hospital setting, where patients wear such bands, it is still essential to verify that you have the correct patient.

The best way to verify a patient's name is to ask him or her to state it. Then ask the patient for his or her birth date. Be sure the medication is the one that the prescriber (who wrote the prescription) intended to give to the patient.

✳❓ CRITICAL THINKING

> You enter the reception area of a medical office to look for the patient whose name is on the medication. How can you be certain of giving the medication to the right patient? Because patients are sometimes confused or hard of hearing, how can you be certain that the patient who responds is the right one?

Right Drug

In a hospital, the pharmacy puts the patient's name on the medicine container and sends it to the nursing unit. In an office or a clinic setting, you will likely be the one to select the medication from a medication closet or cabinet, so no patient name will be on the bottle. In both cases, you must be sure to select the correct drug. This is not always easy because many drug names look alike and many pills look alike. To avoid mistakes, compare the order in the patient's medical record to the label on the container.

In an office or clinic, three simple steps can help ensure that you have the correct medication.

1. Check the label before you take the bottle from the shelf.
2. Check the label before you pour the drug out.
3. Check the label before you put the bottle back on the shelf.

Drug cabinets in medical offices are arranged with both convenience and safety in mind. Placing drugs on shelves alphabetically may seem more organized, but you are more likely to select the wrong drug if similar names are organized together. Instead, arrange medications by classification or manufacturer.

In a hospital, scanning a bar code to double-check a medication with a computer system may help reduce medication errors. The prescriber enters the order into the computer, and the scan checks the bar code on the drug against the original prescription. This technology may soon be available in the medical office.

✳❓ CRITICAL THINKING

> What is the safest way to arrange drugs in a drug cabinet to avoid medication errors?

⬤ *Fast Tip 1.1* Safe Medication Storage
_____

Most people know that medications should be safely locked up away from young children but fail to think about others in the household. This can lead to tragic consequences when individuals lack knowledge about drug safety. For example, teenagers can abuse vitamin pills, cough syrup, cold medications, and inhalable drugs. Older people who are confused may take medications that are left, for example, on the counter. Emphasize to patients the need to store medications safely no matter what the age of others in the household.

When you verify that you have the correct drug, keep the following in mind:

- If the drug does not seem to match the diagnosis of the patient in the chart, double-check with the prescriber that you have been given a correct order.
- The pharmacist dispensing the medication may not know the patient and may not be aware of any special needs he or she has. For example, a liquid formulation may be necessary if the drug must be given through a feeding tube. In such cases you need to alert the person dispensing the medication of your patient's individual needs.

Right Dose

You must ensure that the patient receives the right dose of the medicine. If you suspect that a prescriber may have ordered an inappropriate dose, do not give the drug until you check with him or her.

It is the role of the allied health professional to instruct patients and their caregivers in safe dosing and medication storage (see Fast Tip 1.1). Keep in mind that most people do not have medical training, so they do not fully understand how drugs act and interact in the body. Thus, it is not surprising that many "play around" with their dosages for reasons of their own. If one pill helps, they think, two should be even better. However, two pills could be an overdose, proving dangerous to the patient. Other reasons for self-adjustment of dosage include level of pain, the degree or appearance of side effects, previous history with the same or similar medication, forgetfulness, and information from family members, friends, neighbors, or even the media.

In addition, remember that what is correct for one patient may not be correct for another. For example, if a patient is elderly or has liver or kidney problems, even the "normal" dose may be too much because the drug may not clear the body well and could accumulate to toxic levels. The patient may also not understand that doses may vary from person to person and may take the same dose as his or her spouse or children. Emphasize the importance of taking the correct dose, as prescribed by the patient's health care provider (see Fast Tip 1.2).

Right Time

When a patient is in the hospital, medications are given according to hospital policy at times that are relatively convenient to the staff. In a typical household, however, drugs are taken on a daily rhythm to suit the patient or caregiver. Morning medications, such as allergy pills, are usually taken with breakfast. Evening drugs, such as seizure medications, are taken at suppertime. Drugs that help patients

---

⬤ *Fast Tip 1.2* Age, Size, and Dosage
_____

Babies and young children require lower dosages because their bodies are small and process drugs faster. A dosage that works on a 150-pound adult is not appropriate for a 75-pound child.

---

sleep at home are taken at the patient's usual bedtime, whereas drugs that help patients sleep in the hospital may be given at a set time.

Some medications, such as antibiotics and antiseizure medications, need to be given a standard number of hours apart around the clock to maintain a constant level in the body. For example, if a patient is taking an antibiotic and omits one of the doses to be taken every 6 hours, the microbes have a chance to reproduce and the body's immune system must work harder to fight the infection.

You may need to suggest that the patient wake up at night in order to stay on a 6-hour regimen, which is when a drug needs to be taken every 6 hours. For example, the patient would take the drug at 8 a.m., 2 p.m., 8 p.m., and 2 a.m. Alternatively, perhaps more conveniently, the patient might choose to take the medication at 6 a.m., 12 noon, 6 p.m., and 12 midnight. The choice depends on the patient's preference.

CRITICAL THINKING

What kinds of drugs are usually prescribed to be given at equal intervals throughout the day? Explain why these drugs must be given at exact intervals.

Abbreviations

Abbreviations abound in medicine, and they are especially important during medication administration (see Fast Tip 1.3). For example, sometimes drugs are taken to coat the stomach before a meal or are taken on a full stomach to reduce the chance of nausea. If a drug is to be given before meals, the prescriber might write a.c. (*ante cibum*). For after-meals administration, the prescription is written p.c. (*post cibum*).

Sometimes a medication can be taken as needed (abbreviated *prn*). Other medications may need to be taken every other day (q.o.d.). For example, a nitroglycerin patch might be worn on one day but removed the next day. This prevents the patient from accumulating too much medicine, as would occur if it was used every day.

Medication schedules

The allied health professional may need to help the patient develop a schedule for taking the medication at home. Sometimes it is helpful to write a clear schedule on a chart for the patient to put on a wall at home, such as that shown in Figure 1.1.

Although most orders are for drugs to be administered, sometimes prescribers order that a drug *not* be given for a period of time or that a drug be discontinued. If a patient is having a test the next day that requires the gastrointestinal system to be clear—for better diagnostic imaging or to prevent aspirating (inhaling into the lungs) vomitus—the prescriber may want the patient to take nothing by mouth (abbreviated *npo*) after midnight. If patients with diabetes are *npo*, they usually should not be given insulin because no food is available to interact with the insulin.

The physician may also order a medication to be discontinued. Perhaps the patient does not need it anymore or the prescriber wants to change the medication to a different one. It is important that you tell the patient *not* to take the medication. For example, when a patient is taking a medication to lower her blood pressure and the physician decides to change to a different medication that also lowers blood pressure, her blood pressure may become dangerously low if both medications are taken. Instruct the patient to throw out old prescription medications that have been discontinued to prevent taking them inadvertently.

◯ *Fast Tip 1.3* **Memory Joggers for Frequency of Drug Administration**

*Bi*cycles have two wheels, so *bid* means twice a day.
*Tri*cycles have three wheels, so *tid* means three times each day.
*Quad*rangles have four sides, so *qid* means four times daily.

Weekly Medicine Record

Your Name _____ Chester Earl

Week of _____ August 1, 2007

Name of Medicine and Dose	Size, Shape and Color of Pill	When to Take	Place an X after each medicine when taken						
			Sun	Mon	Tues	Wed	Thurs	Fri	Sat
1. Digoxin 0.125 mg	Round, 1/4 in diameter, white	Daily	X	X	*need refill*				
2. Coumadin 3-4 mg 4-5 mg	Round, 5/16 in diameter, blue	Daily	X	X	X				
3. Furosemide 40 mg -Lasix-	Round, 5/16 in diameter, white	Daily (morning)	X	X	X				
4. Nitroglycerin (trans-dermal system) 0.4 mg	Patch	Daily (12-14 hours)	X	X	X				
5. Monopril 20 mg	Elongated, 3/8 in diameter, white	Daily							
6. Oyster Shell Calcium 1500 mg	Round, 1/2 in diameter, gray	Daily (morning)	X	X	X				
7. Potassium (K-DUR 20 mEq tablet SA Sch)	Large 13/16 x 3/16 x 3/16, white	Daily (morning)	X	X	X				
8. Tylenol 650 mg caplets	Caplet	As needed for headache		X					
9. Chlorpheniramine maleate (allergy tablets) 4 mg	Round tablet, 3/16 diameter yellow	As needed for sleeplessness	X		X				

FIGURE 1.1. Sample medication schedule for patient's use at home.

CRITICAL THINKING

Rachael Smith has been told to be *npo* after midnight before an x-ray series of her bowels. She calls to see if she should take her morning dose of insulin. An office assistant says she should take it because insulin is not given by mouth. If you had taken her call, what would you have said or done?

Right Route

Where the medication enters the body is important. If a prescription calls for a certain drug to be injected into fat and absorbed slowly, it would be dangerous to give it into a vein. Most of the time, medications are given by mouth (PO). Sometimes drugs are put directly into other openings such as the ears, eyes, nose, vagina, or rectum. Other times they are injected into a vein (IV, or intravenously), a muscle (IM, or intramuscularly), skin (ID, or intradermally), or fat (SC, or subcutaneously). Table 1.1 summarizes common abbreviations related to medication administration. As with other abbreviations covered earlier, some are based on Latin words.

Take a few minutes to study these abbreviations. Then, test yourself in the Check Up that follows. How did you do? If you missed any, you might want to make flash cards to help you learn. Put the abbreviation on one side of a 3 × 5 inch index card and write its definition on the other side. Take these cards with you and study whenever you get a chance. You will be able to learn them quickly.

TABLE 1.1 Abbreviations for Drug Administration

a.d.	Right ear	PO	By mouth (orally)
a.s.	Left ear	ID	Intradermal (into skin)
a.u.	Both ears	IM	Intramuscular (into a muscle)
o.d.	Right eye	IV	Intravenous (into a vein)
o.s.	Left eye	$\bar{c}$	With
o.u.	Both eyes	$\bar{s}$	Without

A CLOSER LOOK: Sinister and Dexter

Latin terms can seem scary unless you can relate them to something your mind finds interesting. Here is a story that can help you learn some abbreviations. In many cultures, both hands are washed after urinating or defecating. However, in some countries, running water is not always easily available to wash the hands. In those cultures, people usually designate their left (in Latin, *sinister*) hand as their "evil" hand. They use the left hand for dirty activities, freeing the right hand for courtesies such as shaking hands or eating food from a communal bowl. This is why we customarily extend our right (in Latin, *dexter)* hand when we shake hands. It would be considered rude to extend the left hand, as that is considered by many cultures to be the dirty hand. The abbreviation in Latin for ear is *a*, and for eye is *o*. So if a prescriber writes a.s., it means left (*sinister*) ear; o.s. would mean the left eye.

CHECK UP

Many abbreviations have been presented so far in this chapter. Check what you know by defining the following:

a.u. _____   a.d. _____   IM _____

IV _____   SC _____   tid _____

bid _____   p.c. _____   a.s. _____

prn _____   o.d. _____   o.u. _____

npo _____   ID _____   o.s. _____

Right Documentation

Although a medical office can get busy, you must take the time for proper documentation whenever you give a medication. Do not document a medication before you give it, as the patient might refuse it and you would have committed fraud. Be sure to document not only the medication but also the dose, route, lot number of the drug, and expiration date of the drug (Fig. 1.2). Do not forget your signature to prove who gave the drug. Document this information on your computer system or in the patient's medical record, according to your facility's policy.

OUTLINE FORMAT PROGRESS NOTES

Patient Name _Bill McDonald_

Prob. No. or Letter	Date	Subjective	Objective	Assess	Plans	Page _____
		10:12 a.m.	Injected 1 mL Vitamin B-12 into patient's left deltoid.			
			Lot number 12345 Expiration date 02/04/2008.			
			Observed patient X 15 minutes. Patient tolerated procedure well.			
			— _Nina Beaman CMA_			

FIGURE 1.2. An example of proper documentation in the patient's medical chart after giving a medication to a patient.

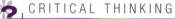 CRITICAL THINKING

Imagine that you gave Cecile Massé 1 mL of a flu shot in the left deltoid muscle. You took it from a container that said lot #1234567, which expires on 12/01/10. How would you document this procedure?

Check with your facility's policy about the abbreviations that are acceptable for use when charting. The Joint Commission on Accreditation of Healthcare Organizations (JCAHO) has stated that some abbreviations are particularly likely to be confused and should not be used (Table 1.2).

ETHICS IN MEDICATION ADMINISTRATION

As an allied health professional, it is your responsibility to see that medications are administered not only safely but ethically. Patients have the right to receive clear information, refuse treatment, and have their privacy respected.

Information

Patients have a right to participate in planning their treatment. Thus it is important to teach patients about their medications on a level they can understand. Although you may understand medical terms, they may not. They may not realize what they are supposed to do. Misunderstandings can lead to injury or overdose.

For example, sometimes patients believe that taking more of a pain medication will relieve their pain better or faster. If a patient is told to take a narcotic every 6 hours as needed for pain, he or she may take it more often, not knowing it could cause confusion, respiratory depression, or death.

TABLE 1.2 Dangerous Abbreviations

ABBREVIATION	POTENTIAL PROBLEM	PREFERRED TERM
Do Not Use		
U (for unit)	Mistaken as zero, four, or cc	Write "unit"
IU (for international unit)	Mistaken as IV (intravenous) or 10 (ten)	Write "international unit"
qd, qod (Latin abbreviations for once daily and every other day)	Mistaken for each other. The period after the "q" can be mistaken for an "i" and the "o" can be mistaken for "i"	Write "daily" and "every other day"
Trailing zero (x.0 mg) (Note: prohibited only for medication-related notations); lack of leading zero (.x mg)	Decimal point is missed	Never write a zero by itself after a decimal point (x mg), and always use a zero before a decimal point (0.x mg)
MS, MSO_4, $MgSO_4$	Confused for one another. Can mean morphine sulfate or magnesium sulfate	Write "morphine sulfate" or "magnesium sulfate"
Avoid		
μg (for microgram)	Mistaken for mg (milligrams) resulting in one thousand-fold dosing overdose	Write "mcg"
hs (for half-strength or Latin abbreviation for bedtime)	Mistaken for either half-strength or hour of sleep (at bedtime). Q.H.S. mistaken for every hour. All can result in dosing error	Write out "half-strength" or "at bedtime"
tiw (for three times a week)	Mistaken for three times a day or twice weekly, resulting in an overdose	Write "3 times weekly" or "three times weekly"
SC or SQ (for subcutaneous)	Mistaken as SL for sublingual or "5 every"	Write "sub-Q," "subQ," or "subcutaneously"

Source: http://www.jcaho.org/. Accessed June 21, 2004.

One way to ensure that patients receive enough information is to teach them to ask the questions in Box 1.1 whenever they start a new medication.

Consent

Patients have the right to refuse treatment, including medications. If they do not understand why they are to take a medication, you should first give them the appropriate information. If they are still reluctant to take a medication, inform the prescriber. To give a medication to someone who refuses it can be considered assault and battery.

A patient may be confused and not understand the treatment. You may need to advocate for the patient. For example, a patient in a hospital emergency department or emergent care clinic may be so frightened and disoriented that she does not clearly understand why she has been told to take a certain medication. She may refuse to allow an injection or to swallow a medication out of fear and ignorance; educating the patient may facilitate understanding.

If the patient is on an experimental drug, he or she has the right to give or not give informed consent. Giving informed consent involves understanding the treatment, its effects, alternative treatments, and what may happen if the treatment is declined. The patient should know whether a drug is experimental and what consequences taking or not taking this drug might create. It is essential to document informed consent, but you must ensure that the patient is comfortable with the decision and that the informed consent is correctly documented. If the patient seems reluctant to sign, notify the physician of your observation.

BOX 1.1   What You Need to Know About Prescription Medicines

As an allied health professional, you should encourage patients to discuss their medication regimen with their health care provider. When a new medication is prescribed, patients can refer to the following list of questions to ask the prescriber or pharmacist.

- What are the various names of the medicine?
- What is it supposed to do?
- Is there a less expensive alternative?
- Why am I taking it?
- How and when do I take the medicine and for how long?
- Should I store it in the refrigerator or cabinet?
- Should I take it with water, food, or with another medication?
- Can it be taken with over-the-counter medicines? Alcohol?
- What do I do if I miss or forget a dose?
- How long should I wait between doses?
- If taken "as needed," how will I know I need it?
- What food, drinks, other medicines, dietary supplements, or activities should I avoid while taking this medication?
- Will any tests or monitoring be required while I am taking this medicine? Do I need to come to the office with a certain regimen?
- What are the possible side effects, and what should I do if they happen?
- When should I expect the medication to start working, and how will I know if it is working?

Privacy

Patients also have rights to privacy. Medication records, like many items in the patient's medical record, are to be kept confidential except for release to pharmacists and other professionals who need the information.

Patients also have a right to receive medications in a quiet, private place. The Health Insurance Portability and Accountability Act (HIPAA) makes allied health professionals accountable to the government to protect the privacy of the patient. Reasonable steps should be taken to ensure that all communications are confidential. For instance, to call a colleague across a waiting room to tell him or her that a drug is ready for a patient whom you've named out loud would be illegal as well as unprofessional.

HIPAA standards also allow patients access to their own medical records and give them more control over how the information in their records is shared. All health care providers must provide a notice to patients alerting them to their rights and that medical information cannot be revealed to other people without the patient's consent. For more information on HIPAA, visit http://www.dhhs.gov/.

CRITICAL THINKING

While entering a crowded reception room, a medical assistant calls back to a colleague that she has to tell a patient that her birth control samples are ready. Immediately afterward, she calls the patient's name aloud. Is this appropriate? How might she have better handled patient confidentiality?

EMERGENCY RESPONSIBILITIES

If a patient comes to your office or facility and shows signs of too much medication in his system, due to either an accident or a deliberate act, you must respond quickly. Refer to office or facility protocols, but usually the first step is to notify the physician immediately and begin the ordered treatment.

If you receive a call from a patient who has ingested a toxic substance, call 911 or ask the patient to do so immediately. Usually when you activate the emergency response system, the dispatcher connects you with a poison control center. Experts at poison control hotlines have training in how to manage toxic substance emergencies. If possible, explain what substance was taken so the staff can better diagnose and treat the problem.

The staff at a poison control center may ask you to do any of the following, depending on the type of toxin:

• Administer activated charcoal, which will bind with the poison. Activated charcoal is usually administered by emergency medical personnel in the field or in emergency departments. The activated charcoal treatment is frequently followed by pumping the patient's stomach to remove the toxin.
• Have the patient drink a large amount of water to dilute the poison.
• Have the patient drink milk to reduce acidity.
• Monitor the patient for certain signs and symptoms.

Follow the directions of the experts carefully, because immediately treating a toxin overdose can save the patient considerable discomfort and harm. Please note that most poison control centers no longer suggest that you induce vomiting with syrup of ipecac because it is not completely effective and can cause complications.

It is also critical to ask patients if they have any allergies *before* giving any medication. Patients who have an allergic reaction to a medication may experience *urticaria* (hives). Their skin may become red, and they may complain of itching. It is important to notify the physician immediately and observe the patient carefully if this reaction occurs.

A severe form of allergy is called *anaphylaxis*. It is especially dangerous if swelling occurs in the neck, which can constrict the trachea and cause death from suffocation. Patients experiencing anaphylaxis have difficulty breathing and may have other symptoms, such as itching, wheezing, anxiety, and light-headedness. The physician may order you to give a medication to reverse the anaphylaxis, such as epinephrine or diphenhydramine (Benadryl). It is safe practice always to observe a patient for 15 minutes after giving an injection, an antibiotic, or an allergy shot to be sure that an allergic reaction is not missed. Be certain to document your observation period, such as "Patient observed for 15 minutes after allergy shot. No signs of anaphylaxis noted."

CRITICAL THINKING

Kendall McGlasson is beginning a new prescription. Before she leaves the office, what would you tell her about potential adverse effects?

SUMMARY

Medication administration is regulated for the public's safety. As an allied health professional, you are responsible for the safe administration of medications. This includes always administering the right drug, in the right dosage, at the right time, by the right route, and to the right patient and then documenting the administration correctly. Always remember that as an allied health professional you must respect patients' rights to receive accurate information, make a truly informed consent, and have their privacy respected.

You also need to be alert to signs of poisoning or anaphylaxis and act appropriately to correct a problem if it exists. Documenting your observation of the patient and your response to any symptoms is vital.

Activities

To make sure that you have learned the key points covered in this chapter, complete the following activities.

True or False
Write *true* if the statement is true. Beside the false statements, write *false* and correct the statement to make it true.

1. If a patient is npo, he or she takes the medication only as needed. _____

2. Drugs that are given a.d. are given in the right eye. _____

3. There are five rights to medication administration. _____

4. You should compare the order with the bottle at least three times. _____

5. In case of anaphylaxis, administer syrup of ipecac. _____

Matching
Write the number for each abbreviation with its definition.

1. bid   _____ after meals

2. c̄   _____ as needed

3. o.s.   _____ before meals

4. tid   _____ both ears

5. s̄   _____ left eye

6. prn   _____ right eye

7. a.u.   _____ three times per day

8. a.c.   _____ twice a day

9. p.c.   _____ with

10. o.d.   _____ without

Multiple Choice
Choose the best answer for each question.

1. Which of the following is a sign of anaphylaxis?
   a. Hallucinations
   b. Bleeding nose
   c. Fixed pupils
   d. Urticaria
   e. Fainting

2. Which abbreviation means "before meals?"
   a. a.c.
   b. a.d.
   c. a.m.
   d. a.s.
   e. a.u.

3. Which of the following routes of administration involves an injection into fat?
   a. Subcutaneous
   b. Intradermal
   c. Intravenous
   d. Intramuscular
   e. Transdermal

4. Which means to put directly into the skin?
   a. Intravenous
   b. Intradermal
   c. Intramuscular
   d. Subcutaneous
   e. Transdermal

5. In an examination room in a medical office, which of the following is the best way to identify a patient?
   a. Check the patient's wrist identification band.
   b. Call the patient by name.
   c. Ask the patient his or her name.
   d. Compare the photo in the patient's chart to the patient.
   e. Ask one of your coworkers who the patient is.

Short Answer
Answer these questions on a separate sheet.

1. What precautions should be taken in a medical office to ensure the safe dispensing of medications? What precautions are taken in a hospital setting?
2. What would you do if a patient began itching after you gave an immunization?
3. What are some possible instructions that a poison control center might give you?
4. What information should you have ready when you call a poison control center?

Application Exercises
Respond to the following scenarios on a separate sheet.

1. The office stores samples from drug representatives in a closet. **What would be the most efficient way to store them—by classification, company, or expiration date? Defend your answer.**
2. You give a measles, mumps, and rubella shot into Brian Dale's left leg. The drug was from lot #2468, expiration date 03/01/08. After you gave the injection, he begins to cry. **How would you document this medication administration in baby Dale's chart?**
3. You go to pull the chart for Walter Roberts and you notice that there are five Walter Roberts seen at this practice. **What information would you need to find the correct chart?**
4. Inger Rimestad frequently forgets to take her medications. She is 77 years old and claims that she cannot remember well. **What would you do to help her learn her medication schedule?**
5. Derrick Pierce is a diabetic who lives with his daughter, who also has diabetes and wonders why they do not take the same dose of insulin. **What would be your response?**
6. Mrs. Valenzuela does not understand English well, but her son, who does understand English, is with her. **How can you be sure that she understands how and when to take her medications?**

7. Robyn Deane begins to itch on her torso after you give her a hepatitis B immunization. **What should you do? How should you document your actions?**
8. Elaine Cote is on an experimental drug. **Write how you would document her informed consent.**

Virtual Field Trips

The following collection of websites can help you learn how to research information on the Internet. If a listed website is not available, see if you can find the information from another website and note where you found it.

1. Go to http://www.drugtopics.com and find the top 50 drugs most frequently associated with medication errors. List the top 10.
2. Visit http://www.aapcc.org (American Association of Poison Control Centers) and find which drug most commonly poisons patients.
3. Surf the Internet to http://www.ismp.org (Institute for Safe Medication Practices) and list what topic this month's alert is about.
4. Find http://www.aapcc.org and note which centers offer TDD/TTY (for the deaf) services.
5. While at http://www.aapcc.org/ collect data to create a brochure on the prevention of poisoning for new parents.

Regulations

To ensure public safety, the U.S. government enacts and enforces laws and regulations related to drugs. The Occupational Safety and Health Administration (OSHA), the Food and Drug Administration (FDA), the Drug Enforcement Agency (DEA), and other government agencies guard the public safety by protecting workers, approving drugs, and enforcing drug laws. This chapter reviews the roles of these agencies. You will also learn the process for developing new drugs to be sold in the United States and how drugs are classified. Finally, you will learn about the illegal use of drugs.

OBJECTIVES

At the end of this chapter, the student will be able to:

- Define key terms.
- Describe the roles of OSHA, FDA, and DEA in patient safety.
- Discuss how drugs are developed.
- Distinguish between brand, generic, and trade names.
- Know the slang street names for illegal drugs.
- Discuss why some drugs are more tightly controlled than others.
- Give an example of a drug from each controlled substances schedule and state why it is classified that way.
- Discuss the role of allied health professionals in recognizing and reporting impaired patients and professionals.

KEY TERMS

Addiction	Chemical name	DEA
Adverse reaction	Clinical trials	Dependent
Blood-borne pathogens	Control group	Double-blind
Brand name	Controlled substances	Efficacy

FDA
Generic name
Habituated
HMO
Impaired provider
IND
Inert

NDA
OSHA
OTC
Placebo
Proprietary name
Random
Street name

Substance abuse
Therapeutic dose
Tolerance
Trade name
USP/NF
Withdrawal

● REGULATORY AUTHORITIES

To protect the health care worker and the public, several governmental authorities regulate and oversee the safe delivery of medications (Table 2.1). Laws and regulations exist to protect the public from dishonest drug sellers, who might claim that the drugs perform some function that they do not. Scientific research is necessary to ensure that drugs are safely and effectively used by the public. You need to be familiar with the regulations so you do not endanger yourself or your patients.

OSHA

The Occupational Safety and Health Administration (OSHA), a branch of the Department of Labor, helps ensure that workers are not exposed to unnecessary job-related risks. As a health care worker, you have a right to be protected from patients' diseases. In turn, you must take steps to protect yourself. OSHA regulations outline some of those precautions.

• Wash your hands before touching patients.
• Do not touch medications with your hands.
• Wear gloves when you might be exposed to a patient's blood or other bodily fluids.
• Put sharp objects (e.g., needles) in specialized sharps disposal containers so you do not accidentally stick yourself with a used needle.

To ensure that health care workers practice safe work habits, OSHA requires that all employees who might have access to blood-borne pathogens (microbes that cause disease) be trained every year on safe practices. OSHA requires that workers learn about workplace safety practices and personal protective equipment (e.g., gloves, face shields). Every practice setting must have protective supplies, such as sharps disposal containers, gloves, masks, and eyewash solutions, readily available. For more information, visit http://www.osha.gov/.

Occupational injuries (those that occur at work) must be reported to OSHA. If an organization has many incidents of occupational injury, the agency may require further training for employees. OSHA is a regulatory agency, so its representatives can inspect a medical organization at any time. Large fines are levied on organizations that do not comply with OSHA regulations.

TABLE 2.1 Federal Agencies

AGENCY	RESPONSIBILITY	ASSOCIATE DEPARTMENT
Occupational Safety and Health Administration (OSHA)	Health care worker safety	Department of Labor
Food and Drug Administration (FDA)	Safety of food and drug supply, approval of new drugs	Department of Health and Human Services
Drug Enforcement Agency (DEA)	Enforces Controlled Substances Act—public safety	Department of Justice

Food and Drug Administration

In the early history of our country, unscrupulous people sold bottles of "miracle" cures to vulnerable patients. These "tonics" frequently did nothing for the patient or, worse, were harmful. The 1906 Pure Food and Drug Act created the Food and Drug Administration (FDA), part of the Department of Health and Human Services, to protect the public from harm by requiring scientific research of drugs before they are approved and regulating how drugs are distributed. Once a drug is approved by the FDA, it is added to the United States Pharmacopoeia/National Formulary, or USP/NF.

All approved drugs must be proven safe and effective before they can be marketed. This means that they must perform the indicated action without causing unacceptable harm. The FDA insists on high standards of scientific research, so it may take 8 years or more for a company to get approval—even if a drug has been approved and sold in another country. However, since 1997, the FDA has had the authority to accelerate the approval process—to as quickly as 6 months—for drugs needed by people who are likely to die waiting for approval. For information about FDA standards, visit http://www.fda.gov/.

A CLOSER LOOK: The Orphan Drug Act

The Orphan Drug Act was passed in 1983 to facilitate the development of drugs for rare diseases, that is, those that affect fewer than 1 in 200,000 people. Pharmaceutical manufacturers had been reluctant to produce these drugs because of poor return on investment; when they did produce them, the drugs were often quite expensive for patients. The Orphan Drug Act encourages the development of these "orphan" drugs. For more information, visit http://www.fda.gov/orphan/.

MedWatch

All drugs have side effects associated with them. A *side effect* is an unintended consequence from a drug. Common side effects include headache, nausea, vomiting, and diarrhea. A side effect that can cause severe harm or death is commonly called an *adverse reaction* or *adverse event*.

As an allied health professional, if you give a drug that causes an adverse reaction, you should report it to the FDA's MedWatch, using the form available at www.fda.gov/MedWatch (Fig. 2.1). Although submission is voluntary, the reporting of problems helps the FDA track trends. If a drug has multiple reports of adverse reactions or a particularly serious event such as death, the manufacturer may voluntarily recall a drug or the FDA may order a recall. The manufacturer of the drug must stop distributing it and contact customers with the product name, size, lot number, code or serial number, reason for recall, and instructions about what to do with the product. Recalled drugs are listed in a weekly FDA Enforcement Report, available on its website. If the adverse event was caused by a vaccine, use the Vaccine Adverse Event Form shown in Figure 2.2.

To continuously monitor public safety, the FDA also holds annual public meetings to hear comments from patients, pharmaceutical manufacturers, and health care professionals about the safety and effectiveness of drugs.

CRITICAL THINKING

Mr. Dupee is upset that he cannot get a drug he has read about. He knows a website in Mexico where he can order this drug. What are the potential dangers if he orders a drug from another country? How might you discuss this with him?

DRUG DEVELOPMENT

Drug development begins after researchers discover, identify, or create agents that show promising effects against a disease or disorder. These agents must go through many stages of development and exploration and meet strict regulatory requirements before they can be tested on humans. The FDA evaluates premarket drugs through its Center for Drug Evaluation and Research (CDER). The Center's

U.S. Department of Health and Human Services

Form Approved: OMB No. 0910-0291, Expires: 10/31/08
See OMB statement on reverse.

MedWatch

The FDA Safety Information and Adverse Event Reporting Program

For VOLUNTARY reporting of adverse events, product problems and product use errors

Page _____ of _____

FDA USE ONLY
Triage unit sequence #

PLEASE TYPE OR USE BLACK INK

A. PATIENT INFORMATION

1. Patient Identifier	2. Age at Time of Event, or Date of Birth:	3. Sex	4. Weight
In confidence		☐ Female ☐ Male	_____ lb or _____ kg

B. ADVERSE EVENT, PRODUCT PROBLEM OR ERROR

Check all that apply:

1. ☐ Adverse Event   ☐ Product Problem (e.g., defects/malfunctions)
   ☐ Product Use Error   ☐ Problem with Different Manufacturer of Same Medicine

2. Outcomes Attributed to Adverse Event
   (Check all that apply)
   ☐ Death: _____ (mm/dd/yyyy)   ☐ Disability or Permanent Damage
   ☐ Life-threatening   ☐ Congenital Anomaly/Birth Defect
   ☐ Hospitalization - initial or prolonged ☐ Other Serious (Important Medical Events)
   ☐ Required Intervention to Prevent Permanent Impairment/Damage (Devices)

3. Date of Event (mm/dd/yyyy)	4. Date of this Report (mm/dd/yyyy)

5. Describe Event, Problem or Product Use Error

6. Relevant Tests/Laboratory Data, Including Dates

7. Other Relevant History, Including Preexisting Medical Conditions (e.g., allergies, race, pregnancy, smoking and alcohol use, liver/kidney problems, etc.)

C. PRODUCT AVAILABILITY

Product Available for Evaluation? (Do not send product to FDA)

☐ Yes   ☐ No   ☐ Returned to Manufacturer on: _____ (mm/dd/yyyy)

D. SUSPECT PRODUCT(S)

1. Name, Strength, Manufacturer (from product label)
   #1
   #2

2. Dose or Amount	Frequency	Route
#1		
#2		

3. Dates of Use (If unknown, give duration) from/to (or best estimate)	5. Event Abated After Use Stopped or Dose Reduced?
#1	#1 ☐ Yes ☐ No ☐ Doesn't Apply
#2	#2 ☐ Yes ☐ No ☐ Doesn't Apply

4. Diagnosis or Reason for Use (Indication)	8. Event Reappeared After Reintroduction?
#1	#1 ☐ Yes ☐ No ☐ Doesn't Apply
#2	#2 ☐ Yes ☐ No ☐ Doesn't Apply

6. Lot #	7. Expiration Date	9. NDC # or Unique ID
#1	#1	
#2	#2	

E. SUSPECT MEDICAL DEVICE

1. Brand Name

2. Common Device Name

3. Manufacturer Name, City and State

4. Model #	Lot #	5. Operator of Device
Catalog #	Expiration Date (mm/dd/yyyy)	☐ Health Professional
Serial #	Other #	☐ Lay User/Patient ☐ Other:

6. If Implanted, Give Date (mm/dd/yyyy)	7. If Explanted, Give Date (mm/dd/yyyy)

8. Is this a Single-use Device that was Reprocessed and Reused on a Patient?
   ☐ Yes   ☐ No

9. If Yes to Item No. 8, Enter Name and Address of Reprocessor

F. OTHER (CONCOMITANT) MEDICAL PRODUCTS

Product names and therapy dates (exclude treatment of event)

G. REPORTER (See confidentiality section on back)

1. Name and Address

Phone #	E-mail

2. Health Professional?	3. Occupation	4. Also Reported to:
☐ Yes ☐ No		☐ Manufacturer
5. If you do NOT want your identity disclosed to the manufacturer, place an "X" in this box: ☐		☐ User Facility ☐ Distributor/Importer

FORM FDA 3500 (10/05)   Submission of a report does not constitute an admission that medical personnel or the product caused or contributed to the event.

FIGURE 2.1. The MedWatch form is completed in the case of serious adverse events from drug administration. (From U.S. Department of Health & Human Services, Food and Drug Administration. Retrieved April 10, 2006, from http://www.fda.gov/MedWatch/SAFETY/3500.pdf)

WEBSITE: www.vaers.hhs.gov   E-MAIL: info@vaers.org   FAX: 1-877-721-0366

VACCINE ADVERSE EVENT REPORTING SYSTEM
24 Hour Toll-Free Information 1-800-822-7967
P.O. Box 1100, Rockville, MD 20849-1100
PATIENT IDENTITY KEPT CONFIDENTIAL

VAERS

For CDC/FDA Use Only
VAERS Number _____
Date Received _____

Patient Name:

Last   First   M.I.

Address

City   State   Zip
Telephone no. (____) _____

Vaccine administered by (Name):

Responsible
Physician _____
Facility Name/Address

City   State   Zip
Telephone no. (____) _____

Form completed by (Name):

Relation   ☐ Vaccine Provider ☐ Patient/Parent
to Patient   ☐ Manufacturer   ☐ Other
Address (if different from patient or provider)

City   State   Zip
Telephone no. (____) _____

| 1. State | 2. County where administered | 3. Date of birth / / mm dd yy | 4. Patient age | 5. Sex ☐ M ☐ F | 6. Date form completed / / mm dd yy |

7. Describe adverse events(s) (symptoms, signs, time course) and treatment, if any

8. Check all appropriate:
☐ Patient died   (date ___/___/___)
                          mm dd yy
☐ Life threatening illness
☐ Required emergency room/doctor visit
☐ Required hospitalization (_____days)
☐ Resulted in prolongation of hospitalization
☐ Resulted in permanent disability
☐ None of the above

9. Patient recovered   ☐ YES ☐ NO ☐ UNKNOWN

12. Relevant diagnostic tests/laboratory data

| 10. Date of vaccination / / mm dd yy AM/PM Time ___ PM | 11. Adverse event onset / / mm dd yy AM/PM Time ___ PM |

13. Enter all vaccines given on date listed in no. 10

Vaccine (type)	Manufacturer	Lot number	Route/Site	No. Previous Doses
a.				
b.				
c.				
d.				

14. Any other vaccinations within 4 weeks prior to the date listed in no. 10

Vaccine (type)	Manufacturer	Lot number	Route/Site	No. Previous doses	Date given
a.					
b.					

15. Vaccinated at:
☐ Private doctor's office/hospital   ☐ Military clinic/hospital
☐ Public health clinic/hospital   ☐ Other/unknown

16. Vaccine purchased with:
☐ Private funds   ☐ Military funds
☐ Public funds   ☐ Other/unknown

17. Other medications

18. Illness at time of vaccination (specify)

19. Pre-existing physician-diagnosed allergies, birth defects, medical conditions (specify)

20. Have you reported this adverse event previously?
☐ No   ☐ To health department
☐ To doctor   ☐ To manufacturer

Only for children 5 and under

22. Birth weight _____ lb. _____ oz.

23. No. of brothers and sisters

21. Adverse event following prior vaccination (check all applicable, specify)

	Adverse Event	Onset Age	Type Vaccine	Dose no. in series
☐ In patient				
☐ In brother or sister				

Only for reports submitted by manufacturer/immunization project

24. Mfr./imm. proj. report no.

25. Date received by mfr./imm.proj.

26. 15 day report?   ☐ Yes ☐ No

27. Report type   ☐ Initial ☐ Follow-Up

Health care providers and manufacturers are required by law (42 USC 300aa-25) to report reactions to vaccines listed in the Table of Reportable Events Following Immunization. Reports for reactions to other vaccines are voluntary except when required as a condition of immunization grant awards.

Form VAERS-1(FDA)

FIGURE 2.2. If an adverse event is due to a vaccine, the allied health professional must use the Vaccine Adverse Event Reporting System form. (From U.S. Department of Health & Human Services, Food and Drug Administration. Retrieved April 10, 2006, from http://www.fda.gov/cber/vaers/vaers.htm)

goals are to ensure that beneficial drug products are safe, available, and labeled with information about risks and benefits. The FDA approves a drug when it judges that the benefits of using the drug outweigh the risks for the intended population and use.

After a drug is on the market and available for use, it is continually monitored and evaluated for its benefits and risks, not only by the FDA but also by health care providers and patients taking the drugs. Figure 2.3 demonstrates the role of the FDA in risk management.

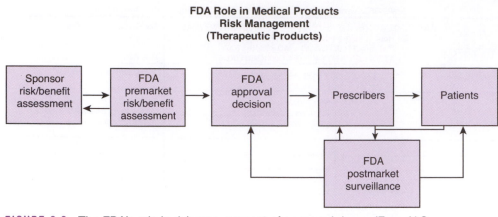

FIGURE 2.3. The FDA's role in risk management of approved drugs. (From U.S. Department of Health & Human Services, Food and Drug Administration. Retrieved March 7, 2007, from http://www.fda.gov/oc/tfrm/executivesummary.pdf)

A large part of drug development requires developers to conduct clinical trials or studies. After testing in laboratories and in animals, a drug must be carefully tested in humans. Researchers use clinical trials to test the effects of a drug in human subjects with the goal of determining effectiveness, side effects, toxicity, and interactions. The effect of the active drug under study is compared with what happens without any drug or with a placebo. A placebo is an inactive (inert) substance that is sometimes given to participants in clinical trials to compare it with an active substance. The study drug may also be compared to a drug already on the market.

Clinical Trials

Study participants are randomly (in no particular order) assigned to one of at least two groups (Fig. 2.4). One group is the placebo or control group. The people in the other group or groups would then receive the active study drug or drugs. The participants do not know whether they are receiving an inactive or active drug; that way, they do not invalidate the study by reporting effects they believe they would have if receiving one or the other. Similarly, if the clinician conducting the study knew which patients were taking the active drug, the scientist might change the results—consciously or subconsciously. Therefore, to be sure the results of the drug trials are accurate, most studies are double-blind, meaning that neither the participants nor the clinicians know who received the active drug. Computers are used to generate random numbers to assign to patients, and the study drug and placebo appear the same.

To encourage volunteers, treatment is usually free, and volunteers may be paid for participating or receive funds to cover transportation costs to and from where the patients are followed. They must also sign a detailed consent form.

Clinical trials are conducted in several phases (Table 2.2). The goal of Phase 1 trials is to determine safety. A small number of healthy participants take a drug for several months to see if it harms them. For example, a drug might give them diarrhea or negatively affect their vital signs. If the drug causes significant harmful effects, the trial stops. Usually the participants are men because of concern about giving experimental drugs to women who might be or become pregnant. One drawback of this practice is that researchers may not see harmful effects that occur only in women until a later research phase.

CRITICAL THINKING

Not all people who volunteer for clinical trials are acceptable for the research. What do you think might eliminate a patient from clinical trials?

Phase 2 clinical trials involve hundreds of patients (all of whom have the disease targeted by the drug) for longer periods of time. Although safety is still important, the main goal is to see if a drug works as desired (efficacy). For example, if a drug is potentially to be used to lower blood choles-

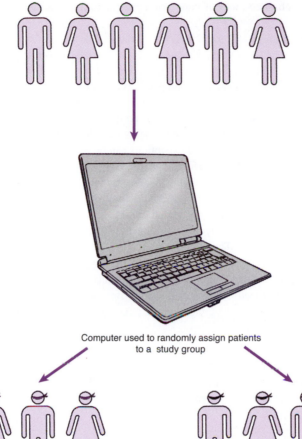

Computer used to randomly assign patients
to a study group

Intervention group
receive study drug

Control group
receive placebo
or
another drug

FIGURE 2.4. In a randomized, double-blind clinical trial, neither patients nor clinicians
know which person is receiving which drug or placebo.

TABLE 2.2 Clinical Trials			
PHASE	**NO. OF PATIENTS**	**LENGTH**	**PURPOSE**
1	20–100	Several months	Safety—does the drug do harm
2	Up to several hundred	Several months to 2 years	Efficacy—does the drug help the patient; also looks at safety
3	Several hundred to thousands	1–4 years	Dosage—how much should the patient take to be helped without overdosing; also looks at safety and efficacy
4 (postmarketing trials)	Thousands	Ongoing	Continuing evaluation through MedWatch

terol, samples of participants' blood are checked to see if their blood cholesterol becomes lower while they take this drug.

Phase 3 trials are for drugs that have been proven to be safe and effective. These trials involve hundreds to thousands of participants and can last 1–4 years. Frequently Phase 3 trials are run in several facilities (e.g., hospitals, physician offices, clinics), each enrolling hundreds of patients. The manufacturer is testing for safety, effectiveness, and dosage. The therapeutic (best) dose is evaluated during this phase; the goal is to give the least amount of drug possible to gain the necessary effect.

During the first three phases of clinical trials the drug is known as an investigational new drug (IND), and its use is limited to those who meet specific criteria for being included in the trial. If the drug is being developed to help critically ill patients, special exceptions can be granted. The FDA allows some physicians the compassionate use of INDs before approval. If a patient is suffering greatly and may die without the drug, a physician can prescribe it before FDA approval. It is important to note, however, that most Health Maintenance Organizations (HMOs) do not cover the costs of experimental drugs because they are expensive to obtain if you are not participating in the research.

If the clinical trials show that the drug is safe and effective, and a therapeutic dose is established, the manufacturer next applies to the FDA for approval. The manufacturer submits a new drug application (NDA), with the results of the scientific testing. Depending on the drug, the approval process can take from 6 months to several years; as many as 12 years might pass from preclinical trials to approval.

Because the process of getting a drug approved is lengthy and expensive, and only about one drug is marketed for every 5000 to 10,000 compounds tested, the manufacturer usually receives a 17- to 20-year patent to recover the cost and make a profit.

CRITICAL THINKING

Canadians are protected by the Health Protection Branch (HPB) of the Department of Health and Welfare. Why might it be important for countries to cooperate in drug research?

Once the FDA approves the drug, it can be marketed and distributed outside the clinical trials groups. However, surveillance for any problems not previously identified continues through the MedWatch program (http://www.fda.gov/medwatch). Additional research may also be conducted. These activities are referred to as postmarketing (or Phase 4) trials.

NAMES OF DRUGS

Drugs are known by chemical, brand (or trade), generic, and "street" names. It is important to understand how these names are derived to avoid confusion.

Chemical Name

When a drug is first developed, it is known as a mix of chemicals. The *chemical* name is meaningful to the scientists who are doing the research but means little to others. It is not necessary for allied health professionals to memorize chemical names.

Brand Name

Once a drug clears Phases 1–3 of clinical trials, it gets a *brand* or *trade* name (also sometimes called a *proprietary* name), to which the company owns the rights. Because the brand name will be used in advertising, the company selects a name that is easy to remember and that may indicate the drug's purpose. For example, Restoril helps patients sleep. The first letters of brand names are capitalized, and the names are usually followed by the letters R or TM with circles around them.

CRITICAL THINKING

Drug names sometimes reflect what the drug does. Without looking them up, guess for what purpose the following drugs are used. Then check them in your drug reference book.

1. Azmacort
2. Bronkaid
3. Elimite
4. Flexeril
5. Glucotrol
6. Lipitor
7. NasalCrom
8. Nicoderm
9. Pepcid
10. Rythmol

How did you do?

Generic Name

Once a drug's patent period has ended, the drug's trademark status is not protected, so other companies may produce the drug under its *generic*, or common, name. No one but the manufacturer that was given the trademark status can use the brand name, but other companies can now manufacture the drug. Because these other companies did not do the research or spend as much on marketing, they can produce the medication much more cheaply than the original manufacturer.

The FDA has specific requirements for manufacturers of generic drugs (Box 2.1). If the company uses the generic name, the drug must have the active ingredient the generic name specifies, but different fillers can be used. In some people, the drug is more effective in the brand-name form than in the generic form, but most people adapt well to a generic brand. Because the generic drug is cheaper, HMOs often require that patients and prescribers use the less expensive version of the drug to receive reimbursement.

Unlike the brand name, the first letter of the generic name is capitalized only if it begins a sentence. The generic name can also provide a clue as to the classification (type) to which a drug belongs (see Fast Tip 2.1). The generic name becomes the official name of the drug.

BOX 2.1 FDA Requirements for Generic Drugs

- Generic drugs must have the same active ingredients and the same labeled strength as brand-name products. They must be just as strong, pure, and stable as brand-name drugs and of the same quality.
- Generic drugs must have the same dosage form (e.g., liquids, capsules) and must be administered in the same way. In the body, they must work the same.
- Generic drug manufacturers must show that a generic drug is bioequivalent to the brand-name drug, which means the generic version delivers the same amount of active ingredients into a patient's bloodstream in the same amount of time as the brand-name drug.
- Generic drug labeling must be essentially the same as the labeling of the brand-name drug.
- Generic drug manufacturers must fully document the generic drug's chemistry, manufacturing steps, and quality control measures.
- Manufacturers must assure the FDA that the raw materials and finished product meet specifications of the U.S. Pharmacopoeia, the organization that sets standards for drug purity in the United States. Both brand-name and generic drug factories must meet the same standards. The FDA inspects about 3500 factories a year to make sure they meet the standards. Often the same factories make both brand-name and generic drugs.
- Before it can be sold, manufacturers must show that a generic drug will remain potent and unchanged until the expiration date on the label.
- Manufacturers must comply with federal regulations for good manufacturing practices and provide the FDA a full description of facilities they use to manufacture, process, test, package, and label the drug. The FDA inspects manufacturing facilities to ensure compliance.
- Generic drugs may look different from the brand-name equivalent but must work in the same way.

Source: Food and Drug Administration Consumer, September–October 2003.

⊙ *Fast Tip 2.1* Drug Suffixes (Endings of Words)

Sometimes drug suffixes provide clues as to the type of drug it is.

DRUGS WITH THESE ENDINGS	USUALLY BELONG TO THIS CLASS
-caine	Local anesthetics
-cillin	Antibiotics
-dine	Antiulcer agents
-done	Opioid analgesics
-ide	Oral hypoglycemics
-iam	Antianxiety agents
-micin	Antibiotics
-mide	Diuretics
-mycin	Antibiotics
-nium	Neuromuscular blocking agents
-olol	Beta blockers (cardiovascular)
-oxacin	Antibiotic
-pam	Antianxiety agent
-pril	ACE inhibitors
-sone	Steroids
-statin	Antilipemics
-vir	Antivirals
-zide	Diuretics

Source: Med Notes. F.A. Davis, Philadelphia, 2004.

Sometimes the prescriber uses shortened names. If the chemical is followed by carbonate, citrate, gluconate, hydrochloride, hydroxide, phosphate, sodium, or sulfate, the prescriber may think that the pharmacist understands the generic name with the second part. For example, potassium chloride is often ordered as potassium. However, the drug label should have the complete name on it. If you have any doubt about the correct name, you should check with the pharmacist or prescriber.

The generic drug may have a different shape and color from the trade drug. A change in the appearance of medications can confuse patients when they suddenly receive different looking pills from the pharmacy. You should encourage patients to contact the pharmacy if they are suspicious of a change in drugs—it may be that the pharmacy purchased the drug from a different manufacturer, but it may also be a drug error.

Street Names

Sometimes both legal and illegal drugs are known by *street*, or slang, names. Although you may not know the names of illegal drugs that are used on the street, your patients may use them; therefore, you should be familiar with them. See Box 2.2 for common street names for drugs that are frequently abused.

⬤ CONTROL OF DRUGS

The Drug Enforcement Administration (DEA) of the U.S. Department of Justice enforces the laws regarding drug use. Although some medications may be obtained without a prescription—called over-the-counter (OTC) drugs—many require a prescription from a licensed health care provider.

Although OTC drugs are generally safe if taken as indicated, prescription drugs require the control of a prescriber to ensure that the best drug is given for the patient's problem. For example, although patients may be able to choose which OTC medications they should use to treat their headaches, they

---

Box 2.2   Street Names for Commonly Abused Drugs

Sometimes both legal and illegal drugs are known by *street* or slang names. The following are street names for selected addictive drugs.

Cannabinoids
Hashish—boom, chronic, gangster, hash, hash oil, hemp
Marijuana—blunt, dope, ganja, grass, herb, joints, Mary Jane, pot, reefer, sinsemilla, skunk, wacky weed, weed, widow

Depressants
Barbiturates—barbs, phennies, reds, red birds, tooies, yellows, yellow jackets
Benzodiazepines—candy, downers, sleeping pills, tranks
Flunitrazepam—forget-me pill, Mexican Valium, R2, Roche, roofies, roofinol, rope, rophies
GHB—G, Georgia home boy, grievous bodily harm, liquid ecstasy
Methaqualone—ludes, mandrex, quad, quay

Dissociative anesthetics
Ketamine—cat Valiums, K, special K, vitamin K
PCP and analogs—angel dust, boat, hog, love boat, peace pill

Hallucinogens
LSD—acid, blotter, boomers, cubes, microdot, red/green dragon, yellow sunshines
Mescaline—buttons, cactus, mesc, peyote
Psilocybin—magic mushroom, purple passion, shrooms

Opioids and morphine derivatives
Codeine—Captain Cody, Cody, door and fours, loads, pancakes and syrup, schoolboy
Fentanyl and analogs—Apache, China girl, China white, dance fever, friend, goodfella, jackpot, murder 8, Tango and Cash, TNT
Heroin—big daddy, brown sugar, dope, H, horse, junk, skag, skunk, smack, tar, white horse
Morphine—M, Miss Emma, monkey, white stuff
Opium—big O, black stuff, block, gum, hop

Stimulants
Amphetamine—bennies, black beauties, crosses, hearts, LA turnaround, speed, truck drivers, uppers
Methamphetamine—chalk, crystal, glass, ice, meth, speed
Cocaine—bump, C, candy, Charlie, coke, crack, dust, flake, flow, girl, nose candy, rock, snow, toot
MDMA—Adam, beans, clarity, E, ecstasy, Eve, lover's speed, peace, STP, X, XTC, zinger

Other
Anabolic steroids—juice, roids
Inhalants—bombers, buzz bomb, laughing gas, poppers, snappers, whippets

Source: National Institute on Drug Abuse. For more information, go to http://www.drugabuse.gov.

---

need health care providers with medical training to select the correct oral contraceptive for their individual circumstances.

Be sure the person ordering the medication is lawfully allowed to do so. In some states, nurse practitioners and physician assistants are allowed to prescribe medications. Some prescriptions are strictly controlled because the drugs, referred to as *controlled substances,* can cause addiction or patient harm if misused. Prescribers must register with the DEA to prescribe drugs, and in the case of controlled substances, the registry number must be printed on the prescription.

Controlled substances are categorized into schedules, which are designated by Roman numerals. It is not necessary to memorize all of the drugs in them, but the categories are important to know. The most highly controlled drugs are Schedule I drugs and the least-controlled are Schedule V drugs (Table 2.3).

TABLE 2.3   DEA Controlled Substance Schedules

SCHEDULE	ABUSE POTENTIAL	MEDICAL USE	SAMPLE DRUGS*
I	High	No accepted medical use in the U.S.	Heroin, marijuana, LSD, methaqualone
II	High; may lead to severe dependence (psychological or physical)	Has a currently accepted medical use; may have severe restrictions	Cocaine, methadone, methamphetamine, morphine, PCP, Oxy-Contin
III	Less than the drugs and substances in schedules I and II; may lead to moderate or low physical dependence or high psychological dependence	Has a currently accepted medical use	Anabolic steroids, codeine and hydrocodone with aspirin or Tylenol, some barbiturates
IV	Low, relative to substances in schedule III; may lead to limited dependence (psychological or physical)	Has a currently accepted medical use	Valium, Xanax
V	Low, relative to substances in schedule IV; may lead to limited dependence (psychological or physical)	Has a currently accepted medical use	Cough medicines with codeine

Source: http://www.usdoj.gov/dea/pubs/abuse/1-csa.htm
*Not a comprehensive list.

Schedule I drugs are considered to be highly addictive, both physically and psychologically, and they have no medical use. These drugs, such as heroin, are considered so dangerous they are illegal; there are jail penalties for even possessing them. Prescribers never write orders for Schedule I drugs except in carefully controlled research facilities. Allied health professionals should never possess these drugs, as criminal prosecution may result.

Schedule II drugs have a high potential for physical and psychological addiction. Their use is heavily restricted because they are popular with drug addicts. These drugs are dispensed through a written prescription only—having an office assistant phone the pharmacy with the prescription is not allowed—and the prescriber must write the prescription. No refills are permitted. The office staff may fax the prescription to the pharmacy, but the patient must give a handwritten prescription to the pharmacist to receive the medicine. In an emergency, the prescriber may phone in an order to a nurse (e.g., if the patient is in the hospital), but a handwritten copy must be submitted within 72 hours. This category includes drugs that depress the central nervous system, as well as amphetamines, which stimulate it. Examples include cocaine, PCP, methylphenidate (Ritalin), and oxycodone (OxyContin).

Schedule III drugs are moderately addicting. Taking these drugs may lead to limited dependence. Refills are allowed up to five times in 6 months. This category includes combination drugs that contain a small amount of a narcotic with a less-addictive medication, such as acetaminophen or aspirin. This means that the patient gets less of the narcotic dose in each tablet, yet the combination of drugs is still powerful. Examples are anabolic steroids, hydrocodone (Hydrocet), and Tylenol 3. Allied health care professionals may write the prescription for the drug, but the prescriber must sign it.

Schedule IV drugs have lower abuse potential but are still controlled. As with schedule III drugs, allied health care professionals may write the prescription (e.g., name, route, dosage), but the prescriber must sign it. A health care worker can fax or phone in these orders to the pharmacy or facility. Refills are allowed up to five times in 6 months in this category. Examples include lorazepam (Ativan), diazepam (Valium), phenobarbital, and alprazolam (Xanax).

Schedule V drugs have the lowest potential for abuse. They include OTC cough suppressants, to which a small amount of codeine has been added, and preparations for diarrhea, such as paregoric and opium tincture. Because the syrup is thick, it is difficult to take enough to overdose; but small children like the taste of the syrup, so advise parents to keep the medicine away from children between doses. Examples are diphenoxylate hydrochloride and atropine sulfate preparations (Lomotil), Robitussin A-C, and Children's Tylenol 3.

Drugs may be prescribed in more than one schedule. For example full-strength codeine is a Schedule II drug because it is a highly addictive narcotic. If a manufacturer adds more acetaminophen or aspirin so that only a small amount of the narcotic is in the medication, it can be classified as a Schedule III drug. If the manufacturer puts a little narcotic in a lot of syrup, the medication can be classified as a Schedule V (e.g., Children's Tylenol with Codeine syrup) because it is less addictive if taken in such a small quantity.

For more information about controlled substances, go to the DEA website: http://www.usdoj.gov/dea/.

MANAGING CONTROLLED SUBSTANCES

If you work in an office that has controlled substances, you need to keep an inventory of them. You must keep a log of when you receive certain controlled medications and to whom you dispensed them. Be sure to sign off as to which patient received what dosage and sign your name to the documentation. Sign your name to the drug count only if you have counted the drugs to show that the count is accurate. Notify the physician immediately if the controlled drug count is not as recorded. These records must be kept for 2 years. See the DEA website for complete information. In the hospital setting, nurses usually count and log out the controlled substances on the unit. For more information about the Controlled Substance Act, visit http://www.usdoj.gov/dea/pubs/abuse/1-csa.htm.

Drug-addicted patients or people who sell drugs may come to the health care office or facility in search of controlled substances. These drugs should be kept double-locked in a safe place whenever they are not in your sight. Patients should not know where they are stored. Be suspicious of a patient who asks you for this information. If controlled substances are stolen or lost, the prescriber who has a DEA number must file DEA Form 106 Report of Theft or Loss of Controlled Substances, which is available on the DEA website.

If you need to dispose of a controlled medication, perhaps because it fell on the floor, you must have someone witness the disposal with you, and it must be destroyed beyond any possible reuse. Many states require that you return unused medications to a pharmacy or state police facility for incineration to ensure complete disposal. Controlled substances must be clearly marked as controlled. The label on the medication bottle shows a "C" for controlled substances. Do not put controlled substances in unmarked containers.

SUBSTANCE ABUSE

Substance abuse is a maladaptive pattern of behavior marked by the use of chemical agents. The key to substance abuse is that the patient does not adapt well under the influence of the substance.

Thousands of lives are lost each year in the United States because of substance abuse. Some substances are commonly and legally used, such as nicotine and alcohol (ETOH). Others are illegal drugs. Still others, such as steroids, are seen as a way to enhance athletic performance (see Fast Tip 2.2). Allied health professionals may see patients who show signs of substance abuse, including tremors (shaking), poor judgment, or slurred speech. It is important to remember that these signs can also be signs of disease states, so include all the facts when documenting such signs in the medical record.

Some drugs are especially addictive. Addiction means that you are compulsively driven to take the drug, often to the exclusion of all other activities. Most patients do not start taking a drug with the thought of becoming addicted, but over time they may become dependent on the drug—craving it either psychologically or physically. For example, a patient experiencing pain after an injury may take more and more of a medication to cope with the pain. Soon more of the drug is needed to produce the same effect because tolerance has developed.

> ### Fast Tip 2.2 Steroid Abuse
>
> The National Institute on Drug Abuse (NIDA) reports that anabolic steroids are frequently abused by people who want to build muscles, reduce body fat, and improve sports performance. Abuse is estimated to be high among competitive body builders and athletes. Men usually abuse steroids to become larger and more muscular, whereas women abuse steroids to become lean and muscular. Doses taken by abusers can be up to 100 times greater than doses used for treating medical conditions, such as the muscle wasting seen with acquired immunodeficiency syndrome (AIDS). Steroids can cause hormonal system disruptions, musculoskeletal system effects, infections, cardiovascular diseases, liver and skin dysfunction, and behavioral effects. (*Source: NIDA Notes*, Volume 15, Number 3, July 2000.)

Other people become habituated to drugs. This means they are psychologically tolerant of the drug and need more and more to achieve the desired effect. They may not physically need the drug but believe that they cannot live without it. For example, a patient may have pain after an injury. As his injury heals, he needs less of the drug for pain relief, but he begins to enjoy the way the drug makes him feel. He may take more of the medication to cope with what he perceives as the pain. Soon he takes increasing amounts of the drug because he has developed tolerance for it. Having the drug in his system becomes "normal."

It is vital to keep patients free of pain when they are in the acute stage of their disease or recovering from surgery. However, prescribers are typically reluctant to increase dosages over the long term for these patients. If patients engage in drug-seeking behavior (constantly requesting more medication out of proportion to physiological needs), the prescriber may reduce the amount of medication allowed and refer the patient for psychological counseling. Sometimes when a patient stops taking the medication, he or she may experience symptoms of *withdrawal,* such as tremors, emotional distress, and hallucinations. Chronic pain is a particular challenge, especially in those who are terminally ill (dying). These patients may experience increasing, not decreasing, pain as the disease worsens. The health care provider may prescribe more painkillers as time goes on but must be careful not to overprescribe drugs that can injure the patient by suppressing breathing.

CRITICAL THINKING

A patient calls frequently and begs for more pain medication. The doctor and staff are frustrated with the repeated requests, which they attribute to drug-seeking behavior. How would you handle this situation?

One of the best treatments for preventing behavior that may lead to tolerance or habituation is education. Frequently, patients do not understand the purpose of the medication or why they must stay within the ordered dose. You can help educate them by teaching them about side effects and cautionary situations (e.g., do not take during pregnancy). Chapter 6 provides you with resources to help your patients.

Perhaps a more difficult situation to handle is learning that a member of your office staff is abusing substances. If a health care provider is *impaired* (not fully functional mentally or physically) when caring for patients, it can have deadly consequences. The provider, under the influence of alcohol or other substances, may prescribe a wrong drug or be unable to safely perform minor surgery. An addicted staff member may steal drugs from the health care provider's stock, a facility's medication cart, or even from patients. Addicted people go to extreme lengths to get their drug(s) of choice and often lie to cover their behavior.

How can you determine if someone is impaired? In addition to the physical signs, certain common behaviors signal substance abuse, as noted in Box 2.3. For example, the health care provider may

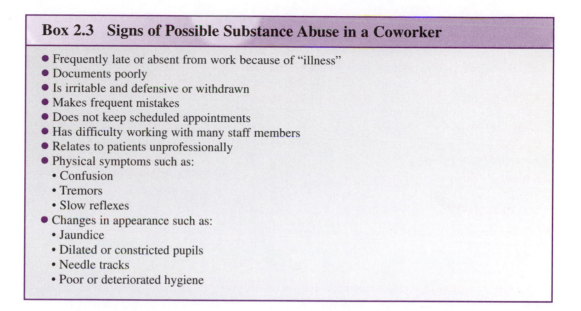

Box 2.3 Signs of Possible Substance Abuse in a Coworker

- Frequently late or absent from work because of "illness"
- Documents poorly
- Is irritable and defensive or withdrawn
- Makes frequent mistakes
- Does not keep scheduled appointments
- Has difficulty working with many staff members
- Relates to patients unprofessionally
- Physical symptoms such as:
  - Confusion
  - Tremors
  - Slow reflexes
- Changes in appearance such as:
  - Jaundice
  - Dilated or constricted pupils
  - Needle tracks
  - Poor or deteriorated hygiene

spend an inappropriate time away from patient tasks and make strange excuses for the absences. Although there may be reasons for these behaviors other than substance abuse, you must protect your patients. If any of your colleagues is impaired, report the behavior to your supervisor or office manager immediately. If the impaired person has a license, your supervisor should report the behavior to the state Board of Medicine, Board of Nursing, or another board, depending on the license. This may seem harsh, but the public depends on you for their safety.

Typically, addicted people may deny substance abuse or minimize the effects of their habit. If you have noticed that someone is impaired, you must focus on getting the person treatment. You do not do people a favor by enabling them to continue with their self-destructive behaviors. Follow your facility's protocol on how impaired employees are referred for treatment. Many employers have employee assistance programs or support groups organized through the human resources department.

Be familiar with local resources for treatment so you can help your colleague by suggesting community resources. It is important that you set boundaries and not accommodate the abuser by covering up the inappropriate behavior. Abusers sometimes lose their families and jobs before they get help. As a health care professional, you have the knowledge and ability to help a person get help.

CRITICAL THINKING

What are the phone number and address for the Board of Medicine and the Board of Nursing in your state? Write them here:

Hint: Licensed individuals post their licenses on the wall. The numbers should be on the licenses. If not, you can go to http://www.ncsbn.org to obtain contact information for the state Board of Nursing and http://www.healthguideusa.org/state_medical_boards.htm for information about your state Board of Medicine.

SUMMARY

Because drugs sometimes harm people, the U.S. government provides regulations and safeguards for their use, sale, and consumption. OSHA enacts laws geared toward protecting health care workers from patient diseases. This agency requires yearly education to ensure the safety of workers. The FDA approves drugs for sale in the United States, and the DEA makes sure that addictive drugs are carefully controlled. It is the professional responsibility of the allied health care worker to know the main laws and regulations related to medications.

Even though drugs can be helpful, they can harm people if used inappropriately. The allied health professional must be alert to signs of addiction in patients and colleagues. If you detect a substance abuser or impaired health care provider, report the facts to your supervisor or the state professional board and suggest that the addicted person obtain treatment.

Activities

To make sure that you have learned the key points covered in this chapter, complete the following activities.

True or False
Write *true* if the statement is true. Beside the false statements, write *false* and correct the statement to make it true.

1. The FDA approves drugs for dispensing in the United States. _____

2. Schedule V drugs are highly addictive. _____

3. The DEA is part of the Department of Health and Human Services. _____

4. OSHA requires yearly education on workplace safety. _____

5. Ativan is a Schedule I drug. _____

6. If the FDA approves a drug, it cannot be recalled. _____

7. Phase 1 clinical trials check for dosage. _____

8. Most drugs that are investigated with clinical trials are eventually approved. _____

9. The trade name becomes the official name of the drug. _____

10. An allied health profession does not need to memorize chemical names. _____

11. HMOs prefer to pay for generic drugs. _____

12. The FDA expects double-blind studies to be submitted. _____

13. FDA approval usually takes less than 6 months. _____

14. An example of a generic name is Restoril. _____

15. An orphan drug is an over-the-counter drug. _____

Multiple Choice
Choose the best answer for each question.

1. The governmental department that regulates workers' safety is:
   a. DEA
   b. DOJ
   c. FDA
   d. DHHS
   e. OSHA

2. Ritalin is a controlled substance in
   a. Schedule I
   b. Schedule II
   c. Schedule III
   d. Schedule IV
   e. Schedule V

3. Illegal drugs are considered to be
   a. Schedule I
   b. Schedule II
   c. Schedule III
   d. Schedule IV
   e. Schedule V

4. How must controlled substances be stored?
   a. In the refrigerator
   b. In the physician's desk
   c. In a double-locked cabinet
   d. With nonprescription medications

5. OSHA requires that:
   a. Controlled substances be logged daily
   b. All drugs be approved before use
   c. Doctors sign all orders
   d. Sharp needles should be disposed of in specially marked containers
   e. Prescription pads contain a special number to authorize the prescriber

6. Which governmental authorities inspect controlled substance logs?
   a. OSHA
   b. DEA
   c. FDA
   d. DHHS
   e. DOL

7. Which word means "more of the drug is needed to create the same effect"?
   a. Addiction
   b. Dependence
   c. Impaired
   d. Tolerance
   e. Withdrawal

8. Which word means "psychologically addicted"?
   a. Dependence
   b. Habituation
   c. Impaired
   d. Tolerance
   e. Withdrawal

9. Which agency determines what goes in the USP/NF?
   a. DEA
   b. FDA
   c. OSHA
   d. DOL
   e. DOJ

10. A drug that you can get without a prescription is referred to as a(an):
   a. IND
   b. OTC
   c. USP/NF
   d. Orphan drug
   e. Controlled substance

11. A placebo is:
   a. An inert ingredient
   b. A clinical trial
   c. A laboratory animal
   d. An FDA form
   e. A common drug name

12. Which is the official name?
   a. Ibuprofen
   b. ($\pm$)-2-(*Para*-isobutylphenyl) propionic acid
   c. Motrin
   d. Pain reliever
   e. Placebo

13. Trademarked drugs are usually protected from other people manufacturing them for:
   a. 1–5 years
   b. 6–10 years
   c. 11–15 years
   d. 17–20 years
   e. 21–25 years

14. Which of the following is the main reason for Phase 2 clinical trials?
   a. Dosage
   b. Efficacy
   c. Safety
   d. Testing on animals
   e. Response to MedWatch complaints

15. To get FDA approval of a drug, the manufacturer must fill out a(an):
   a. MedWatch form
   b. NDA
   c. IND
   d. Form 300

Short Answer
Answer these questions on a separate sheet.

   1. Why does the FDA require double-blind clinical trials before it approves a drug?
   2. Why does the FDA have a public hearing about drugs after they are approved?
   3. Why do some prescribers insist on brand-name drugs and do not allow generic substitutes?
   4. Why do HMOs prefer the purchase of generic drugs?
   5. Do you think it is safe to buy drugs from other countries on the Internet? Why or why not?
   6. Why is OSHA part of the Department of Labor?
   7. Why was the FDA established?
   8. What is the difference between physical and psychological dependence?
   9. What would you need to do if the controlled substance count did not match what was documented?
   10. Why are some prescription drugs controlled and others are not?

Application Exercises
Respond to the following scenarios on a separate sheet.

1. Bonny Glidewell calls to refill her prescription for birth control pills. She complains that she cannot get an appointment with the primary care provider until after her last pill pack will be used. **What would you do?**

2. You notice that a patient is wandering around the area where drugs are stored and later notice that several drugs are missing. **What would you do?**
3. Create a "controlled substance record" as though you were in a physician's office. **What information is important?**
4. You suspect that a colleague is addicted to painkillers. You report it to the office manager, and she says to document your suspicions. **What evidence might support your claim?**
5. **What would you do if you thought your physician employer was impaired and was about to perform surgery?**
6. You are an allied health worker conducting clinical trials on a new drug to lower blood pressure. The participants come in monthly for checkups. **What is the physician likely to order to check on the effectiveness of the drug?**
7. One of your patients, Kayla Christianson, is participating in clinical trials regarding a drug for depression at a local research facility. During a regular checkup at your dermatology office, she confides that she is suicidal. She says "Even this experimental drug does not work for me." **What do you think is happening? What should you do or say?**
8. In animal trials, clinicians fed mice hair dye and determined that eating hair dye was bad for mice. **Does that mean that all women should stop dyeing their hair? Defend your position.**

Virtual Field Trips

Go to the following websites to find the information. If a website is not available, try to find the information through another source.

1. Go to http://www.fda.gov and download a MedWatch Form 3500. Fill it out as though you were reporting adverse effects of a medication.
2. Go to http://www.fda.gov and list the latest products approved by the FDA.
3. Find http://www.deadiversion.usdoj.gov/. Using the DEA controlled substances schedules, list under which level of scheduling each of the following is classified: lysergic acid diethylamide, Marinol, Kaolin Pectin PG, meperidine, and midazolam.
4. Return to http://www.fda.gov and find out what drugs are currently experiencing shortages.
5. In case of bioterrorism, you may need to find information on anthrax vaccinations. Go to http://www.fda.gov and list how you can get information.
6. At http://www.fda.gov, search for a new drug and print its description.
7. Go to http://www.nlm.nih.gov and find out if marijuana is legal for use in the United States.
8. Visit http://www.naadac.org and find a list of clinicians who treat impaired professionals in your area.
9. Go to http://usdoj.gov/dea and find how to get information to teach children not to misuse drugs.
10. Explore http://www.ndmac.ca and find where McNeil Pharmaceuticals is located in Canada.
11. Go to http://www.fda.gov and give all the names for furosemide.
12. Visit http://www.ndmac.ca/. How many forms of naprosyn sodium are there?
13. Go to http://www.hc-sc.gc.ca/. Note the medications used for type 2 diabetes.
14. Go to http://www.nida.nih.gov and write a paragraph on rave drugs.
15. Find http://www.rxlist.com/script/main/hp.asp and find the generic names for the following drugs.
    a. Tylenol
    b. Coumadin
    c. Lanoxin
    d. Ritalin
    e. Vicodin

Sources and Actions

This chapter discusses where medications come from and how they act in our bodies. Pharmacodynamics involves the ways specific drugs produce changes in the body. These changes can be biochemical or physiological. Pharmacokinetics involves how a drug is absorbed, distributed, metabolized, and excreted. These mechanisms, pharmacodynamics and pharmacokinetics, help us understand the fundamental principles of pharmacology.

OBJECTIVES

At the end of this chapter, the student will be able to:

- Define all key terms.
- List five sources of drugs.
- List 10 drugs and record their sources.
- Describe what happens to drugs in the body.
- Discuss how aging affects the absorption of drugs.
- List three diseases that would prevent the excretion of drugs.
- Explain how drugs can adversely affect a fetus in the womb.
- Discuss how culture affects drug use.

KEY TERMS

Absorption
Adverse reaction
Agonists
Antagonists
Biotransformation
BUN
CrCl
Cumulation

Curative
Destructive
Diagnostic
Distribution
Excretion
Half-life
Idiosyncratic
Metabolism

Ototoxicity
Palliative
Pharmacodynamics
Pharmacokinetics
Polypharmacy
Potency
Prophylactic
Psychotropic

Replacement   Systemic   Toxic
Synergism   Teratogenic   Toxins
Synthetic

● SOURCES OF DRUGS

Our ancestors commonly used substances in their environment for medicinal effects. Although drugs are now manufactured in sterile clinical laboratories, many are derived from natural substances such as plants, animals, minerals, and toxins (Fig. 3.1). Some drugs are made by combining chemicals with natural products, such as adrenaline (epinephrine), whereas others are completely and artificially created in a laboratory (synthetic). Barbiturates are an example of synthetic drugs.

Plants

Many drugs come from plants. Digoxin (Lanoxin), a drug used to treat heart failure, is made from the foxglove plant. Epinephrine comes from the ephedra shrub. It is used today, as it was in ancient China, as a bronchodilator. Most estrogen hormone replacements come from yams. The drug Accutane, used for severe acne, contains soybean oil. Rosehips are a rich source of vitamin C.

One problem with plants as a source of medicine is that, as less farmland is available for growing plants, fewer plants are available for making medications.

 CRITICAL THINKING

If we rely on plants for medication, what effect does the increasing population have on our potential supply of medications?

Animals

Domesticated animals also provide a source for some drugs. To ensure the purity of the drugs, donor animals are generally well cared for.

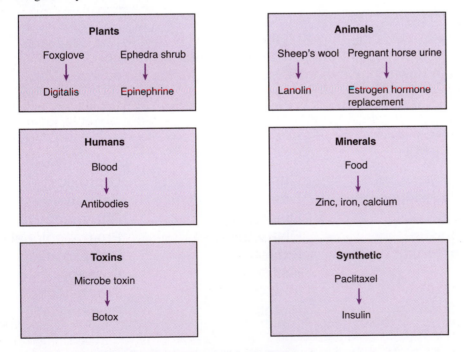

FIGURE 3.1. Examples of drugs and their sources.

Lanolin, a topical skin drug, comes from sheep's wool. No sheep have to die in the process. Cows (bovine) and pigs (porcine) are good sources of hormone replacements. If a patient cannot manufacture a hormone, an animal's hormone can be substituted for the patient's. Horses provide us with the replacement hormone Premarin (conjugated estrogen), which comes from a pregnant mare's urine.

CRITICAL THINKING

Cows and pigs are good sources of hormones. Why do you think animals may be better sources than humans? Why do you think they might not?

Humans

In rare cases, humans are sources for drugs. For example, human antibodies found in blood and breast milk can be given to other humans. People who donate substances from their bodies are carefully screened for health problems beforehand.

Minerals

In the past, people consumed minerals in food grown on farms with mineral-rich soil. Many people now, however, need supplements of common minerals, such as calcium, iron, zinc, magnesium, copper, and selenium.

Mineral replacement is key for patients on certain medications. Diuretic drugs such as furosemide (Lasix) cause the body to lose excess water through the kidneys; minerals such as potassium are lost along with the water. Potassium is needed for the heart to function normally, so supplemental potassium chloride is frequently prescribed as an adjunct. Patients can also get potassium by eating sweet potatoes, bananas, and oranges.

Toxins

Chemical and biological toxins are commonly used in medicine. For instance, certain radioactive chemicals are used to diagnose and treat illnesses. Radioactive iodine, for example, in small dosages can help pinpoint problems in a patient's thyroid, a small gland in the neck. In higher dosages, radioactive iodine is used to shrink thyroid tumors.

Biological toxins can also be used in medicine. For example, botulinum toxin, which comes from a bacterium called *Clostridium botulinum,* is used to reduce skin wrinkling.

Synthesis

Synthetic drugs can be created by genetic engineering or by altering animal cells. Often drugs first obtained from another source can be synthesized in the laboratory, thus saving natural resources. For example, paclitaxel (Taxol), a drug for patients who have cancer, was first made from the bark of the Pacific yew tree and then later developed as a synthetic drug. Insulin can be obtained from pigs or cows, but a synthetic source is most commonly used.

Because we can now map the human genome, we may be able to make drugs specifically tailored to a patient. Thus, prescribers can choose drugs that work better for a one population than for others. Research is also being conducted on the use of existing drugs in targeted populations. For example, BiDil is a combination of two generic drugs—hydralazine HCl and isosorbide dinitrate—that is used to treat African American patients with heart failure.

REASONS FOR MEDICATIONS

No matter what the source, patients take medications for different reasons. *Pharmacodynamics* refers to how a drug produces biochemical or physiological changes in the body. This includes both negative effects and desired effects. Drugs fall into six catagories of desired effects.

Some drugs are *curative*. They are made to cure the problem, such as a diuretic, which helps the body rid itself of excess fluid. Some prevent problems, such as antibiotics given before surgery to prevent infection. These are said to be *prophylactic*. If a drug is used to help diagnose a disease, such as barium that patients swallow to help highlight problems on a radiograph, it is *diagnostic*. Palliative drugs, such as pain relievers, do not cure disease, but they make patients more comfortable. Some drugs replace missing substances and are called *replacements*. Synthroid, for example, is a drug that replaces a thyroid hormone. *Destructive* medications destroy tumors and microbes. *Antineoplastic* (anticancer) drugs are an example of destructive, toxic drugs.

CRITICAL THINKING

Identify the following drugs as curative, prophylactic, diagnostic, palliative, destructive, or replacement.
- Synthroid
- Diuretic ("water pill")
- Flu vaccine
- Radiopaque dye
- Fever reducer
- Anticancer drugs

● A MEDICATION'S JOURNEY

Whenever someone takes or receives a medication, the drug embarks on a journey through the body, referred to as *pharmacokinetics*. The primary stops on this journey are absorption, distribution, metabolism, and excretion (Fig. 3.2). How fast the journey is completed depends in part on the drug itself, how it is given (e.g., swallowed vs. injected), and the patient's metabolic rate.

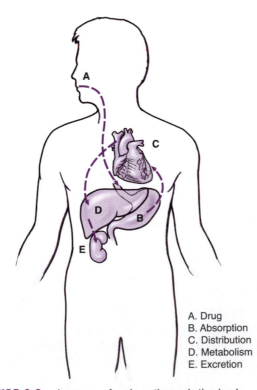

A. Drug
B. Absorption
C. Distribution
D. Metabolism
E. Excretion

FIGURE 3.2. Journey of a drug through the body.

Absorption

Absorption is the process of a substance moving from where it was administered into the bloodstream. The speed of absorption and how fast the drug works partly depends on whether the drug is *topical* or *systemic*. Topical drugs act locally; systemic drugs act in large areas of, or throughout, the body.

An example of a topical medication is ointment for a skin rash. The ointment works quickly in the local area of the rash. Most drugs that are swallowed are systemic. They act faster in liquid than pill form. Intramuscular injections, given into a muscle, provide fairly quick action because muscles have a rich supply of blood. Intravenous injection is the fastest way to the blood supply, as the drug is injected directly into the vein. The route by which a drug is given does not necessarily determine if it produces a topical or a systemic effect. For example, rectal suppositories can work locally (rectal suppositories used to treat hemorrhoids) or systemically (rectal suppositories used to treat nausea).

As an allied health professional, you can take steps to facilitate absorption. For instance, when administering a rectal suppository you can ensure that the rectum is free of feces. If a prescriber orders an intramuscular injection, you can choose which muscle to use. If the patient has a tattoo on the right arm, you may choose to give the injection in the left arm instead. The area with the tattoo may have decreased blood flow and thus slower absorption because of scar tissue and tattoo paint.

? CRITICAL THINKING

How does each of the following factors affect absorption?
- Length of time on the skin
- Food in the stomach
- Acidity of drug
- Tattoo on the skin
- Depth of respirations
- Drug concentration
- Blood supply to the site

Distribution

The second step is distribution. Once a drug is absorbed through a membrane, the bloodstream carries the drug to the site where it is needed. Sometimes the target area is close, and at other times it is far from the site. For example, if a patient inhales a drug, it may work effectively to open up the bronchi, or it may work to decrease pain elsewhere in the body.

Sometimes it is difficult for a drug to get from the blood to an organ because of physiological "barriers." These barriers generally consist of densely packed cells that let nutrients and certain other chemicals pass through but not others. They include the blood–placental barrier, blood–brain barrier, and blood–testicular barrier. Many drugs, such as psychotropic (mind-altering) drugs, can cross the

---

A CLOSER LOOK: The Absorption Factor

Several factors affect medication absorption:

- **Time.** The longer a topical medication is on the skin or mucosa, the more is absorbed. If a patient sucks on a lozenge until it dissolves, more medication is released in the mouth than if the patient chews and swallows it.
- **Food.** A large amount of food slows absorption of systemic medications. Stomach acid in the stomach facilitates absorption; therefore, if there is increased acid in the stomach, the medication is absorbed faster.
- **Depth of breathing.** For inhaled medications, the deeper patients breathe, the more medication they inhale. Ask patients to inhale deeply to get maximum benefit from the medication treatment.

blood–brain barrier. However, antibiotics and other drugs that may be easily absorbed in the stomach cannot cross the blood–brain barrier.

 CRITICAL THINKING

> **Why do drugs that cross the blood–brain barrier tend to have strong negative effects?**

To protect the vulnerable fetus, the blood–placental barrier regulates drugs and other substances passing from mother to fetus. However, alcohol, cocaine, and even some over-the-counter medications can cross this barrier easily and cause harm to the fetus. The use of medications in pregnant women is covered in more detail later in the chapter.

 CRITICAL THINKING

> **Why should a pregnant woman consult her physician before taking an over-the-counter medication?**

The blood–testicular barrier protects the male reproductive organs from toxins that could damage sperm. This barrier also makes certain male reproductive diseases difficult to treat. Many psychotropic drugs have negative sexual effects, such as decreased libido, because they cross both the blood–brain barrier and the blood–testicular barrier.

Metabolism

Metabolism is the third step on the medication journey. This is the process whereby drugs become either more or less active, depending on their chemical makeup. The liver, intestines, and kidneys metabolize drugs to change them in a process called *biotransformation*.

 CRITICAL THINKING

> **David Marchefka has liver damage. How might that damage affect the way his body metabolizes drugs?**

Excretion

Once a medication has acted in the body, it is excreted from the body. Most drugs are removed by the kidneys, although some are released as a gas by the lungs, and a few are excreted via bile. Saliva and sweat glands excrete a small amount of drugs, and breasts excrete some drugs in breast milk.

CRITICAL THINKING

> **Why should a nursing mother contact her doctor before using herbal therapies?**

Drugs that are not excreted well tend to build up in the body. This is called *cumulation*. If drugs accumulate in the body, the patient may become very ill.

Therapeutic Levels

The efficacy of a medication depends on its therapeutic level—the point at which the drug has the maximum desired effect. Giving too little of a drug makes it less than effective. Giving too much can be toxic, or poisonous, to the patient. To be sure the drug level is in the therapeutic range, blood levels may need to be monitored.

Potency, the drug's power or strength, typically increases and then decreases over time (see Fast Tip 3.1). Taking more than one drug can affect potency. A drug is called an agonist when it is taken

⬤ *Fast Tip 3.1* Half-Life

The *half-life* is the length of time required for the concentration of a drug to decrease by one-half in the plasma. The half-life affects the duration of potency for a medication. Drugs with a long half-life may need to be taken less frequently than those with a shorter half-life. The effects of drugs with shorter half-lives tend to wear off faster. For example, an anesthetic with a short half-life may be chosen if the patient plans to drive home from the facility soon after treatment.

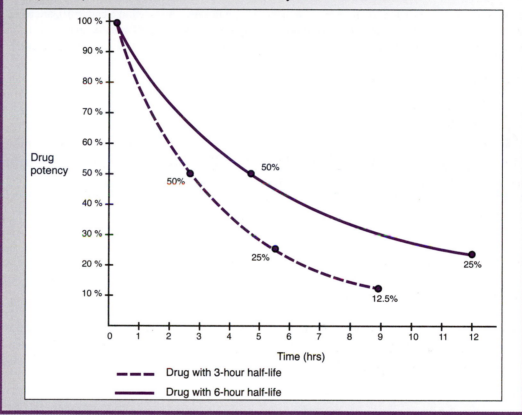

with another drug so the two can work together. This makes the combination of the drugs more powerful than either of them separately (synergism). Antagonists do the opposite—they can make another drug less powerful.

Several factors affect the therapeutic blood level of a drug: other drugs, nutritional factors, body size, environmental factors, sex, and culture.

Drug interactions

If a patient is taking several drugs, adjustments may need to be made in the dosages of each drug. Some drugs potentiate (strengthen) the effects of other drugs, and some weaken their effects. Natural and herbal remedies can also interact with drugs and affect dosing. Always ask the patient if he or she is taking natural or herbal remedies.

Anytime a combination of drugs is ordered, you must check your drug handbook to verify whether the drugs can be given together.

Nutritional factors

A poor diet can reduce therapeutic levels because some nutrients are needed for absorption. Dehydration can cause medication levels to be higher than normal. Laxatives may cause poor absorption from the gastrointestinal tract. Exercise can increase the metabolism and cause medications to be absorbed more quickly. Exercise also decreases the need for insulin and is used to control blood glucose in patients with diabetes. Chewing gum increases saliva, which increases food breakdown and absorption.

Some foods can alter a drug's effect. Administering tetracycline (an antibiotic) with calcium prevents tetracycline's absorption. Most antibiotics work best when taken on an empty stomach. Foods high in vitamin B_6 can impair the actions of drugs use to treat Parkinson's disease. Grapefruit juice inhibits some drugs if taken at the same time.

Body size

Drug dosing is usually based on total body weight. Normal dosages, as noted in Chapter 10, are based on an average adult body weight of 70 kg (about 150 pounds). However, size and distribution of fat in the patient can change the way the drug is processed. In obese patients, if a drug that does not penetrate fatty tissues is used the dosage may have to be adjusted.

Extremely underweight patients usually need lower amounts of drugs because of their lower body weight. Patients with amputated limbs also require lower dosages because of lower body weight.

CRITICAL THINKING

How can the following affect therapeutic levels?
• Poor diet
• Fluid intake
• Laxatives
• Exercise
• Chewing gum
• Antibiotics
• Weight

Environmental factors

Smoking cigarettes induces liver enzymes to metabolize drugs more rapidly. For this reason, patients who smoke cigarettes may need larger doses of liver-metabolized drugs. The effects of active and second-hand smoke may persist for months.

Sex differences

On the whole, men have more muscle and less fat than women. This means that medications are absorbed and distributed in the body more quickly in men than in women.

Cultural effects

The mind is powerful—it can aid or hinder health through deep-rooted cultural beliefs. Different cultures view the use of medications differently. Some cultures have a belief system grounded in scientific research. People in these cultures find comfort in knowing that medicines have gone through rigorous testing before being approved. They are more likely to be dependent on their primary health care provider to choose drugs for them.

More holistic cultures believe that an imbalance in the patient's life causes disease. People with a holistic outlook may be less likely to use conventional drugs and more inclined toward herbal remedies.

Some cultures believe illness comes from magic. There is a belief that if taboos (rules) are broken, evil sprits hurt people. People in these cultures may search for alternative healers, with or without continuing to take medications prescribed by their primary health care provider.

CRITICAL THINKING

Seth Eaton comes to the office with a wound that does not seem to be healing. As he is leaving, he states, "I am going to see my herbalist. Your drugs can't help me!" What would you do or say?

SIDE EFFECTS

Every medication carries a risk of side effects. An adverse effect is a serious side effect such as shock or death. Side effects are usually mild, such as nausea, constipation, or sensitivity to light. Often the patient can continue to take the drug and manage the side effect with medication, taking the drug with food, or some other intervention. Adverse effects are severe and may cause the prescriber to change the medication to a different one.

Not surprisingly, a topical drug has fewer side effects than a systemic one. For example, putting an anti-inflammatory drug such as diphenhydramine (Benadryl) directly onto the skin that is itching reduces the chance of systemic side effects. Swallowing the medication gets rid of inflammation throughout the body but causes more side effects such as drowsiness.

As an allied health professional, you should always check a drug resource for the side effects of the medications your patient is taking so you can watch for them. However, even though a side effect is not listed, a patient can have a unique, or *idiosyncratic*, reaction to any drug. This effect may not have shown up in clinical trials because it is so rare, but it is a real symptom in your patient and must be managed. If it is a serious reaction, report it through the MedWatch program.

SPECIAL PATIENTS

Certain patients require special care related to medication dosage: pediatric patients, the elderly, pregnant women, and patients with diseases related to the liver, kidney, and heart.

A CLOSER LOOK: Side Effects

Side effects are usually classified by body system or organ. Please review the following examples.

Central nervous system—Side effects related to this area include agitation, hallucinations, confusion, delirium, disorientation, depression, drowsiness, sedation, decreased respiration and circulation, dizziness, and coma.

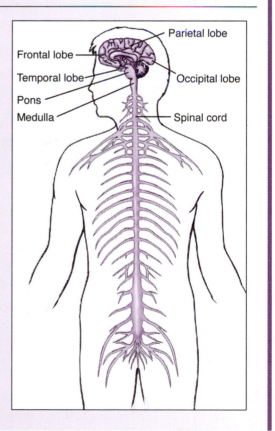

(box continued on page 46)

A CLOSER LOOK: Side Effects *(continued)*

Liver—The liver metabolizes drugs and can be damaged if drugs accumulate. Alcohol, acetaminophen, isoniazid, and aspirin can cause liver damage. Early side effects are detected only by the presence of high liver enzyme levels in the blood. If liver damage is undetected, jaundice (yellowing of the skin and eyes) can occur.

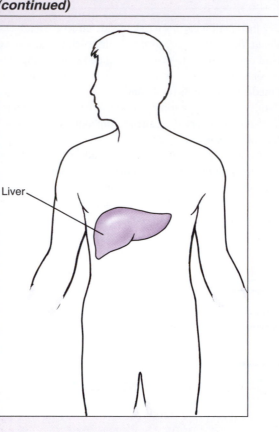

Gastrointestinal system—Examples include anorexia, nausea, vomiting, constipation, and diarrhea. With prolonged use of some drugs, stomach ulcers and colitis (inflammation of the intestines) can occur.

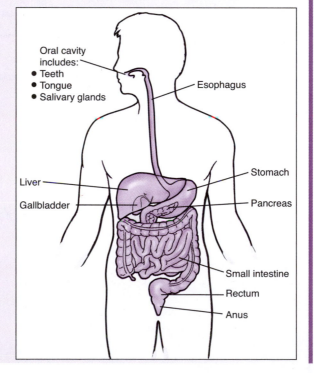

Kidney—The kidneys excrete most medications, so certain kinds of drugs (e.g., ibuprofen and other nonsteroidal anti-inflammatory medications) can impair kidney function. Patients may experience fluid and electrolyte imbalance and abnormally high potassium levels, among other problems.

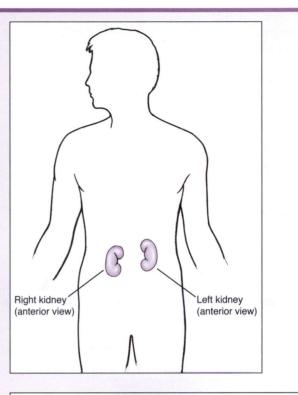

Right kidney
(anterior view)

Left kidney
(anterior view)

Eyes, ears, nose, and throat—Some medications, such as certain types of antibiotics and anticancer drugs, can cause ototoxicity ("ear poisoning"), resulting in loss of hearing or balance.

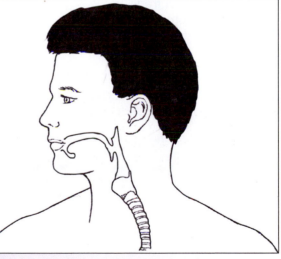

Hematologic—Drugs can cause problems such as poor coagulation of the blood, bleeding, clotting, and bone marrow diseases. Anticancer drugs are especially toxic to bone marrow. Any patient on an anticoagulant to decrease clotting should be carefully monitored for signs of bleeding, such as dark, tarry stools. Blood levels should be monitored to ensure that the drug level is therapeutic but not toxic.

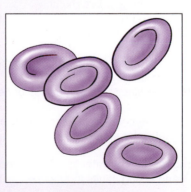

Pediatric Patients

Pediatric patients are not just small adults. They usually have higher metabolism but decreased weight so they need less medication.

A neonate or premature baby has special needs. This baby has a different gastric pH and gastrointestinal motility from adults. Liver and kidney function may not be mature enough to function well in clearing the medication from the patient. Because weight changes rapidly in infants, frequent dosage adjustments must be made.

Infants have poorly developed arm muscles, so medications are injected into the infant's leg if they are to be given into muscle. Infants' and children's blood vessels are more fragile than in adults, and these patients can easily become overhydrated if intravenous therapy is not carefully monitored. Children are frequently afraid of injections and other interventions, so you may have to give age-appropriate explanations about the procedures to these patients.

Most drugs are not tested on pediatric patients, and a drug tested in adults may not act in the same way in a child (Table 3.1). Be especially alert to side effects, and fill out a MedWatch form if there is an adverse reaction.

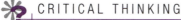

CRITICAL THINKING

How do pediatric patients differ from adult patients regarding the following?
- Amount of dosage
- Site of administration
- Length of needle for parenteral administration
- Fat/muscle body composition
- Metabolism of medication
- Blood vessel fragility
- Blood volume
- Cooperating with therapy

TABLE 3.1 Pharmacology in Neonates, Infants, and Young Children

Because their bodies are not fully developed, it is especially important to monitor drug effects in these age groups.

DEVELOPMENTAL FACTOR	EFFECT
Gastric pH is higher in neonates and infants; adult levels at 20–30 months	Decreased absorption in younger patients
Irregular emptying time for stomach; adult functioning at 6–8 months	Absorption is unpredictable
Decreased lipase secretion in infants	Lipid-formulated drugs are not well absorbed
Thin stratum cornea in infants	Increased absorption of topical medications applied in the eye
Rectally administered drugs absorbed more quickly in infants	Increased absorption can lead to toxicity
Variable blood flow to muscles of neonate	Absorption of drugs injected into muscle is unpredictable
Larger percentage of extracellular and total water in the body in neonates and infants	Wider distribution of drugs
Higher ratio of water to lipid in neonates and young adults in adipose tissue	Lower level of drug in bloodstream

Source: Moser Wood, T. *Advance for Nurse Practitioners* (http://nurse-practitioners.advanceweb.com/common/EditorialSearch/AViewer.aspx?AN=NP_04jun1_npp22.html&AD=06-01-2004).

Geriatric Patients

In patients older than 55 years, decreased absorption occurs because of diminished gastrointestinal function and congestion of abdominal blood vessels. Distribution can also be altered because of low plasma protein levels, particularly if the patient is malnourished. When plasma proteins are decreased, a larger amount of unbound drug results in increased drug action. Thus toxic drug levels can be found in elderly patients, even at normal dosages. The aging process also alters liver and kidney function, resulting in the accumulation of medications. In addition, body composition changes as we age. Elderly patients have increased fatty tissue and decreased skeletal muscle and water, which slows drug absorption and distribution.

Because of these factors, dosages may be lower for elderly patients. Of special concern are sedative-hypnotics, anticoagulants, nonsteroidal anti-inflammatory drugs (NSAIDs), antihypertensives (drugs that lower blood pressure), and thrombolytics (drug that break up blood clots).

Another concern for geriatric patients is *polypharmacy*—taking several medications for more than one problem. As patients take more medications, their risk of drug interactions and side effects rises. You may have to spend more time on education with elderly patients because of the complexity of drug regimens and because decreased patient memory may necessitate repetition of information.

Pregnant Patients

The blood–placental barrier shields the fetus by stopping some medications from crossing from the mother to the fetus. Severe malformations or death of the fetus can occur if a *teratogenic* (literally, monster-producing) drug crosses the placenta.

The fetus is especially vulnerable to medications during the first trimester (when vital organs are forming) and the last trimester (when the baby is prone to accumulating drugs before birth). The FDA classifies drugs as to how safe they are in pregnant women (Table 3.2). Always check your drug handbook before giving a drug to a pregnant woman to ensure that it is not a teratogen.

✱? CRITICAL THINKING

If an obstetric patient calls and asks what over-the-counter drugs she can take for a cold, where would you find that information?

Patients with Organ Dysfunction

Great care must be taken when administering drugs to patients with organ dysfunction, particularly of the liver, kidneys, and heart, because drugs can easily build up to undesirable levels.

TABLE 3.2 FDA Drug Safety Categories for Pregnancy

CATEGORY	RISK	DESCRIPTION	EXAMPLES
A	Lowest	Studies have not shown a risk to mother or fetus.	Levothyroxine (Synthroid)
B	Slight	Animal studies have not shown a risk to the fetus; or if they have, human studies have not.	Insulin (Humulin R)
C	Moderate	Animal studies have shown a risk to the fetus, but controlled studies have not been performed on women.	Furosemide (Lasix)
D	Risky	Studies show these drugs may cause harm to the fetus, so prescriber must weigh risk vs. benefit. May use if another, safer therapy is not available.	Warfarin (Coumadin)
X	Highest	Studies have shown significant risk to mother and fetus.	Castor oil (Purge)

Source: Deglin JH. and Vallerand AH. *Davis's Drug Guide for Nurses*. Philadelphia, F.A. Davis, 2003.

Because the liver metabolizes drugs, poor functioning leads to a buildup of drugs and toxic effects. Patients who chronically abuse alcohol may have destroyed much of their liver's ability to function. Decreased serum protein levels can alter a drug's ability to bond. More unbound medication is therefore available to exert its effect, which can lead to side effects. Unfortunately, no laboratory test adequately predicts appropriate dosages when the liver is not working properly.

CRITICAL THINKING

How does liver disease affect the accumulation of drugs in the body?

Most drugs are metabolized in the liver and excreted through the kidneys. Others are excreted unmetabolized through the kidneys. Not only can this destroy the kidneys, it puts patients with kidney disease at risk for accumulating toxic amounts of drugs. To determine the proper dosing of drugs in patients with kidney disease, blood specimens are drawn for laboratory tests, such as blood urea nitrogen (BUN) and creatinine clearance (CrCl).

In patients with heart failure, the heart fails to pump fluid adequately. This can cause congestion of blood vessels in the gastrointestinal tract, which results in decreased drug absorption and decreased delivery of the drug to the liver. Kidney function is also compromised by the congestion, leading to delayed excretion and thus drug accumulation in the patient. For these reasons, patients with heart failure usually take decreased doses of medications.

SUMMARY

Medications come from several sources: plants, animals, minerals, and the laboratory. When drugs enter our bodies, they are absorbed across membranes, distributed to a site of action, metabolized at that site, and finally excreted. If disease processes exist, drugs can accumulate and cause toxicity.

Even though drugs can be helpful, they can also cause side effects and serious adverse effects. It is vital that you use a drug handbook to look up any drug about which you need more information.

To make sure that you have learned the key points covered in this chapter, complete the following activities.

True or False

Write *true* if the statement is true. Beside the false statements, write *false* and correct the statement to make it true.

1. Cumulation means a drug causes disease. _____

2. An antagonist blocks a drug from being effective. _____

3. Efficacy means the strength of the drug. _____

4. A drug's half-life is the time needed to decrease the drug's plasma concentration by 50%. _____

5. Psychotropic drugs cross the blood–brain barrier. _____

6. A prophylactic drug prevents illness. _____

7. Synthetic drugs are created in a laboratory. _____

8. Anticancer drugs cross the blood–placenta barrier. _____

9. Ototoxicity can damage the eyes. _____

10. Idiosyncratic means safe for children. _____

Multiple Choice

Choose the best answer for each question.

1. Where does lanolin come from?
   a. Animal
   b. Plant
   c. Mineral
   d. Human
   e. Synthesis

2. Where does potassium chloride come from?
   a. Animal
   b. Plant
   c. Mineral
   d. Human
   e. Synthesis

3. Where does digoxin (Lanoxin) come from?
   a. Animal
   b. Plant
   c. Mineral
   d. Human
   e. Synthesis

4. Where do barbiturates come from?
   a. Animal
   b. Plant
   c. Mineral
   d. Human
   e. Synthesis

5. Which means leaving the body?
   a. Absorption
   b. Biotransformation
   c. Distribution
   d. Excretion
   e. Metabolism

6. Which means moving through membranes?
   a. Absorption
   b. Biotransformation
   c. Distribution
   d. Excretion
   e. Metabolism

7. Which is a replacement drug?
   a. Digoxin
   b. Lasix
   c. Accutane
   d. Synthroid
   e. Plavix

8. Which is a diagnostic drug?
   a. Estrogen
   b. Barium
   c. Flu vaccine
   d. Anticancer drug
   e. Vitamin C

9. Which is a destructive drug?
   a. Antibiotic
   b. Insulin
   c. Diuretic
   d. Psychotropic
   e. Potassium chloride

10. Ototoxicity occurs in the:
   a. Eyes
   b. Ears
   c. Liver
   d. Kidneys
   e. Brain

Short Answer Questions
Answer these questions on a separate sheet.

1. Why might the physician order you to give an antagonist?
2. Why are drugs not tested on children during clinical trials?
3. Are animals good sources for drugs? Explain your answer.
4. Why can a drug be toxic to a fetus without hurting the mother?
5. If a patient is scheduled for surgery, why would the doctor order a prophylactic antibiotic?

Application Exercises

Respond to the following scenarios on a separate sheet.

1. Mary Jessie Tyler is on a blood-thinner. She does not understand why she needs to have blood drawn monthly. **How would you educate her?**
2. Daniel Gilbert has cirrhosis of the liver. **How might this affect his metabolism of drugs?**
3. Butler DePoy is coming in for a flu shot into the muscle. He insists that he wants it in his arm, not his buttocks. Both arms are covered in tattoos. **What would you do?**
4. Roelofs Seeber has diabetes. Because of her diabetes, she has increased blood pressure and kidney problems. **How does this affect the distribution and elimination of drugs from her body?**
5. Thomas Nelson just turned 65. **What aspects of the aging process might cause his physician to reevaluate the dosage of the medication he has taken for 20 years?**
6. Jerry Gill, an elderly patient, comes in with a paper bag containing assorted pills. He is not sure which he is supposed to be taking. **What would you do?**
7. You draw blood from Gary Gledhill, to check compliance with drug therapy, but the laboratory results show none of that drug in his blood. **What might be happening? What would you do?**
8. Muhammed Al-Doost is a devout Muslim. He does not eat pork. **Can he have porcine insulin?**
9. Azeeza Wood was born prematurely. **How might her prematurity affect the way drugs work in her little body?**
10. Patrick Snow is 72 years old. He complains that normal dosages of antidepressants make him feel sleepy. **How does his age affect his body's use of the drug?**
11. Beth Rollins is pregnant. She calls the office to see what drugs she can use for cold symptoms. **Where would you look to find out which drugs are safe for her?**
12. Mickie Scanlon is a diabetic with impaired vision. **How should an allied health worker make sure he can take his medications safely?**
13. Valentina Artomovich wants to know why she needs less of a medication as she ages. Because her liver is getting sicker, she insists she should be taking more medication, not less. **What would you say to her?**
14. Vera Bishop complains that she hears ringing in her ears since starting a new drug. **What is this called, and what might be causing this?**
15. Leta Hardwick is going in for dental surgery. Her physician prescribes an antibiotic even before the surgery. **How would you explain to her why she needs to take the antibiotic?**

Virtual Field Trips

Go to the following websites to find the information. If a website is not available, try to find the information through another source.

1. Go to http://www.mdadvice.com/. List the adverse effects of too much vitamin A (beta-carotene, retinol).
2. Visit http://www.nlm.nih.gov/medlineplus and find the side effects of:
   Coumadin
   Ritalin
   Valproic acid
   Lithium
   OxyContin
3. Go to your search engine and research *fetal alcohol syndrome*. What are the teratogenic effects of alcohol ingestion during pregnancy?
4. Surf to http://www.nlm.nih.gov/medlineplus/. Methotrexate kills cancer cells. What are its side effects?
5. Go to http://www.rxlist.com/. Research *lithium*. Why is it important to obtain frequent blood specimens from lithium patients?

Forms and Routes of Drugs

Medications come in different forms and can be delivered in different ways. Some drugs need to be quickly absorbed and are injected or inhaled. Others are absorbed more slowly through the gastrointestinal system. In some cases, localized treatment is needed and is performed by placing the medication on the skin or mucosa. Other medications are needed systemically and are therefore administered into the bloodstream. This chapter reviews common routes and forms for delivering medications.

OBJECTIVES

At the end of this chapter, the student will be able to:

● Define all key terms.
● List the forms in which medications are distributed.
● Discuss how the different forms of drugs affect the body.
● List the possible routes for administering medications.
● Describe why prescribers choose certain forms and routes over others.
● Cite the resource where you can determine if you are allowed to administer IV therapy.

KEY TERMS

Buffered	Enteric-coated	Intradermal
Caplets	ETOH	Intramuscular
Capsules	Gels	IUD
Creams	Implanted devices	IV push
Delayed action	Induration	Jellies
Effervescent	Infusion	Liniments
Elixirs	Inhalation	Lotions
Emulsions	Inhalers	Lozenges
Enemas	Inserts	Magmas

Nebulizer
Ointments
Ophthalmic
Oral
Otic
Parenteral
Patch
Piggyback
Plasters

Powders
PPD
Salves
Scored
Solutions
Subcutaneous
Sublingual
Suppositories
Suspensions

Syrups
Tablets
Timed-release
Topical
Transdermal
Troches
Viscous

● ROUTES AND FORMS

The form of a medication relates to the desired route. The main routes are gastrointestinal, parenteral, nasal, ophthalmic, otic, and topical (Box 4.1). More specifics about how to administer drugs are given in Chapter 7.

Gastrointestinal Route

By far, the most common route is the gastrointestinal system. Although absorption is slower by this route compared to others, it is less invasive and tolerated well by most patients. Gastrointestinal routes include buccal, sublingual, oral, and rectal.

Buccal route

The buccal, or cheek, route is good for applying medication in the mouth or throat to ease local inflammation. Troches or lozenges can be held in the cheek. They are usually pleasant-tasting and melt slowly over time, coating the throat and mouth. For a sore throat, this is the ideal route. It is important to tell the patient not to swallow or bite the buccal medication, as it would then not work as planned. The patient may need to refrain from drinking for 15 to 20 minutes after taking the buccal medication to maximize the effect and prevent the medication from being washed away.

Sublingual route

Sublingual means under the tongue. The many capillaries under the tongue provide a rich blood supply for quick absorption of a medication. For that reason, nitroglycerin, which improves heart function, is placed there for immediate relief of heart pain or during a heart attack. Although slower than an injection into a vein, the sublingual route delivers medication quickly, without it having to pass completely through the digestive system.

Oral route

The oral (swallowing) route is the easiest for the patient, but medications must go through the digestive system for absorption. Several drug forms can be given via the oral route.

BOX 4.1 Medication Routes	
Gastrointestinal	Subcutaneous (SC)
Buccal	Intravenous (IV)
Sublingual	**Inhalation**
Oral	**Nasal**
Rectal	**Ophthalmic**
Parenteral	**Otic**
Intradermal (ID)	**Topical/transdermal**
Intramuscular (IM)	**Vaginal**

Gelatin-coated *capsules* containing drugs are easier to swallow than tablets. They can be easily pulled apart to mix the contained drug into food for those who have difficulty swallowing. Capsules can be made to release medication quickly or a little at a time (timed-release or delayed action), which allows the patient to take it less often. Of course, timed-release capsules cannot be opened or crushed lest they release the drug all at once and overdose the patient. They must therefore be swallowed whole.

Effervescent salts are granules or coarse powders containing one or more medicinal agents, as well as tartaric acid or sodium bicarbonate. When dissolved in water or other liquids, effervescent salts produce bubbles. An example is Alka-Seltzer.

Elixirs contain alcohol (ETOH) in the preparation and so should not be used in children or alcoholics. They must be kept tightly capped to prevent evaporation. Elixirs are used less often than in the past because of the detrimental effects of alcohol, the potential for interaction with many other medications, and the development of new medication delivery systems. Elixirs are usually not given to diabetics because the liver converts the alcohol to sugar.

Emulsions are liquid drug preparations that contain oils and fats in water. They must usually be shaken to mix them. *Magmas* are also liquid and contain fine particles in milk. An example is Milk of Magnesia.

Powders are finely rounded forms of an active drug. Sometimes powders, such as BC Powder or Goody's Powder for pain relief, are placed on the tongue and absorbed into the bloodstream. Other medications, such as bulk laxatives, are added to large amounts of water and are taken orally.

Solutions are medications evenly distributed throughout a liquid. You do not need to shake solutions, and the medication amount should be equally distributed whether you withdraw from the top or the bottom. An example is normal saline solution.

Suspensions are medications dispersed in a liquid, but the medication may not been evenly distributed. For that reason, you usually have to shake a suspension. They are easier to swallow than tablets for patients who have trouble swallowing. An example is Pepto-Bismol.

Syrups, as the name suggests, are medications added to highly sweetened liquids. They are especially popular with children. Caution should be exercised in diabetics because of the high sugar content. An example is Robitussin cough syrup. It is important for children to understand that they are taking a medicine, not a type of candy.

Tablets, disks of compressed medication, may be the most popular form of medication. They come in a variety of shapes and colors that distinguish them from other tablets (see Fast Tip 4.1). Tablets can be scored (marked in half) for easy separation if half of a tablet is needed. Tablets are rarely cut by more than half.

Rectal route

Some medications can be given by the rectal route, directly into the rectum (the end of the digestive system). This route is sometimes necessary because the patient has severe nausea or vomiting. Liquids placed in the rectum to encourage bowel movement are called enemas. Suppositories are medications suspended in a waxy substance such as cocoa butter that melt at body temperature.

⚪ *Fast Tip 4.1* Special Forms of Tablets

Tablets can be coated to improve swallowing or prevent release in the stomach (enteric-coated), or they can be in a timed-release form. Enteric-coated drugs are released not in the stomach but in the intestines, so they are especially useful for people with stomach ulcers or sensitivity. Buffered tablets have antacids added to them to prevent stomach irritation. Caplets are similar to tablets but may be easier for some patients to swallow.

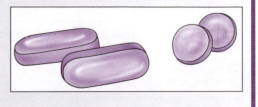

CRITICAL THINKING

Why is the gastrointestinal route so popular for taking medications?

Parenteral Route

Parenteral, meaning given by a route other than the digestive system, is another route for medications. Many medications are injected in solutions. Sometimes powders are ordered, but bacteriostatic sodium chloride solution or aqueous (water) solution must be added so the drug can be injected. Although the injection may hurt when the needle is inserted, the patient does not usually experience great pain at the injection site if care is taken to select the correct site and inject the solution slowly.

Intradermal route

Using the intradermal (ID) route, the medication stays mostly in the dermis of the skin. Injected just underneath the skin at a 15° angle, this route is primarily used for allergy testing and to check for exposure to tuberculosis.

A CLOSER LOOK: Tuberculosis Testing

To see if a patient has been exposed to tuberculosis (TB), a small amount of purified protein derivative (PPD) is injected just under the skin. If a patient has already been exposed to TB, a hard swelling (induration) appears within several days. Redness without swelling is not indicative of a positive PPD. If you notice induration on a patient, you must measure and document it. Usually the local Public Health Department needs to be notified.

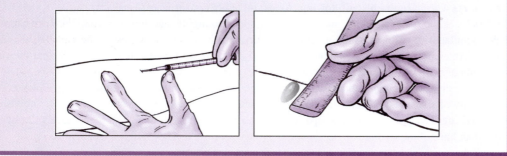

Implanted devices can be placed intradermally or into a body cavity to release a medication over time. An example is an implanted device that releases contraceptive hormones, such as Norplant, which is implanted in the arm.

Intramuscular route

With an intramuscular (IM) injection, medication is quickly absorbed into the bloodstream because of the plentiful blood supply to muscles. The onset of drug action usually occurs within 10 to 15 minutes. IM injections are inserted at a 90° angle into a muscle. Sites for IM injections must be identified accurately. Damage to major blood vessels and nerves could occur if an inappropriate site is used. Also, sites should be rotated to avoid damaging the muscle.

CRITICAL THINKING

Is it professional to tell a child that an injection will not hurt? Explain.

Subcutaneous route

Fat does not have a good blood supply, so a medication injected by the subcutaneous route is absorbed slowly over time. Subcutaneous injections are medications in solution injected at a 45° angle into the fatty layer below the skin. Insulin is destroyed in the gastrointestinal tract and is most commonly given by this route. Heparin, which prevents blood clots, may also be given subcutaneously. Site rotation is important to promote absorption and to avoid the development of nodules in the subcutaneous tissue.

Intravenous route

The fastest way to get medication into the bloodstream is by the intravenous (IV) route, which means injecting the drug directly into a vein. IV injection causes immediate absorption and availability. This can be good for quick relief of symptoms and in an emergency, but it is also the most dangerous route because there is little time to correct any errors in administration. In addition, the patient receives the full dose of the drug.

In the modern world, where technology changes quickly and there is a shortage of nurses, the role of the allied health professional is a dynamic one. In some states and some facilities, allied health professionals can insert IV lines, hang IV bags of fluid, disconnect IV lines, or flush ports in IV lines. In other facilities and localities, this is considered solely a nursing function. It is important that you understand what your state and facility permit you to do, so you do not practice nursing without a license. It is helpful for you to at least understand IV therapy, however, and you should be prepared to assess patients for signs and symptoms of infection and problems with their IV lines. More detail about IV infusions is provided in Chapter 7.

Intravenously administered drugs are given one of three ways. A drip, or *infusion*, means that a large volume of medication in fluid is administered over time through an IV line. A *piggyback* line holds a small amount (50–100 mL) of solution given at certain ordered intervals, along with an IV infusion. *IV push* refers to a small volume of drug injected through a syringe into a special lock in the IV line, which has been inserted into a vein. Because of the high potential for harm to the patient if an IV push is done incorrectly, only nurses, physicians, and other health care professionals are normally permitted to give drugs this way.

Veins for insertion of an IV are not always the ones most prominent visibly. A better vein may be the one that can be felt after a tourniquet is applied. The health care professional inserting an IV must consider several factors (Table 4.1). It is ideal to use the nondominant arm or hand and one that has not been recently injured. The hand is preferred so that, if the IV has to be placed in another vein, it can be placed in a vein above the original site. Just as important as where to place an IV is where not to place it. The health care professional should not use a site in a swollen arm, in an arm that is not functioning normally because of stroke, or in an arm on the same side as a mastectomy (removal of breast tissue). The Infusion Nurses Society recommends rotating IV sites every 72 hours.

Complications of IV therapy include bleeding, infection, phlebitis, infiltration, catheter dislodgement, occlusion, vein irritation, severed catheter, hematoma, venous spasm, thrombosis, thrombophlebitis, circulatory overload, nerve or tendon or ligament damage, systemic infection, air embolism, allergic reaction, incompatibility of medications, and irreversible medication error.

TABLE 4.1 Advantages and Disadvantages of IV Insertion Sites

VEIN	ADVANTAGES	DISADVANTAGES
Metacarpals	Easily accessed	Decreased wrist movement
Accessory cephalic	Does not impair mobility because it is a large vein	Discomfort at bend of wrist
Cephalic	Does not impair mobility because it is a large vein	Makes it more difficult for patient to move wrist and difficult to stabilize vein
Basilic	Large, straight vein	Uncomfortable insertion, difficult to stabilize vein
Antecubital	Large, easily seen vein	Frequently used for blood drawing, so often vein is scarred. Patient has to keep arm straight, which is uncomfortable

Inhalation Route

Inhalation (breathing in) allows rapid absorption of a medication. Respiratory system medications can easily be inhaled and begin working where they are most needed. Sometimes powders or drugs in solution are added to special equipment to introduce the medication via forced air. With a *nebulizer*, a patient learns how to add the medication in a chamber with water to be inhaled with forced air. Metered-dose *inhalers* are used to deliver specific doses through a hand-held inhalation device. Anesthetics, insulin, and the influenza vaccine can be administered by inhalation.

Nasal Route

Nasal medications are administered as fine droplets inhaled from droppers or small spray bottles. For localized treatment of nose problems, medications are pulled into droppers and placed in the nose with the patient's head tilted backward.

Ophthalmic Route

Ophthalmic medications are placed in the eye. They can be given as drops or ointments. Eye drops may be used to lubricate the eye or treat other conditions through absorption in the inner canthus of the eye. Ophthalmic ointments are thickened drug solutions that are applied to the inside lower eyelids. Ocular *inserts* are small transparent membranes that contain medication. They are placed between the eye and lower conjunctiva and release medications over a period of time. Remember always to keep ophthalmic preparations sterile to avoid infection.

Otic Route

Otic preparations, usually in the form of drops, are for the ear. These are fairly easy to administer and usually work locally and quickly. They must be given at room temperature to prevent pain or fainting.

Topical/Transdermal Route

Sometimes it is easier to deliver a medication across membranes. Medications given by the topical or transdermal route are absorbed locally into the skin. Some drugs, such as nitroglycerin, are given topically to achieve a systemic effect. Topical drugs come in several preparations. Semisolid preparations include *creams, ointments*, *gels*, and *plasters*. Because ointments sink into the skin more than creams, dosage orders for the two may differ even for the same drug. Usually if the skin is wet, use a cream. If the skin is dry, use an ointment. An example of a cream is aloe vera cream for burns. Gels are semisolid suspensions; an example is Metrogel for acne. Plasters are medicated preparations that adhere to the body skin with materials such as paper, linen, moleskin, or plastic. An example is a salicylic acid plaster.

Other semisolid preparations include *liniments* (or *salves*) and *lotions*. Liniments are rubbed on the skin to irritate it. They may cause a burning or tingling sensation but relieve underlying pain. An example is Ben Gay for sore muscles. Lotions are used externally for skin disorders. They are patted on, not rubbed into, the skin. An example of a lotion is calamine lotion for itching.

Fine-granulated *powders* are sometimes applied to the skin to reduce moisture or to treat fungal diseases. An example is a powder to put on toes to prevent athlete's foot.

A transdermal *patch* is an amazing form of drug delivery (Fig. 4.1). Patches contain medication that is delivered over time. Patches were used in the space shuttles at the end of the last century to reduce nausea. Since then, patches have grown in popularity and are used, for example, for pain relief, vasodilation, and hormone replacement, and as part of a smoking cessation program. Transdermal patches apply medication in a specific amount over a specific area, so they should never be cut. An example of a transdermal patch is a NicoDerm patch to reduce the craving to smoke tobacco.

CRITICAL THINKING

What would be the effect of cutting a transdermal patch? Is it advisable?

Vaginal Route

Vaginal medications are usually used for a local effect. *Foams* use aerosol to place the substance into the vagina. *Gels* and *jellies* are solid particles of medication in *viscous* (thick) suspensions. The thick-

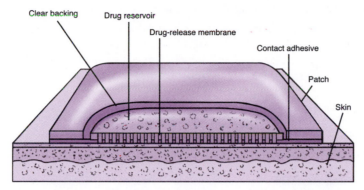

FIGURE 4.1. In a transdermal delivery system, the medication is contained in a drug reservoir, which is released through a membrane when the patch is applied to the skin by an adhesive backing.

BOX 4.2　Medication Forms

Solids	**Foams**
Capsules	Creams
Implanted devices	Gels
Lozenges	Liniments
Patches	Lotions
Plasters	Magmas
Powders	Ointments
Suppositories	Salves
Tablets	Solutions
Troches	Suspensions
Liquids	Syrups
Elixirs	**Gases**
Emulsions	Aerosols
Effervescent salts	Mists
Enemas	Sprays

---

ness of the suspension prevents the medication from leaking. An example is a contraceptive lubricant. *Creams* (*lotions*), jellies, and gels are all products that can release hormones for contraceptive purposes. For example, foam may be placed in a diaphragm and inserted into the vagina or applied with a specialized applicator. An *intrauterine device* (IUD) is a contraceptive device implanted into the uterus; some devices are coated with and release the hormone progesterone.

Box 4.2 summarizes the various types of medication.

 S U M M A R Y

Medications come in different forms and are given by different routes. It is important to give drugs in the correct route, as ordered, because dosages vary depending on where the drug is given.

Activities

To make sure that you have learned the key points covered in this chapter, complete the following activities.

Multiple Choice

Choose the best answer for each question.

1. PPD is given by which route?
   a. IV
   b. ID
   c. IM
   d. SC

2. Flu vaccination is given by which route?
   a. IV
   b. ID
   c. IM
   d. SC

3. A 45° angle is used with which of the following injections?
   a. IV
   b. ID
   c. IM
   d. SC

4. Large amounts of fluid can be given only by:
   a. IV
   b. ID
   c. Inhalation
   d. IM

5. Which of the following is the fastest route for medication to get to the bloodstream?
   a. SC
   b. Inhalation
   c. ID
   d. Transdermal

6. Which of the following is parenteral?
   a. IV
   b. Buccal
   c. Oral
   d. Rectal

7. Gases are administered through which of the following routes?
   a. IV
   b. Inhalation
   c. ID
   d. Vaginal

8. Which of the following contains alcohol?
   a. Capsule
   b. Magma
   c. Emulsion
   d. Elixir

9. Which must be added to a liquid before administering?
   a. Effervescent salts
   b. Magmas
   c. Foams
   d. Troches

10. Which of the following is given rectally?
   a. Syrups
   b. Emulsions
   c. Suppositories
   d. Suspensions

Application Exercises

Respond to the following scenarios on a separate sheet.

1. To aid your memory, you decide to make a chart to help you remember the content of this chapter. **Use books and resources as needed to complete the chart in Table 4.2.**
2. Your patient does not understand why his medication cannot be given orally. **Discuss the advantages and disadvantages of the gastrointestinal route.**
3. Your physician has asked you to assemble the following drugs in case of an emergency and store them in the crash cart. **By what route is each drug given, and for what is it used?**
   a. Adrenaline (epinephrine)
   b. Aminophylline
   c. Benadryl
   d. Compazine
   e. Dextrose
   f. Digoxin
   g. Diuril
   h. Hydrocortisone
   i. Narcan
   j. Nitroglycerin
   k. Valium

4. You have assembled the above medications in the crash cart. **What other supplies might be necessary to put with these medications for administration during an emergency.**
5. You notice that your colleagues at work do not wear gloves when handling medications. **For what routes must gloves be worn? Defend your answer.**

Virtual Field Trips

Go to the following websites to find the information. If a website is not available, try to find the information through another source.

1. Visit http://www.apha.org and link to your state health department. Determine who you should notify if you notice a positive PPD.
2. Go to http://www.ask.com and search dictionaries for "parenteral." Go to at least three of these sites and write down how the word is pronounced, its function, and its definition. Why do you think there are different definitions for this word?
3. Surf to http://www.rxlist.com or a similar website and find the forms and routes of the following drugs:
   a. Milk of Magnesia
   b. Colace
   c. Phenergan
   d. Prolixin
   e. Estrogen

4. Find the website for your state's Board of Medicine (can be found on http://www.ama-assn.org) and find out if IV therapy can be delegated to unlicensed professionals in your state.

TABLE 4.2 Reference Guide for Routes

Complete the table below.

ROUTE	WHEN USED	EXAMPLE
Buccal		
Inhalation	Used when quick absorption is needed	Anesthesia, bronchodilators
Intradermal		
Intramuscular		
Intravenous		
Oral		
Rectal		
Subcutaneous		
Sublingual		
Transdermal		
Vaginal		

Prescriptions and Labels

A key part of keeping the patient safe is ensuring the accuracy of prescriptions for medications. Drugs have a variety of names, come from several sources, are given by different routes, and act in various ways; hence, the prescriber must give specific information to avoid mistakes when filling or administering medications. This chapter discusses types of prescriber orders, parts of prescriptions, and medication labels.

OBJECTIVES

At the end of this chapter, the student will be able to:

- Define key terms.
- Discuss precautions to ensure patient safety.
- Identify the parts of a legal prescription.
- List which health care providers are able to write prescriptions in your state.
- Define abbreviations used in prescriptions.
- Interpret labels safely.

KEY TERMS

Automatic stop order	mEq	Subscription
Cap	mL	Superscription
d/c	mg	T
Elix	oz	t
gm	OTC	Tab
gr	Rx	Telephone orders
gtt	Signature	Verbal orders
Inscription	Standing orders	
mcg	Stat orders	

⬤ PRESCRIPTIONS

The prescription is a written record of the prescriber's order. Be sure you know who can prescribe medications in your state. In addition to physicians, nurse practitioners and physician assistants are also allowed to prescribe. On every prescription pad, the prescriber is identified by name and DEA number.

Prescriptions are dispensed only by health care professionals licensed to do so, and only patients whose name is on the prescription should take the medication. Drugs are ordered in facilities and prescriber offices. You will probably have the most contact with prescriptions in an office setting, so the information in this chapter focuses more on that practice area.

Types of Orders

Written, verbal, or standing orders can be the basis for a prescription. The orders are then written on a prescription form that usually is preprinted with the prescriber's name, address, and telephone number. *Stat* orders are one-time orders, usually for drugs given in an emergency situation. If a physician says to give a medication *stat*, it means immediately.

Written orders

Obtain a written order for a prescription whenever possible to decrease chances of misunderstanding and subsequent errors. As an allied health professional, you must make sure the prescriber writes or types the prescription accurately. Time pressures are no excuse for sloppy handwriting. If prescribers have poor handwriting, offer to write or type the prescription, then have them read and sign it. The exception is a prescription for a Schedule II drug, which must be written by the prescriber.

Verbal orders

A prescriber occasionally gives a verbal order. When this happens, it is important to write words and numbers carefully. Check with your supervisor to see if you are allowed to take a verbal order. If you are, be sure to read what you have written back to the prescriber to ensure that you have it correct. Some offices require that the prescriber also repeat the information back to you. The prescriber must sign the order as soon as possible. Remember that verbal orders are not permitted for Schedule II drugs.

Standing orders

A prescriber may leave a list of standing orders to be used in specific circumstances that routinely occur. Before a diagnostic test, for example, a prescriber may require the patient to be *npo* (nothing by mouth) after midnight, have an enema, follow a clear liquid diet, and take an antibiotic. One physician in a practice may prefer one brand of antibiotic, whereas another physician might prefer a different one. It is important to verify standing orders with the prescriber.

Stop orders

Automatic stop orders are orders given only for a limited period of time. For an example, an antibiotic may be taken twice a day for 10 days. The order stops after 10 days and is not refilled without the prescriber renewing it. To *d/c* an order is to discontinue it; this can also be an abbreviation for discharge.

No matter what kind of order is given, it is important that the prescription is clear. Patients can die if a pharmacist cannot read what the prescriber wrote and gives the wrong medication or the wrong dose. Before giving a written prescription to a patient, check to see if it is correct and legible. If not, return it to the prescriber to be rewritten or typed.

❋❓ CRITICAL THINKING

You review a prescription and find you cannot determine if the medication is Trileptal (an antiseizure medication) or Tylenol 3 (a narcotic pain reliever). What would the difference be to the patient if the wrong drug were given? What should you do in this situation?

BOX 5.1	**Abbreviations Related to Medication Administration**
cap	capsule
elix	elixir
gm	gram
gr	grain
gtt	drop
mcg	microgram
mEq	milliequivalent
mL	milliliter
mg	milligram
oz	ounce
tab	tablet
T, Tb	tablespoon
t, tsp	teaspoon

● WRITTEN PRESCRIPTION

You must understand the parts of a prescription to prevent errors and to teach patients important facts about their medications. You may need to translate the complicated Latin terms that are written as a fast notation because they are not usually understood by the patient. Before proceeding, you might want to review the abbreviations you learned in Chapter 1. Box 5.1 lists the common abbreviations related to medication administration you need to know. Abbreviations can vary from one setting to the next, so be sure to check which are—and are not—accepted where you work.

Parts of a Prescription

Every prescription must include several parts: name, address, phone number, and DEA number of the prescriber; name and address of the patient; date of order; *Rx* (which means "take thou" and is an abbreviation for prescription or treatment—also called the *superscription*); *inscription* (name of drug, dosage, and quantity to be dispensed); directions for taking the drug (*signature*); refill numbers (*subscription*); whether a generic can be used; and the signature of prescriber (Fig. 5.1). In a large medical group, there may be one prescription form with all the legal prescribers listed. Let us take a closer look at some of these parts.

Be sure the current address of the patient is on the prescription form. It would be helpful to the pharmacist if you would write it on the form. Asking the patient for the current address also double-checks that you have the correct address on file for the patient.

The date of the order is important for filing insurance claims and because it links the drug therapy with the office visit. It is best for the date to match the office visit even though patients may wait to fill the prescription because they have received free samples at the office or emergency department.

The drug name must be clearly identified. The prescriber may write the generic or brand name. The prescriber also notes whether a generic drug can be substituted for a brand-name drug. As we learned in Chapter 2, insurance companies and HMOs usually prefer paying for the cheaper drug. However, some patients are allergic to dyes or fillers found in certain generic drugs. In that case, the brand-name drug is the best choice.

The dosage is a crucial piece of information. Make sure the strength is clearly indicated. Missing a decimal point or a zero (e.g., 25 mg instead of 2.5 mg) can harm a patient. If a dosage seems inappropriate, check your drug resources before giving the patient the prescription.

The quantity to be dispensed is indicated by a number after a pound sign (#). For an acute problem, the drug may be given for only a short time. Thus, perhaps only 1 week's or 1 month's supply is given. A chronic problem may require a 90-day supply plus three refills to continue the drug treatment for a year.

The prescriber may specify how many refills are allowed without the patient retuning to the office to be seen again. For chronic conditions, the patient may not return to the office for a while. Refill

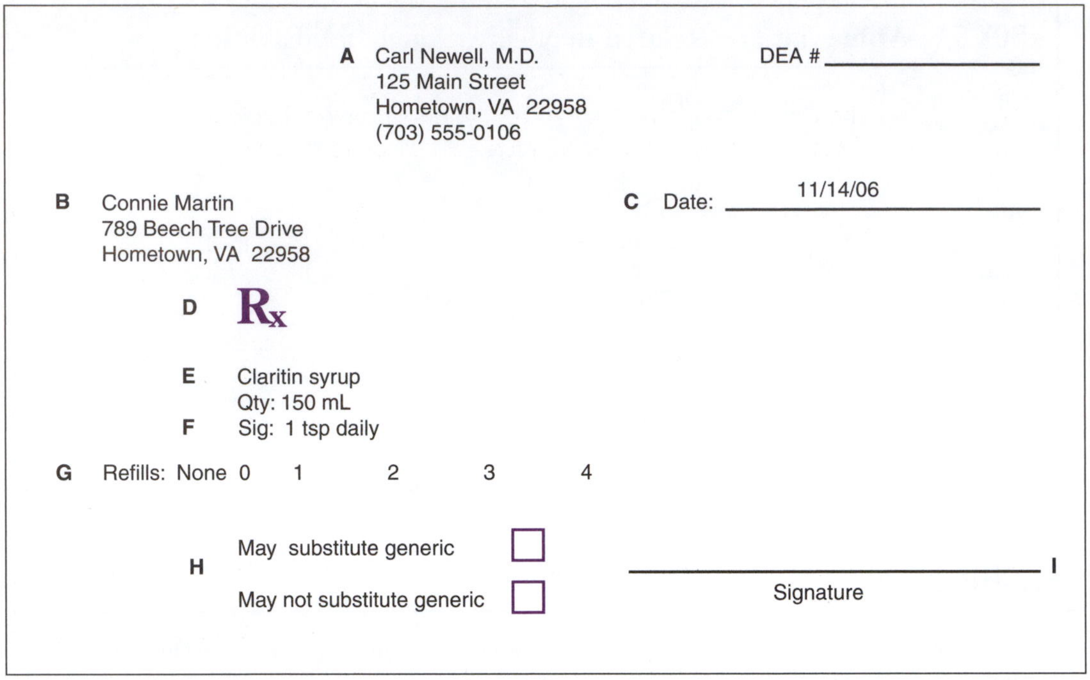

A Carl Newell, M.D.
125 Main Street
Hometown, VA 22958
(703) 555-0106

DEA # _____

B Connie Martin
789 Beech Tree Drive
Hometown, VA 22958

C Date: _____11/14/06_____

D **R**x

E Claritin syrup
Qty: 150 mL
F Sig: 1 tsp daily

G Refills: None   0   1   2   3   4

H May substitute generic   ☐

May not substitute generic   ☐

_____ I
Signature

FIGURE 5.1. Sample prescription. A prescription has several parts: (A) name, address, phone number; and DEA number of prescriber; (B) patient's name and address; (C) date; (D) Rx (abbreviation for prescription or treatment); (E) inscription (name of drug, the dosage, and the quantity to be prescribed); (F) signature (directions to the patient); (G) number of refills; (H) whether a generic can be used; and (I) prescriber's signature.

orders facilitate the continuity of care for chronic illnesses, because the patient does not need to return for more prescriptions.

The signature is from *signetur*, a Latin word for "write on the label." It gives directions to the patient for when and how to take the drug. Prescribers use standardized abbreviations when writing prescriptions. For example, a prescriber may write "1 tab every 4h prn." This Latin is not understood by most patients, so the pharmacist writes, "Take 1 tablet every 4 hours as needed" for the patient.

CRITICAL THINKING

If most patients do not understand Latin, why do you think physicians write the signature in Latin?

If a patient calls for a refill, the prescriber may refill the prescription without asking to see the patient again, especially for patients with chronic conditions or those taking birth control pills. After the refill has been approved, the allied health professional must document in the patient's medical record that it was phoned into the pharmacy.

CRITICAL THINKING

You work in a busy gynecologist's office. Many women run out of birth control pills before you can schedule them to come in to be seen. Create a protocol for refilling oral contraceptives without seeing the patient.

● LABELS

The prescriber writes the prescription, and the pharmacist types up a label with vital information for the patient. A valid label includes the pharmacy's name, address, and telephone number (Fig. 5.2). This

---

⬤ CHECK UP

Before completing the rest of the chapter, test yourself on the following abbreviations. If you do not know some of them, make flashcards to help you memorize them.

$\overline{a}$ _____   gtt _____   o.u. _____

a.c. _____   hs _____   oz _____

a.d. _____   ID _____ $\overline{p}$ _____

a.s. _____   IM _____   p.c. _____

a.u. _____   IV _____   prn _____

bid _____   mcg _____ $\overline{s}$ _____

$\overline{c}$ _____   mEq _____   SC _____

cap _____   mg _____   stat _____

d/c _____   mL _____   Tb _____

elix _____   npo _____   tid _____

gm _____   o.d. _____   tsp _____

gr _____   o.s. _____

---

helps the patient contact the pharmacist in case of problems or questions. For accuracy, the prescriber's name and perhaps license classification (MD or FNP, for example) are also on the label. The label must include the patient's full name and the medication's name, strength, dosage form, quantity, and manufacturer (if generic).

The dispensing date, which may differ from the date the prescriber wrote the prescription, is also on the label, along with refill information. The pharmacist notes when the medication will expire or lose its potency.

The pharmacist originates an Rx number that identifies this unique prescription in the computer system and on the label. The patient can refill the prescription using this number.

The pharmacist translates the Latin abbreviations into English for the patient (compare Fig. 5.1 with Fig. 5.2). It is important that the patient understands the order, but he or she may be hesitant to ask a pharmacist about it. Therefore, before the patient leaves the medical office, be sure that the patient understands how to take the drug. Also instruct the patient to carefully read the label that the pharmacist puts on the bottle (see Fast Tip 5.1).

Labels are not found only on prescription drugs. Over-the-counter (OTC) drugs can be purchased without a prescription. The FDA has determined that, if the consumer takes an OTC medication as directed on the label, the drug is safe for the general population. However, that does not mean these drugs are without side effects. As with prescription drugs, it is important for patients to read the label, including the dosage and side effects that may occur. OTC drugs can interact negatively with prescription drugs. For example, some cold medicines increase the action of sedatives, so a person taking both medications would be sleepier than expected.

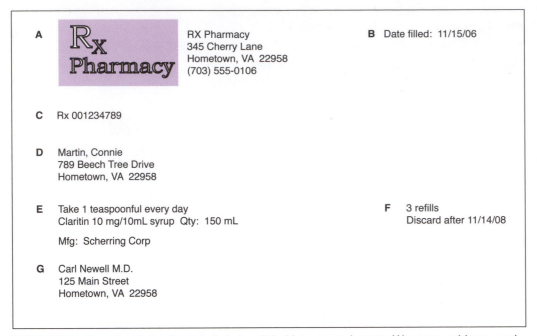

A RX Pharmacy
345 Cherry Lane
Hometown, VA 22958
(703) 555-0106

B Date filled: 11/15/06

C Rx 001234789

D Martin, Connie
789 Beech Tree Drive
Hometown, VA 22958

E Take 1 teaspoonful every day
Claritin 10 mg/10mL syrup Qty: 150 mL

Mfg: Scherring Corp

F 3 refills
Discard after 11/14/08

G Carl Newell M.D.
125 Main Street
Hometown, VA 22958

FIGURE 5.2. Sample medication label. A drug label has several parts: (A) name, address, and phone number for the pharmacy; (B) the date when the prescription was filled; (C) Rx (prescription) number; (D) name and address of the patient; (E) drug name, dosage, frequency, and quantity (Latin terms are translated into English for the patient) and the manufacturer for generic drugs; (F) number of refills and when the medication expires; and (G) name of prescriber.

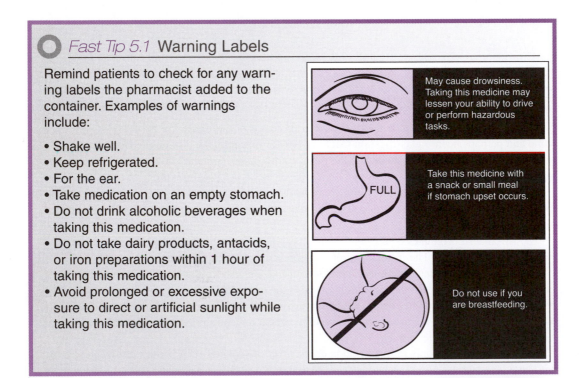

Fast Tip 5.1 Warning Labels

Remind patients to check for any warning labels the pharmacist added to the container. Examples of warnings include:

• Shake well.
• Keep refrigerated.
• For the ear.
• Take medication on an empty stomach.
• Do not drink alcoholic beverages when taking this medication.
• Do not take dairy products, antacids, or iron preparations within 1 hour of taking this medication.
• Avoid prolonged or excessive exposure to direct or artificial sunlight while taking this medication.

May cause drowsiness. Taking this medicine may lessen your ability to drive or perform hazardous tasks.

Take this medicine with a snack or small meal if stomach upset occurs.

Do not use if you are breastfeeding.

SUMMARY

To safely prescribe drugs, the prescriber must write clearly and accurately. The allied health professional must ensure the safe transfer of information from the prescriber through the patient to the pharmacist. To do so, you must memorize abbreviations and understand the parts of the prescription. You also need to be able to read labels and educate patients about them.

Activities

To make sure that you have learned the key points covered in this chapter, complete the following activities.

True or False

Write *true* if the statement is true. Beside the false statements, write *false* and correct the statement to make it true.

1. Sometimes people other than a physician can legally write prescriptions. _____

2. The FDA issues a prescriber number for physicians. _____

3. OTC medications are never dangerous. _____

4. A pharmacist can decide whether a generic drug can be used for a brand-name drug. _____

5. A stat order is a standing order. _____

Multiple Choice

Choose the best answer for each question.

1. **Which of the following is the explanation of how to take a medication?**
   a. Inscription
   b. Superscription
   c. Subscription
   d. Signature

2. **The abbreviation for three times per day is:**
   a. bid
   b. od
   c. hs
   d. tid

3. **Which abbreviation means without?**
   a. $\overline{ss}$
   b. x
   c. $\overline{c}$
   d. $\overline{s}$
   e. w

4. **Which means a drop?**
   a. gm
   b. gr
   c. gtt
   d. mg

5. **Which means to give the drug immediately?**
   a. prn
   b. stat
   c. npo
   d. d/c

Application Exercises

Respond to the following scenarios on a separate sheet.

1. **What standing orders might be necessary for Henry Krause to have a barium enema diagnostic test?**
2. **Write a prescription for Brittany Mays for:** Feldane 20 mg capsules. Quantity = 30. Take 1 every day with food or milk. Before breakfast.
3. Your physician frequently misplaces prescription pads. **How should they be stored to ensure that they are not misused?**
4. Prednisone is ordered: 4 pills today, 3 tomorrow, 2 the day after tomorrow, 1 the day after that, then stop. **How many are dispensed?**
5. **How does the label read for the following prescription?**
   Warren Short. Nitroglycerin tablets. 0.4 mg sublingually every 5 minutes, up to 3 tablets for chest pain. Dr. Clark Castillo wants him to have 60 tablets. The prescription may be refilled as needed, but once the bottle is opened it should be used for only 6 months.
6. Donna Peachy is prescribed doxycycline 100 mg tablets. This prescription is for 20 tablets, with 2 taken as an initial dose, then 1 tablet every 12 hours until the supply is exhausted. **How would you document the above prescription in Ms. Peachy's chart?**
7. **Create a prescription for the following.**
   Dr. Duncan Campbell wants Peter Burton to have Tylenol 3 (a controlled substance) for pain: 1–2 tablets every 4–6 hours as he needs the medication. He wants him to have 30 tablets. No refills.
8. Theresa Harp, a nurse practitioner, wants Sharon Wheeler to take potassium tablets daily. **Write the prescription for** K-Dur, 20 mEq once daily in the morning for 90 days. The prescription can be refilled 3 times.

Virtual Field Trips

Go to the following websites to find the information. If a website is not available, try to find the information through another source.

1. Go to http://www.walgreens.com and print a label in Russian and Spanish.
2. Surf to http://www.health.umd.edu and print a patient education brochure on How to Take Medication the Right Way. If you cannot access this site, create your own teaching aid.
3. Go to http://www.fda.gov/cder/consumerinfo/otc_text.htm and review the educational materials related to OTC drugs.
4. Search http://www.nlm.nih.gov for an article on prescription drug labels and print it.
5. Go to http://www.noprescriptionneeded.com or a similar website. What do you think about patients ordering medications without prescriptions?

Resources

The previous chapters discussed how an allied health professional must use great care when giving patients medications. Do you have to memorize all the drugs on the market to achieve your goal of patient safety? No. Even if you could remember them, soon there would be a new batch to memorize, then another and another. Instead, you can turn to a drug information resource. Some are books; others are electronic. This chapter reviews the many resources you can access to find information about medications.

OBJECTIVES

At the end of this chapter, the student will be able to:

- Define key terms.
- Compare the usefulness of different drug resources.
- Differentiate between the printed resources of drugs approved by the FDA and computerized sources.
- List 10 websites where you can find information about pharmacology.
- Discuss what features make a reliable website.
- Bookmark selected websites for easy computer access.

KEY TERMS

ADI
Compendium of Drug Therapy
Drug Facts and Comparisons
Drug Information
Drug Topics Red Book
Orange Book
PDR
USP/DI
USP/NF

● DRUG RESOURCES

Health care professionals can turn to many resources for drug information. Some contain massive amounts of information, and others focus on only a few drugs. Some resources use medical terms extensively; others keep it simple so patients can understand the information. Resources can be divided into two categories—comprehensive and clinically based—and include print and online formats.

Comprehensive Resources

Seek out comprehensive resources when you need in-depth information about medications. Many of these resources are available only in print form, whereas others are available only online.

The government produces two major comprehensive resources. *The United States Pharmacopoeia/National Formulary* (USP/NF) is the official source of information for drugs approved by the FDA. It is revised every 5 years, with frequent supplements in between. The USP/NF also provides standards for identification, quality, strength, and purity of substances. The *United States Pharmacopoeia/Dispensing Information* (USP/DI) is published by the United States Pharmacopeial Convention (Rockville, MD). The first of this two-volume set is *Drug Information for Health Providers* and is written primarily for prescribers. The other volume, *Advice for the Patient*, is written in language that is easy for patients to understand. It gives tips for proper use of drugs and includes a pronunciation key. These books must be purchased but are also available in many medical libraries.

A much more widely used comprehensive resource is the *Physician's Desk Reference* (PDR), which is available in most health care settings. It is published annually by Medical Economics Publishing and is financed by pharmaceutical manufacturers. The PDR contains information about thousands of drugs and is indexed by trade name, generic name, classification, and manufacturer. Color photographs of some drugs are also included, which helps identify medications when patients are unsure of what they are taking. There is also a volume for over-the-counter (OTC) drugs.

A CLOSER LOOK: Organization of the *Physician Desk Reference* (PDR)

The PDR is organized as follows:

Section 1 (white): Manufacturer's Index. This is an alphabetical listing of manufacturers with their addresses and phone numbers.

Section 2 (pink): Brand and Generic Name Index. This is an alphabetical listing of medications by generic and trade names.

Section 3 (blue): Classification Index. This section lists drugs by classification (e.g., antibiotics, analgesics)

Section 4 (gray): Product Identification Guide. Manufacturers display photographs of medications. The drugs are listed by manufacturer.

Section 5 (white): Product Information Section. This section contains the detailed information you would find on package inserts, alphabetized by manufacturer and then product.

Section 6 (white): This is a catch-all section that includes:

- Controlled substances categories
- FDA use-in-pregnancy ratings
- FDA telephone directory
- Poison control centers
- Drug information centers
- Look-alike, sound-alike drug names
- Adverse event report forms

The PDR is a large volume that cannot be carried in a laboratory coat pocket but can be stored on a bookshelf in an office or a facility. To keep prescribers current, supplements are published and distributed free of charge throughout the year. The cross-referencing provides multiple ways to find drugs. The lengthy, medically oriented descriptions are often too in-depth for most patients.

> ### CRITICAL THINKING
>
> **What are the advantages and disadvantages of comprehensive books such as the PDR?**

Several other detailed resources are typically available in a medical library or in some facilities. *Drug Facts and Comparisons* is updated monthly. It compares and evaluates medications and is used frequently by pharmacists. The drugs are grouped by their classification, so similar drugs are indexed together.

The *Compendium of Drug Therapy* is published yearly by the Biomedical Information Corporation (New York, NY). These volumes are distributed to prescribers: *Compendium of Patient Information* and *Compendium of Drug Therapy*. They include photographs of some drugs and phone numbers of poison control centers and pharmaceutical companies.

The *American Drug Index* (ADI) is an alphabetical listing of drugs. You use it just like a dictionary, and it shows trade and generic names and drug classifications. It is useful if you need to know just the correct spelling, what a drug was, or its other names.

The *Drug Topics Red Book* is used primarily for pricing. It includes both prescription and OTC drugs.

The *Drug Information* of the American Health-System Formulary Service is a volume published annually for the Health-System Pharmacists (Bethesda, MD). It is concise and more general than the PDR, but it contains no photographs.

Clinically Based Resources

In the daily clinical setting, the allied health professional turns to more "user-friendly" resources. Having a book that fits in your laboratory coat pocket for easy access is optimal. These books are frequently called drug handbooks and may give information in terms a patient can understand. Sometimes a book is supplemented by an electronic resource such as a CD-ROM. Other clinically based resources include the package insert for the drug and electronic resources, such as the personal digital assistant (PDA) and the many websites on the Internet.

Drug handbooks

A partial example of a monograph in a drug handbook is shown in Box 6.1. You must have access to the Internet or a drug guide, such as *Davis's Drug Guide for Nurses*, which also contains a CD-ROM with a dosage calculator. Although you may use any drug handbook, exercises in this book reference this guide.

> ### CRITICAL THINKING
>
> **What are the characteristics of a good reference handbook?**

Whatever handbook you choose, take some time to become familiar with the features of the book (see Fast Tip 6.1).

Package insert

Each medication comes with a special insert prepared by the manufacturer according to FDA guidelines. It is good to know what information your patient receives when the drugs are picked up at the pharmacy so you can answer any questions the patient might have. Package inserts frequently contain the following information:

- Drug names—trade, generic, and sometimes chemical
- Classifications—what the drug does
- Clinical pharmacology—how the drug works
- Indications and usage—why it was prescribed
- Contraindications—coexisting diseases and symptoms that increase the risk of problems or reactions
- Warnings—dangers associated with this drug
- Precautions—special circumstances relating to this drug
- Adverse reactions—harmful side effects
- Drug abuse and dependence—information about abuse risk
- Overdosage—symptoms and signs if you take too much
- Dosage and administration—how it is given and the usual dose
- How supplied—what forms it comes in (e.g., capsules, tablets)
- Drug company—name of the manufacturer and how to reach the company
- Date of packet insert—date the insert was printed

BOX 6.1 Partial Monograph from a Drug Handbook

High Alert
Digoxin (di-**jox**-in); Digitek, Lanoxicaps, Lanoxin

CLASSIFICATION(S)

Therapeutic: antiarrhythmics, inotropics
Pharmacologic: digitalis glycosides
Pregnancy Category C

INDICATIONS

- Treatment of CHF
- Tachyarrhythmias
  - Atrial fibrillation and atrial flutter (slows ventricular rate)
  - Paroxysmal atrial tachycardia

ACTION

- Increases the force of myocardial contraction
- Prolongs refractory period of the AV node
- Decreases conduction through the SA and AV nodes
- **Therapeutic effects**
  - Increased cardiac output (positive inotropic effect) and slowing of the heart rate (negative chronotropic effect)

PHARMACOKINETICS

Absorption: 60–80% absorbed after oral administration of tablets; 70–85% absorbed after administration of elixir. Absorption from liquid-filled capsules is 90–100%; 80% absorbed from IM sites (IM route not recommended due to pain/irritation)
Distribution: widely distributed; crosses placenta and enters breast milk
Metabolism and excretion: excreted almost entirely unchanged by the kidneys
Half-life: 36–48 hours (increased in renal impairment)

TIME OF ACTION

Antiarrhythmic or inotropic effects, provided that a loading dose has been given

Route	Onset (minutes)	Peak (hours)	Duration* (days)
Digoxin—PO	30–120	2–8	2–4
Digoxin—IM	30	4–6	2–4
Digoxin—IV	5–30	1–4	2–4

*Duration listed is that for normal renal function; with impaired renal function, the duration is longer.

BOX 6.1 Partial Monograph from a Drug Handbook (continued)

CONTRAINDICATIONS/PRECAUTIONS

Contraindicated in the presence of
- Hypersensitivity
- Uncontrolled ventricular arrhythmias
- AV block
- Idiopathic hypertrophic subaortic stenosis
- Constrictive pericarditis
- Known alcohol intolerance (elixir only)

Use cautiously in the presence of

- Electrolyte abnormalities (hypokalemia, hypercalcemia, and hypomagnesemia may predispose to toxicity)
- Hypothyroidism
- *Geri:* Geriatric patients (very sensitive to toxic effects, dose adjustments required for age-related decrease in renal function and body weight)
- Myocardial infarction (MI)
- Renal impairment (dose reduction required)
- Obesity (dose should be based on ideal body weight)
- *OB:* Pregnancy (although safety has not been established, digoxin has been used during pregnancy without adverse effects on the fetus). *Lactation:* Similar concentrations in serum and breast milk result in subtherapeutic levels in infant, use with caution.

ADVERSE REACTIONS/SIDE EFFECTS

Note: CAPITALS indicate life-threatening; <u>underline</u> indicates most frequent.

CNS: <u>fatigue</u>, headache, weakness
EENT: blurred vision, yellow or green vision
CV: ARRHYTHMIAS, <u>bradycardia</u>, ECG changes, AV block, SA block
GI: <u>anorexia</u>, <u>nausea</u>, <u>vomiting</u>, diarrhea
Endo: gynecomastia
Hemat: thrombocytopenia
Metab: hyperkalemia with acute toxicity

INTERACTIONS

Drug–Drug
- *Thiazide* and *loop diuretics, piperacillin, ticarcillin, amphotericin B*, and *corticosteroids* and excessive use of *laxatives* may cause hypokalemia, which may increase the risk of toxicity.
- *Amiodarone,* some *benzodiazepines, cyclosporine, diphenoxylate, indomethacin, itraconazole, propafenone, propantheline, quinidine, quinine, spironolactone,* and *verapamil* may increase serum levels and may lead to toxicity (serum level monitoring/dose reduction may be required).
- Blood levels may be decreased by oral *aminoglycosides, some antineoplastics (bleomycin, carmustine, cyclophosphamide, cytarabine, doxorubicin, methotrexate, procarbazine, vincristine), activated charcoal, cholestyramine, colestipol, kaolin/pectin, metoclopramide, penicillamine, rifampin,* or *sulfasalazine.*
- In a small percentage (10%) of patients, gut bacteria metabolize digoxin to inactive compounds; *gatifloxacin, macrolide anti-infectives (erythromycin, azithromycin, clarithromycin),* and *tetracyclines,* by killing these bacteria, cause increased digoxin levels and toxicity; dose may need to be decreased for up to 9 weeks.
- Additive bradycardia may occur with *beta-blockers* and other *antiarrhythmics (quinidine, disopyramide).*
- Concurrent use of *sympathomimetics* may increase the risk of arrhythmias
- *Thyroid hormones* may decrease therapeutic effects.

Drug–Natural
- *Licorice* and stimulant natural products (*aloe*) may increase the risk of potassium depletion.
- St. John's wort may decrease both the digoxin level and its effect.

(box continued on page 78)

BOX 6.1 Partial Monograph from a Drug Handbook (continued)

Drug–Food
- Concurrent ingestion of a *high-fiber meal* may decrease absorption. Administer digoxin 1 hour before or 2 hours after such a meal

ROUTE AND DOSAGE

For a rapid effect, a larger initial loading/digitalizing dose should be given in several divided doses over 12–24 hours. Maintenance doses are determined for digoxin by renal function. All dosing must be evaluated by individual response. In general, doses required for atrial arrhythmias are higher than those for an inotropic effect. When determining the dose, consider that the bioavailability of gelatin capsules (Lanoxicaps) is greater than that of tablets.

- **IV** (Adults): *Digitalizing dose*—0.5–1 mg given as 50% of the dose initially and one-quarter of the initial dose in each of two subsequent doses at 6- to 12-hour intervals
- **IV** (Children >10 years): *Digitalizing dose*—8–12 mcg/kg given as 50% of the dose initially and one-quarter of the initial dose in each of two subsequent doses at 6- to 12-hour intervals
- **IV** (Children 5–10 years): *Digitalizing dose*—15–30 mcg/kg given as 50% of the dose initially and one-quarter of the initial dose in each of two subsequent doses at 6- to 12-hour intervals
- **IV** (Children 2–5 years): *Digitalizing dose*—25–35 mcg/kg given as 50% of the dose initially and one-quarter of the initial dose in each of two subsequent doses at 6- to 12-hour intervals
- **IV** (Children 1–24 months): *Digitalizing dose*—30–50 mcg/kg given as 50% of the dose initially and one quarter of the initial dose in each of two subsequent doses at 6- to 12-hour intervals
- **IV** (Infants—full term): *Digitalizing dose*—20–30 mcg/kg given as 50% of the dose initially and one-quarter of the initial dose in each of two subsequent doses at 6- to 12-hour intervals
- **IV** (Infants—premature): *Digitalizing dose*—15–25 mcg/kg given as 50% of the dose initially and one-quarter of the initial dose in each of two subsequent doses at 6- to 12-hour intervals
- **PO** (Adults): *Digitalizing dose*—0.75–1.5 mg given as 50% of the dose initially and one-quarter of the initial dose in each of two subsequent doses at 6- to 12-hour intervals. *Maintenance dose*—0.125–0.5 mg/day as tablets or 0.35–0.5 mg/day as gelatin capsules, depending on patient's lean body weight, renal function, and serum level
- **PO** (Geriatric patients): Daily dosage should not exceed 0.125 mg except when treating atrial fibrillation
- **PO** (Children >10 years): *Digitalizing dose*—10–15 mcg/kg given as 50% of the dose initially and one-quarter of the initial dose in each of two subsequent doses at 6- to 12-hour intervals. *Maintenance dose*—2.5–5 mcg/kg given daily as a single dose
- **PO** (Children 5–10 years): *Digitalizing dose*—20–35 mcg/kg given as 50% of the dose initially and one-quarter of the initial dose in each of two subsequent doses at 6- to 12-hour intervals. *Maintenance dose*—5–10 mcg/kg given daily in two divided doses
- **PO** (Children 2–5 years): *Digitalizing dose*—30–40 mcg/kg given as 50% of the dose initially and one-quarter of the initial dose in each of two subsequent doses at 6- to 12-hour intervals. *Maintenance dose*—7.5–10 mcg/kg given daily in two divided doses
- **PO** (Children 1–24 months): *Digitalizing dose*—35–60 mcg/kg given as 50% of the dose initially and one-quarter of the initial dose in each of two subsequent doses at 6- to 12-hour intervals. *Maintenance dose*—10–15 mcg/kg given daily in two divided doses
- **PO** (Infants—full term): *Digitalizing dose*—25–35 mcg/kg given as 50% of the dose initially and one-quarter of the initial dose in each of two subsequent doses at 6- to 12-hour intervals. *Maintenance dose*—6–10 mcg/kg given daily in two divided doses
- **PO** (Infants—premature): *Digitalizing dose*—20–30 mcg/kg given as 50% of the dose initially and one-quarter of the initial dose in each of two subsequent doses at 6- to 12-hour intervals. *Maintenance dose*—5–7.5 mcg/kg given daily in two divided doses

AVAILABILITY

- *Tablets:* 0.125 mg, 0.25 mg, 0.5 mg
- *Cost: Lanoxin*—0.125 mg, $21.32/100; 0.25 mg, $21.32/100. *Generic*—$8.79/100
- *Capsules:* 0.05 mg, 0.1 mg, 0.2 mg
  Pediatric elixir (lime flavor) 0.05 mg/ml
- *Injection:* 0.25 mg/ml
- *Pediatric injection:* 0.1 mg/ml

Source: Deglin JH. and Vallerand AH. *Davis's Drug Guide for Nurses*, ed. 10. F.A. Davis, Philadelphia, 2007, pp 386–388, with permission.

◯ *Fast Tip 6.1* Drug Handbook Features
_____

Be sure you can easily find all of these features. To make it easy, next to each feature put the page number where it is found in your drug handbook.

- Abbreviations
- Anaphylaxis management
- Body surface area nomogram (a reference for easily determining the body surface area of a patient, which can affect drug dosage)
- Combination drugs
- Compatibility of drugs in syringes and IV bags
- Controlled substance chart
- Dietary guidelines and RDA (Recommended Daily Allowance) for vitamins
- Dosage calculations formulas
- Herbal and natural products
- Immunization schedules
- Measurement conversions
- Medication error and adverse reaction reporting forms
- Photographs of drugs
- Pregnancy categories
- Other helpful features

🖉 CHECK UP

Answer the following using your drug handbook or PDR.

1. What color is Zoloft 50 mg? _____

2. Can children take Bactrim? _____

3. What are two side effects of phenobarbital? _____

4. What is the usual adult dosage of Depakote? _____

5. What is a precaution when taking Coumadin? _____

6. For what purpose is caffeine prescribed? _____

7. Can you mix adrenaline (epinephrine) HCl with potassium in an intravenous (IV) drip? _____

8. What is the generic equivalent of Restoril? _____

9. Does morphine sulfate interact with alcohol? _____

10. What is the therapeutic effect of lithium? _____

11. What is an adverse reaction to penicillin? _____

(box continued on page 80)

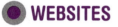 **CHECK UP** (continued)

12. What allergic precautions are assessed before giving a hepatitis B vaccination? _____

13. Can oral polio vaccination be given to people with cancer? _____

14. By what routes can Colace be given? _____

15. What forms of Tylenol exist? _____

16. Is nitroglycerin available in a transdermal patch? _____

17. Can you break a Calan SR tablet? _____

18. Is Demerol given IM? _____

19. What is the trade name for naprosyn sodium? _____

20. What is NPH insulin? _____

Electronic resources

In most offices and facilities, electronic resources are readily accessible to allied health professionals. They include websites on the Internet, special software on a computer, and palm-sized computers, such as a personal digital assistant (PDA) on which is loaded information. You can download programs onto a PDA and have a lot of drug information available in a small space. In addition, you can keep current on new drugs by programming the PDA to access the most recent information.

WEBSITES

This section focuses on websites, encouraging you to visit many Internet sites, compare them, and select your favorites for future use (Table 6.1).

To get the most benefit from your Internet surfing, you should know how website addresses (URLs) are named. URLs include educational institutions, governmental agencies, professional organizations, and commercial enterprises. The ending of the URL indicates to which category it belongs.

- .gov—governmental agency
- .edu—educational institution
- .org—professional organization
- .com—commercial enterprise

Governmental Agencies. Websites with .gov are sponsored by the U.S. government and are designed to get information directly to the public. They are funded by taxpayers and so do not usually require a password or fee for access. The FDA and DEA, for example, are accessed through government websites.

Educational Institutions. Educational institutions, such as colleges and universities, sponsor websites that are usually signified by .edu at the end of the URL. For example, Baylor College of Medicine is found at http://www.bcm.tmc.edu/. Some institutions give information about the university only, whereas others post research findings that can be accessed by the public. Universities are good sources of information about the current use of drugs and treatment of diseases. Some professors or students have pages on the website that may or may not be endorsed by the college. These may appear with a ~ to signify a personal page. For example, http://www.mycollege.edu~Smith would be a professor's personal site.

TABLE 6.1 Sample Websites

Many websites are available on the Internet. Visit at least one site from each section and bookmark your favorites. Compare how they are written and the type of information they provide. You may have your own favorite sites related to this topic that you want to share with your classmates.

NAME AND URL	DESCRIPTION
Government Websites	
National Center for Complementary and Alternative Medicine—http://www.nccam.nih.gov/	Good resource for studies on nontraditional therapies; part of the National Institutes of Health.
National Institute on Drug Abuse—http://www.nida.nih.gov/	Good resource on drug abuse for patient and community education.
U.S. Centers for Disease Control and Prevention—http://www.cdc.gov/	Tracks outbreaks of diseases and keeps the public informed. Good site for anthrax and smallpox vaccination information.
U.S. Department of Health and Human Services—http://www.healthfinder.gov/	Excellent health resource for patients and other consumers; has Spanish section.
U.S. Drug Enforcement Administration—http://www.usdoj.gov/dea/	Tells how to handle and classify controlled substances. Also has teaching information about drug abuse and statistics on drug misuse.
U.S. Food and Drug Administration—http://www.fda.gov/	Approves drugs and runs MedWatch—to keep track of adverse drug effects. Lists standards for drug approval. Site where manufacturers apply for IND applications.
U.S. Food and Drug Administration, Center for Drug Evaluation and Research—http://www.fda.gov/cder/	Includes information (in English and Spanish) about drug research in the United States. Also has MedWatch reports, lists of drugs in short supply, and the important drug resource the *Orange Book* of the FDA.
U.S. National Institutes of Health—http://www.nih.gov/	Good resources and articles on drug topics. For status of clinical trials go to http://www.ClinicalTrials.gov
U.S. National Library of Medicine—http://nlm.nih.gov/	Catalogs and publishes research through PubMed (http://www.ncbi.nlm.nih.gov/PubMed) and MEDLINE (http://www.nlm.nih.gov/medlineplus)
Educational Websites	
Harvard Medical School—http://www.intelihealth.com/	Provides consumer health information. Sponsored by Aetna.
Johns Hopkins Medicine—http://www.hopkinsmedicine.org/	Good source of health information and information about results of studies conducted by Johns Hopkins researchers.
Medical College of Wisconsin—http://www.intmed.mcw.edu/drug.html/	Has flashcards of drugs to train its medical students. Has hyperlinks to drugs.com and other sites you may not be able to easily access on your own. Other hyperlinks include PharmWeb and NeedyMeds (to help fund medications for needy patients). It has an online self-assessment about pharmacology that you might like to try.
Professional Organization Websites	
American Pharmacists Association—http://www.aphanet.org/	Fosters research on pharmacology topics.
American Society of Health-System Pharmacists—http://www.safemedication.com/	Includes excellent information about safety and vaccines.

(table continued on page 82)

TABLE 6.1   Sample Websites (continued)

NAME AND URL	DESCRIPTION
Dr. Pen—http://www.drpen.com/	Information about current drugs, including the ICD-9 diagnostic codes with the drug names. Dr. Pen also comes in a pocket-sized printed version.
Institute for Safe Medication Practices—http://www.ismp.org/	Website for the organization that audits MedWatch reports and works with the FDA to reduce medication problems. Provides excellent safety information.
Librarian's Index—http://www.lii.org/	Site's motto is "Information you can trust." Good first stop because librarians have indexed a lot of information from many sources.
Mayo Clinic—http://www.mayohealth.org/	Cutting-edge research from this research center.
Medem—http://www.medem.com/	Site is sponsored and reviewed by many medical societies. Has a special section for patients to obtain information in lay terms.
RX Assistance—http://www.rxassist.org/	Provides information about resources for patients who cannot afford their prescriptions.
United States Pharmacopeial Convention, Inc.—http://www.usp.org/	Website for the organization that writes the USP/NF. Includes fascinating statistics on the top 50 drug products associated with medication errors and standards for more than 3000 medicines, dietary supplements, and health care products.

Commercial Websites

AIDS Educational Global Information System—http://www.aegis.com/	Describes treatment of AIDS in easy terms to understand.
Drug Facts and Comparisons—http://www.factsandcomparisons.com/	Has an online version of *Drug Facts and Comparisons* and drug databases for downloading, as well as hyperlinks to many good resources.
Dr. Koop—http://www.drkoop.com/	Former Surgeon General Koop's website. Has lots of information aimed at disease prevention.
Drug Topics—http://www.drugtopics.com/	Audits the number of prescriptions filled, so it is a good source for the list of the top prescribed drugs.
Drugs—http://www.drugs.com/	You can search for information about drugs, find FDA alerts, and obtain information on more than 24,000 drugs.
Getting Well—http://www.gettingwell.com/	A consumer-oriented version of the PDR.
Giant Food—http://www.giantfood.com pharm_ask_pharmacist.cfm/	Good information for consumers from this grocery and pharmacy chain.
Medscape—http://www.medscape.com/	Need to register (it is free and worth it). Many excellent resources and articles.
Palmgear—http://www.palmgear.com/	Source of drug information you can purchase and download on a PDA.
Rite Aid—http://www.riteaid.com/	Gives information on drugs and helps locate the nearest Rite Aid Pharmacy.

NAME AND URL	DESCRIPTION
Rxlist—http://www.rxlist.com/	Created by a hospital pharmacist, this excellent site is user-friendly with information arranged in a logical order. Good source for quickly finding drug information relating to pharmacology.
Walgreens' Pharmacy— http://www.walgreens.com/	Another informative site for the public that includes how to find the nearest Walgreens Pharmacy.
WebMD—http://www.my.webmd.com/	Source of a wealth of information on health, drugs, and medical conditions.

Pharmaceutical Websites

Bayer—http://www.bayer.com/ Boehringer-Ingelheim—http://www. boehringer-ingelheim.com/ corporate/home/home.asp/ Berlex—http://www.berlex.com/ Glaxo Wellcome and Wyeth— http://www.gsk.com/ Merck—http://www.merck.com/ and http://www.merckmedicus.com/ Ortho McNeil—http://www. orthomcneil.com/	Provide drug-specific information from manu-facturer.

Professional Organizations. Professional medical, nursing, and pharmacological organizations also have websites. Some sites are available only to their members, but others are dedicated to educating the public and therefore offer information free of charge to patients and other health care workers. Some organizations create a dot-com address to help the public and use a dot-org address for their members. Allied health care workers may choose to join some of these professional organizations to continue their education in their area of practice.

Commercial Enterprises. Commercial enterprises need to make money to support a website. For that reason, they may try to sell products to visitors or might charge for information. If you wanted to download drug information for your PDA, for example, you would probably have to pay for it. Be careful about information you read on commercial sites. Whereas governmental agencies, colleges, and professional organizations hold authors accountable for information on their sites, commercial sites are usually accountable only to themselves. Thus, their information might be slanted. In the same way that reputable newspapers differ in quality from "tabloids," some commercial sites are more reputable than others.

A special category of commercial websites is *pharmaceutical companies*. These websites can be rich sources of free information; however, they usually highlight only the drugs they manufacture. Many of these sites are user-friendly, as they are trying to inform patients as well as health care professionals. Although companies must follow FDA guidelines when presenting drug information, it is important to realize that there are still ways to "slant" the information. For example, the main page may show people in carefree activities as a result of the drug's effects, with the side effects in small print below or on a secondary page. The FDA does not have the resources to monitor all websites to ensure adherence to its guidelines.

Many websites you have explored so far have been created by companies, organizations, or agencies in the United States. Other countries have information about drugs too. You can even buy drugs without a prescription from other countries, usually less expensively than you could in the United States. If the origin of the website is not in the United States, another set of letters is added. For instance, dot-uk indicates the United Kingdom, and dot-ic indicates Iceland.

CRITICAL THINKING

Which kinds of websites do you think would provide the most reliable information?

Search Engines. Search engines can help you find information more easily on the Internet. Unlike websites that provide "homes" with lots of different "rooms" to explore, search engines narrow your search for information, so you tour only the rooms that have important information for you. The search engines look for web pages with the information for which you ask. However, you must be specific (using something called Boolean logic) regarding what you ask to avoid getting thousands of responses to a query (see Fast Tip 6.2).

For example, do not type "drugs" in the search window when you really want only drugs that are for gastrointestinal problems. You might add "stomach" to "drugs" to narrow the search. You might broaden a search by thinking what other words mean the same thing. For example, you might not get much by searching for "pot"; but adding "marijuana" or "weed" might increase your yield. You can narrow your search by using "near," "…", +, −, and "fields." Fields are used to specify where to locate your search in each document to increase the relevance of the results—for example, *title: Viagra*.

Examples of search engines are the following:

- http://www.alltheweb.com
- http://www.altavista.com
- http://www.ask.com
- http://www.dogpile.com
- http://www.excite.com
- http://www.goodsearch.com

◯ *Fast Tip 6.2* Quick Reference for Boolean Logic

Today's search engines are powerful tools that scour the Internet for websites and then, after you conduct a search, present the most suitable websites for that search. Some search engines, though not all, allow searchers to use Boolean logic to explain more precisely what they're looking for. Boolean logic refers to using connecting words so the search engine "thinks" the way you want it to.

1. For instance, if you searched for "stomach" *AND* "drugs":

    AND used between two or more search terms means that *all* the words must appear on a web page for it to be included in the search results.

2. If you searched for "drugs" *OR* "pharmaceuticals":

    OR used between two or more search terms means that *any* of the words on either side of "OR" must appear on a web page for it to be included in the search results.

3. You could also search for "controlled AND drugs *NOT* illegal":

    NOT used between two or more search terms excludes what follows it. In the example, the search results would include web pages with the words "controlled" and "drugs" but *not* the word "illegal."

Other Ways to Search

1. "National Institutes of Health"

    Quotation marks ("…") used around words means all of those words must appear *in the exact order* on a web page for it to be included in the search results.

2. "Alcohol *NEAR* abuse"

    NEAR used between two or more search terms means that one word must appear in close proximity to another on a web page for it to be included in the search results.

3. "Drugs + abuse"

    A *plus sign* used in front of a word or phrase means that the word or phrase must appear on a web page for it to be included in the search results.

4. "Vaccinations − animals"

    A *minus sign* used in front of a word or phrase means that the word or phrase must not appear on a web page for it to be included in the search results.

- http://www.google.com
- http://www.live.com
- http://www.medmatrix.org
- http://www.webcrawler.com
- http://search.yahoo.com

EVALUATING A WEBSITE

It is important that you evaluate websites for your own education and to help patients evaluate sites. Box 6.2 lists some criteria for deciding whether a website is a reliable source of information. Other websites with resources that educate professionals and patients on how to choose a good website include:

- American Medical Association (http://www.jama.ama-assn.org)
- Johns Hopkins Center for Communications Programs (http://www.jhuccp.org)
- VirtualSalt (http://www.virtualsalt.com)
- World Wide Web Virtual Library (http://vlib.org)

CRITICAL THINKING

What are the top three most important qualities of a website? Why?

Patients may order medications through a disreputable source on the Internet instead of through reputable ones. Allied health professionals should teach patients to be suspicious of pharmacies online that dispense medications without prescriptions, do not have a toll-free number and a street address

---

BOX 6.2 Evaluating a Website

Although access to the Internet gives you an unlimited number of resources, you must exercise care when trusting websites. Here are some criteria for evaluating websites.

Reputable source—Is the content on the site based on well-researched principles or just one author's opinions? Is the author well trained and well educated? What are the credentials of the author?

Established organization—Is this organization "here today, gone tomorrow"; or has it been representing the profession for years? Does the site have a good reputation among your colleagues? Is it an established source of health care information or just a general website?

Peer-reviewed—Have reputable authorities, such as colleagues or librarians, reviewed this site?

Objectivity—Does the author have an issue that he or she feels so strongly about that objectivity is lost? Is the writing slanted to one opinion?

Current—How current is the information? How frequently is it updated?

Scientific—Is it a research institution or company that is using proven scientific methods to support its claims? How large was the patient sample size in research studies?

Depth—Does the site publish the opinions of a single author, or does it gather large amounts of information before making decisions?

Credible—Is this information believable? Have you read other research that contradicts it? Is it so far out of the mainstream of knowledge as to be unbelievable?

Other Important Criteria
- Is the site easy to find?
- Does it have a name that is easy to remember and spell?
- Is the browser frequently unavailable?
- Is the site down for editing more than it is up for reading?
- Does the site load quickly?
- Is it easy to navigate in the site?
- Can you find what you want quickly?
- Is it well organized?

posted on the site, do not allow consumers to contact the pharmacist if they have questions, or sell only a limited number of medications.

SUMMARY

Allied health professionals have many resources they can use to find information about medications. Although it is exciting to have so much information online, it is important to evaluate websites carefully using set criteria. You cannot endorse websites as totally reliable, but you can guide your patients to reputable ones, such as those sponsored by professional organizations. Many of your patients learn unreliable information from websites and chat rooms. You can help them by sharing criteria for evaluating websites and explaining how the type of sponsor can affect how objective the site is.

Activities

To make sure that you have learned the key points covered in this chapter, complete the following activities.

True or False
Write *true* if the statement is true. Beside the false statements, write *false* and correct the statement to make it true.

1. The PDR easily fits into your laboratory coat pocket. _____

2. The USP/DI is useful for patients to read. _____

3. The USP/NF is the official drug resource of the U.S. government. _____

4. The blue section of the PDR lists drugs by classification. _____

5. The PDR does not contain photographs. _____

Multiple Choice
Choose the best answer for each question.

1. Which term means "harmful side effects?"
   a. Warnings
   b. Overdosage
   c. Adverse reactions
   d. Precautions
   e. Contraindications

2. Package inserts contain all of the following information *except*:
   a. Date of package insert
   b. Contraindications
   c. Name of drug
   d. Pharmacies that carry the drug
   e. Clinical pharmacology

3. The correct ending for the website http://www.fda is:
   a. .edu
   b. .com
   c. .gov
   d. .org

4. The correct ending for the website http://www.bayer is:
   a. .edu
   b. .com
   c. .gov
   d. .org

5. The National Library of Medicine is part of the:
   a. FDA
   b. CBC
   c. OSHA
   d. NIH
   e. DOJ

Application Exercises

Using a drug handbook, PDR, or the Internet, answer the following.

1. What is the infant dosage of bacitracin IM?

2. What color pill is acyclovir 200 mg?

3. What is the classification of spironolactone?

4. What are five side effects of tamoxifen?

5. What are the routes of methylprednisone?

6. What is the primary side effect of loratidine?

7. What special concerns are involved with testosterone?

8. What drugs does Dopar interact with adversely?

9. Does Os-Cal 500 come in tablets or patches?

10. Should a child take BuSpar?

11. What drugs are combined in Vicodin?

12. Can pregnant women safely take interferon beta-1a?

13. What color is Zantac 300 mg?

14. What are the administration routes of Dalacin?

15. Is meperidine compatible with KCl in an IV drip?

16. What is the brand name of divalproex sodium?

17. What is meclizine hydrochloride used for?

18. What is the duration of atropine sulfate p.m.?

19. How does hydrocodone bitartrate affect laboratory tests?

20. What are the routes of Prolixin?

21. What is the generic name of Restoril?

22. What is Narcan used for?

23. Can someone on Coumadin take aspirin?

24. What is the primary side effect of Feosol?

25. What is the child's dosage of ibuprofen?

Application

Using drug resources, respond to questions in the following scenarios on a separate sheet.

1. You remember that your pharmaceutical representative, Chuck Collins, brought some new antibiotics when he last visited the office. The physician you work for cannot remember the name of the new drugs. **How can you get this information?**
2. A physician is speaking to the local medical society on "Pharmaceutical Treatment of Diabetes." **How might you search for information on this topic?**
3. You do the coding and billing for a small physician's office. If would be nice if you could find a pocket-sized book with a list of drugs and the ICD-9 codes that went with them. **Where would you find one?**
4. Debbie Glazer, one of your patients, bought a PDR at the local wholesale warehouse. She has now read about the drugs she has been taking and calls your office to complain that they all have huge side effects that she does not want. **How would you respond?**
5. Jackie Soucier confides that she has very little money to pay for medications. **How can you help her?**

Virtual Field Trips

Go to the following websites to find the information. If a website is not available, try to find the information through another source.

1. Go to http://www.rxlist.com and print the top 50 prescribed drugs for last year.
2. Access http://www.jhuccp.org and go to the Johns Hopkins Center for Communication Programs. Create your own template with at least 10 criteria for evaluating whether sites are good or bad.
3. Surf to at least 10 of the sites mentioned in this chapter. Print the home pages, and bookmark the sites you liked the best.
4. Visit http://www.needymeds.com/. Do you think this is a reputable site? Why or why not?
5. Go to http://www.nabp.net/vipps and discuss the VIPPS seal on Internet sites. What does it mean, and who oversees the program?

Administration
of Medicines

Medication Administration

This chapter describes the supplies needed and the correct procedure for each route of medication administration. Choosing the correct supplies saves time and ensures patient safety. Different supplies are needed depending on the route of administration. These routes are oral, nasal, ophthalmic, otic, inhalation, transdermal, vaginal, rectal, intramuscular (IM), subcutaneous (SC), intradermal (ID), and intravenous (IV). Many factors determine the route of administration, including the chemicals in the drug, how fast a response is needed, and if a local or a body-wide effect is desired.

The chapter first discusses the supplies and then how to administer medications correctly. The prescriber orders a specific route, but you need to know which supplies to use.

OBJECTIVES

At the end of this chapter, the student will be able to:

- Define all key terms.
- Explain what supplies are needed for medication administration.
- Select the correct needle and syringe for parenteral injections.
- Describe the solutions used in IV therapy.
- Describe blood products.
- Describe how to safely administer oral medications.
- Discuss the methods for administering medications through nasogastric or gastric tubes.
- Discuss how to inject IM, SC, and ID medications safely.
- Describe how to administer ophthalmic and otic medications correctly.
- Discuss precautions for the safe administration of inhalation therapy.
- Describe how to apply transdermal patches correctly.
- Describe how to insert vaginal and rectal medications safely.
- Discuss how to prepare the patient for IV therapy.

KEY TERMS

Additive	Infiltration	Primed
Ampule	Lactated Ringer's	Protective cap
Barrel	Lipids	Reconstitute
Blister pack	Lumen	Saline
Bulk	Meniscus	Spacers
Calibrated	Mortar	Spike
Cannula	NSS	Thrombus
CPAP	Osmosis	Tip
Crystalloid	Packed cells	TPN
Deltoid	Particulate	Tuberculin
Dextrose	PCA	Units
Dialysis	Pestle	Vastus lateralis
Dorsogluteal	Phlebitis	Ventrogluteal
Drip chamber	Piggyback	Vial
Electrolytes	Plasma	Vitamins
Filter	Platelets	Wheal
Flow regulator	Plunger	Whole blood
Gauge	Polymerized	Z-track
Hub	hemoglobin	
Hypodermic	Port	

⬤ SUPPLIES

Health care settings are busy places, with many patients who have many different needs. It is important to work safely and efficiently to be sure patients do not have to wait a long time for treatment and that they receive the proper care. Gathering the right supplies before starting drug preparation and administration saves time. In addition, an item needed for one route of administration may not be correct for another, so having the right supplies helps keep the patient safe. This section describes the supplies needed for parenteral (given by a route other than the alimentary canal) and nonparenteral medicines.

Nonparenteral Supplies

Supplies for nonparenteral drugs include bottles, unit dose packages, droppers, inhalation delivery systems, patches, and suppositories. The supplies needed depend on how the drug will be administered.

Bottles and unit-dose packages

Most medications are taken by mouth. Oral drugs are frequently poured out of a *bulk* (multiple-dose) bottle first into the cap (if they are pills) of the bottle and then into a medicine cup (Fig. 7.1). Frequently, pills come prepackaged in individual doses, referred to as unit-dose. A group of unit-doses may be contained in a *blister pack,* which must be gently opened by pressing on the tablet so that the pill falls into the medicine cup. Always wash your hands beforehand, and do not touch the pill so microbes are not transferred from your hands to the pill to the patient.

Sometimes the prescriber orders the tablets to be crushed before they are administered (see Fast Tip 7.1). Often this is so the tablets can be mixed with food or a liquid to make it easier for patients to swallow. Not all pills can be crushed. For example, pills coated to slow down the release of the drug (enteric-coated) and timed-release capsules should not be crushed.

Droppers

A dropper is used to administer small amounts of a drug into the nose (the nasal route), eye (ophthalmic route), ear (otic route), or mouth (oral route). Insert the open end of the tube into the liquid

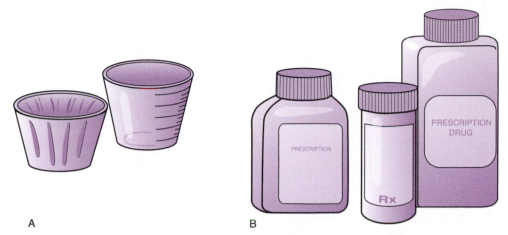

A   B

FIGURE 7.1. Supplies for oral administration: (A) medication cups; (B) bulk container.

drug and gently squeeze the rubber bulb at the top to draw up the liquid (Fig. 7.2). Droppers are sometimes calibrated for exact dosing. Be sure to inspect the dropper visually for holes. If the dropper enters a body opening or cavity (e.g., the nose), you must clean the dropper after use in soap and water.

Inhalation delivery systems

Sometimes it is important for a medication to be directly applied to the lungs or to be absorbed directly into the body through the lungs. Special devices are used to ensure that, as the patient breathes in (inhales), the medicine enters the lungs. The medicine is inhaled in the form of droplets in compressed air or a gas such as oxygen, meaning the drug is aerosolized. This quick method of administration is ideal for delivering certain kinds of anesthesia and drugs that break up congestion in the lungs. Because patients with asthma have inflammation in parts of their lungs, inhalation is a good way to deliver asthma medications where they are needed. Powders are more easily inhaled if sterile water or sodium chloride is added to be aerosolized with the medication.

○ *Fast Tip 7.1* Crushing Tablets

A mortar and pestle can be used to crush tablets. The mortar is a bowl, usually made of glass, in which tablets (not enteric-coated or timed-release) may be placed to be crushed. The pestle, a club-shaped tool usually made of glass, is used to crush the tablets. Do not crush a tablet unless the prescriber has given you permission to do so, because some tablets have been coated to be timed-release and crushing would disrupt this.

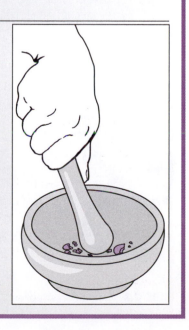

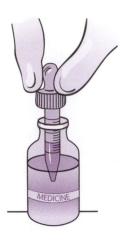

FIGURE 7.2. Using a dropper to dispense medication.

Two portable inhalation delivery systems are inhalers and spacers (Fig. 7.3). Hand-held *inhalers* fit easily into a patient's pocket or purse. *Spacers* help a patient hold an inhaler. They are especially good for children and cognitively impaired (unable to think clearly) or disabled adults. Spacers have an extension tunnel, so the medication is held and administered whenever the patient inhales—rather than escaping into the air if the patient exhales instead of inhaling. *Nebulizers* are manual or electronic devices that force medication-laced air into the lungs. Nebulizers are also fairly portable and use compressed air or oxygen to force medication into the lungs. These devices are especially good for children and patients who tire easily.

Not as portable as a nebulizer is a *CPAP* machine, which forces room air or oxygen into the lungs, even when the patient forgets to breathe (Fig. 7.4). It is ideal for patients with sleep apnea, a situation where the patient stops breathing for short periods of time while asleep. Remember that oxygen from a tank or out of a special wall port is considered a medication and requires an order from a prescriber for the number of liters to be delivered each minute. This is usually written as L/minute.

Oxygen can be given to the patient through a nasal cannula or a mask (see Fig. 7.4). The prongs of the nasal cannula fit into a patient's nose. Although this is more comfortable for a patient than a mask, only lower concentrations (levels) of oxygen can be delivered.

A mask is used to deliver high concentrations of oxygen, but it can be frightening to small children and patients who are disoriented and do not know where or who they are. These patients may feel like they are being suffocated. Teaching the patient what to expect or placing the mask near, but not on, the face may help ease the fear.

CPAP, nasal cannula, and mask (also used with a CPAP machine) used over periods of time require the air to be moisturized to avoid drying out the skin and mucosa. Patients should add distilled water to special chambers in the CPAP machine to humidify the air; distilled water does not have the chemicals that are in tap water and so does not add chemicals to the machine.

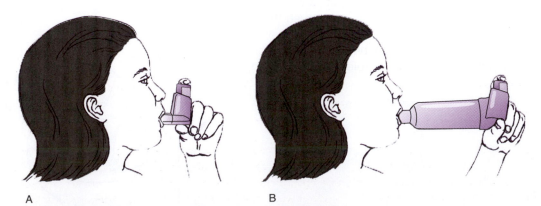

A   B

FIGURE 7.3. Inhalation supplies: (A) inhaler; (B) inhaler with spacer.

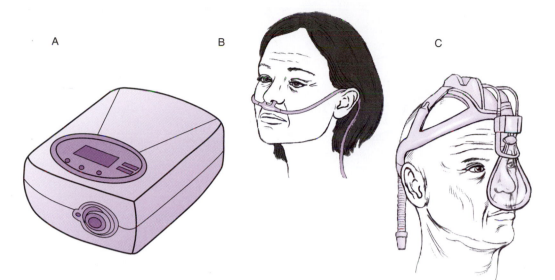

FIGURE 7.4. (A) CPAP machine. (B) Nasal cannula. (C) Mask.

CRITICAL THINKING

What would happen if a patient used a CPAP machine with a mask for 30 minutes without having added water to the inhaled air?

Patches/suppositories

Sometimes a drug is delivered across skin or mucosa (transdermal). This may be done when patients have a difficult time swallowing or are too nauseated to take medicine by mouth.

The most common method of transdermal delivery is to apply a patch that has the medication in it. Patches usually come prepared, although they can be made. The advantages of the transdermal patch are that it is easy to apply to the skin, it remains effective over long periods of time, it is easy to remove, and it results in reliable, even drug distribution in the body. Uses of transdermal patches include treatment of chronic pain, motion sickness, smoking cessation, hormone replacement, birth control, blood pressure, heart conditions, allergies, and angina.

Suppositories are another way to deliver medicine across mucosa. Drugs are mixed with a firm substance such as glycerine and then molded so the form can be easily inserted into a body cavity, such as the rectum or vagina. Most suppositories are packaged in foil.

Parenteral Supplies for Injectable Medications

Supplies used for preparing medicines that are injected include ampules, vials, needles, syringes, and IV-related items, including bags or bottles of solutions, tubing, needles, and catheters.

Ampules and vials

An *ampule* is a small glass container that holds only one dose of a medication in solution for injections (Fig. 7.5). The ampule is broken by placing gauze around the neck to protect the hand and keep glass from falling into the medicine. It is best to draw the solution from the ampule into a syringe with one needle, then change to a different needle to inject the solution into the patient; this reduces the chance of broken glass entering the patient. Sometimes filtering devices are used with the needle to remove any broken glass.

Most injectable solutions are supplied in vials instead of ampules (see Fig. 7.5). Vials are glass or plastic containers sealed on the top with rubber stoppers. This makes the inside of the container sterile (without bacteria) as it does not have to be opened or broken. Occasionally, powder is in the vial, and fluid, such as bacteriostatic sodium chloride or water, is added to it to mix, or *reconstitute*, the solution. Once reconstituted, the vial should be used fairly quickly, according to the instructions of the

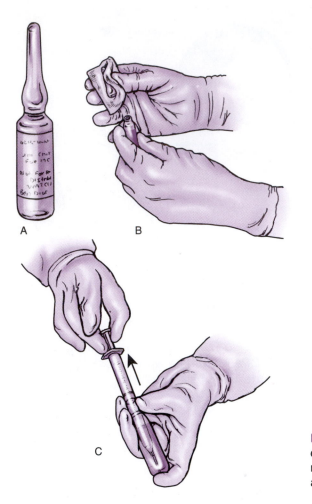

FIGURE 7.5. An ampule is a small glass container that holds only one dose of a medication (A). To use: break off the top (B) and draw the contents into a syringe (C).

manufacturer of the drug. The reasoning behind this practice is that the powder is more durable when stored without the fluid.

CRITICAL THINKING

Why do you think vials are used more than ampules?

Needles

Choosing a needle is based on two measurements—length and width. Needle length ranges from $\frac{3}{8}$ inch to 2 inches (Fig. 7.6). A smaller needle is used for ID injections and a longer one for IM injections. Small lengths are used for small children and small muscles.

The width of the inside of a needle (lumen) is measured by *gauge* (Fig. 7.7). Gauges vary from 18 (largest) to 27 (smallest). The higher the number, the smaller is the lumen.

A CLOSER LOOK: Medication Vials

Vials are either multiple- or unit-dose. Multiple-dose vials contain several doses. After the first dose, the top of the stopper should be cleaned with an alcohol swab or other disinfecting swab before inserting a needle into the vial for another dose. Unit-dose vials contain just one dose of medicine and are thrown away after use.

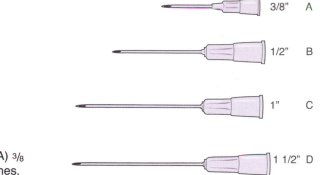

FIGURE 7.6. Various needle lengths: (A) ³/₈ inch; (B) ½ inch; (C) 1 inch; (D) 1½ inches.

The viscosity (thickness) of the fluid being given determines which gauge is chosen. A drug resource or the instructions that come with the medication help determine the proper gauge of needle for the fluid. A thin fluid could pass through a 27-gauge needle, whereas for a thick fluid (e.g., blood) a 20-gauge needle might be used.

Syringes

Figure 7.8 shows the parts of a syringe. There are three basic types of syringe—TB, insulin, and standard (Fig. 7.9). For TB (tuberculosis) testing or other ID injections, little fluid is injected. This situation calls for a narrow, finely calibrated syringe known as a *tuberculin* syringe. Every tenth line is longer to make it easier to see 0.1-mL increments (see Fast Tip 7.2).

An insulin syringe is calibrated in *units* instead of milliliters (Fig. 7.10). It can hold no more than 1 mL. The standard U-100 insulin syringe has 100 units calibrated on the barrel, and each line usually equals 2 units. For small children or small amounts, insulin syringes are available in 30- and 50-unit capacity syringes. Because they have less capacity, each mark equals 1 unit, not 2 (see Fast Tip 7.3).

Standard, or *hypodermic*, syringes are available in sizes ranging from 3 mL to 50 mL. Even if the needle is attached or packaged together with the syringe, it may be better to use a different gauge or length needle—especially if the patient is small or is a child. Prepackaged needles can be replaced with smaller ones. The calibration of these syringes depends on the size.

Syringes are available without needles to deliver medication into the mouth. They also can be purchased without needles, so separate needles can be attached according to the length and gauge desired for the specific task.

The various types of syringe are summarized in Table 7.1.

Safety devices

Because the Occupational Safety and Health Administration (OSHA) of the Department of Labor requires that employers protect employees from accidental needle-sticks, safety devices are frequently attached to needles. These devices make needles more costly, but safer. Accidental needle-sticks can

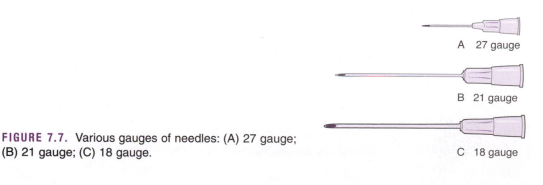

FIGURE 7.7. Various gauges of needles: (A) 27 gauge; (B) 21 gauge; (C) 18 gauge.

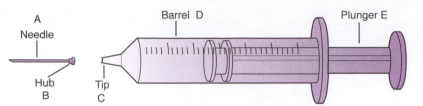

FIGURE 7.8. Parts of a syringe: (A) needle; (B) hub; (C) tip; (D) barrel; (E) plunger.

result in the transfer of blood-borne pathogens (bacteria and viruses) from the patient to the person administering the medication.

Needle protectors either retract the needle before it is pulled out of the patient or cover the needle after usage (Fig. 7.11). The easiest way to become familiar with the various types of needle protectors is to practice with them on a manikin or piece of food (hot dog, orange, or turkey leg, for example). OSHA requires that medical offices use safe needle protectors.

Ideally, a needle is never recapped by hand. After the injection, the needle and syringe should immediately be thrown away in a biohazard sharps container (Fig. 7.12). However, after medication has been withdrawn from a vial, the needle may be recapped so it can be taken to the patient for administration of the medicine. It is best to recap a needle by pressing the needle cap against a firm object or placing it in a special recapping device to recap with the pressure of the device—not the hand (Fig. 7.13).

CRITICAL THINKING

Why is it dangerous to recap a needle? With so many safety devices available, why do you think there are still so many needle-sticks?

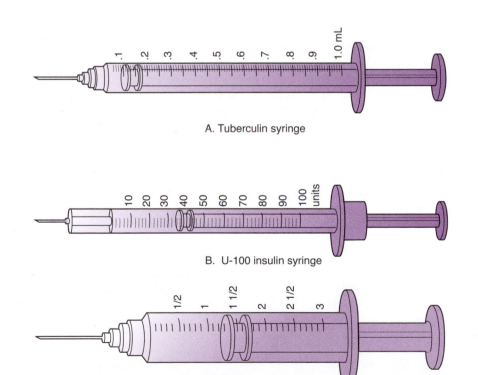

A. Tuberculin syringe

B. U-100 insulin syringe

C. 3 mL syringe

FIGURE 7.9. Types of syringe: (A) tuberculin; (B) insulin; (C) hypodermic.

TABLE 7.1 Syringes and Uses

SYRINGE TYPE	CALIBRATION AND CAPACITY	SAMPLE USE
Tuberculin	One line = 0.1 mL Capacity = 1 mL	Tuberculin testing or other ID injections Newborn and pediatric dosages
Insulin	One line = 2 units Capacity = 100 units	Insulin administration
Standard	Varies with size	IM injections

⊙ *Fast Tip 7.2* TB syringes

Tuberculin (TB) syringes are also frequently used for newborns and pediatric dosages because doses of medicine for these patients are usually quite small.

Prefilled syringes

An emergency leaves little time to prepare medication for injection. For speed and accuracy in an emergency situation, drugs can be placed in a preloaded cartridge that can quickly be attached in a special cartridge plunger (Fig. 7.14). After the cartridge is used, do not throw the holder away. Simply dispose of the glass or plastic cartridge and retain the holder for future use.

IV supplies

A licensed health care professional such as a registered nurse is responsible for starting and managing IV lines. However, other members of the health care team need to be familiar with IV supplies in

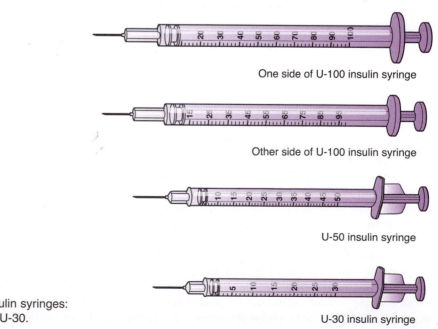

One side of U-100 insulin syringe

Other side of U-100 insulin syringe

U-50 insulin syringe

FIGURE 7.10. Insulin syringes: U-100, U-50, and U-30.

U-30 insulin syringe

⊙ *Fast Tip 7.3* Checking Insulin

Because an overdose or underdose of insulin can kill a patient, facilities may have a policy that all insulin doses must be double-checked by two people before administering them.

---

case they are asked to help prepare them. These supplies include special bags filled with solutions that may or may not contain *additives* (medications, electrolytes, vitamins), tubing, IV needles, and IV catheters.

IV solutions

Sometimes a patient just needs fluids, and other times the patient may need additives, total parenteral nutrition, or blood. Types of fluids, or *solutions,* are dextrose, saline, and lactated Ringer's (see Fast Tip 7.4).

A *dextrose* solution is a sugar and water solution. Dextrose 2.5% in water (D-2.5-W), 5% in water (D-5-W), and 10% in water (D-10-W) are the most popular. Dextrose can also come in combinations of 20%–70%, but these are for patients with extremely low blood sugar levels, such as diabetics, infants, and severely malnourished patients.

If sugar is not needed, a *saline*, or sodium chloride (salt), solution may be prescribed. Sodium is a vital *electrolyte* (substance carrying an electrical charge). The usual solution, 0.9% sodium chloride (NaCl), is called *normal saline solution* (NSS). Also available is $\frac{1}{2}$ NSS, which is 0.45% NaCl. Normal saline solutions can be added to dextrose solutions, such as D5NS or D10/0.45 NaCl. *Crystalloids* are IV solutions that provide NSS with or without other electrolytes.

A CLOSER LOOK: Electrolytes

Electrolytes are substances that carry either a positive or negative electrical charge. They are important for helping cells function normally. Common electrolytes include sodium, potassium, and magnesium.

Lactated Ringer's solution was created by Sidney Ringer, an English physiologist who mixed dextrose, potassium, chloride, sodium, lactate, and calcium to form an especially healthful mixture for patients. Ringer's lactate (RL) and dextrose 5% in lactated Ringer's (D5LR) are other names for these mixtures.

Sometimes medications or electrolytes need to be given several times per day over short periods of time. In this case, a *piggyback* solution is used. This is a separate IV bag and tubing that is connected to the primary IV tubing. The piggyback might contain, for example, an antibiotic or potassium that is given every 4 hours in 100 mL of fluid.

Vitamins can be added to IV solutions, especially when patients cannot process vitamins in their gastrointestinal system. Vitamins help with many body processes and can give the patient more energy.

Total parenteral nutrition (TPN) is given when the patient's digestive system needs a complete rest. A nutritional solution is infused (flowed) directly into the veins to give the patient complete nutrition. TPN fluids are made to be placed directly into a large vein. They provide the patient with a well-rounded supply of fluid and electrolytes plus calories from fats, protein, and vitamins. TPN fluids require the use of special long-term IV catheters that a physician places usually in the subclavian vein. The end of the catheter lies in the superior vena cava.

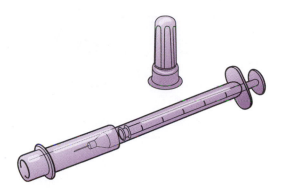

FIGURE 7.11. A syringe with a needle protector covering the needle after use.

Lipids, or fats, may also be added to IV solutions. Sometimes soybean or safflower oil is added to water, glycerin, and egg yolks. This increases the caloric source for patients who need it. Lipids, like TPN, usually require a special line.

Blood and blood products can also be administered through an IV line. A licensed health care professional gives blood, but it is important for everyone on the team to understand the types of blood products.

Whole blood provides complete correction of blood loss. One unit of whole blood is 500 mL. *Packed red blood cells* are concentrated preparations of red blood cells with most of the plasma removed. Removing the plasma cuts the amount of fluid. The smaller amount of fluid means less chance of fluid overload in certain patients, such as infants and patients with heart failure. *Platelets* are removed from whole blood and have a small amount of plasma added. They have a short shelf life of only 5 days and are used for patients who have low platelet levels.

Polymerized hemoglobin solution is a bag of natural hemoglobin that has been chemically changed and is used to provide concentrated hemoglobin. It is used only when other blood products are not available.

Before blood or any blood products are given, the patient's blood type must be checked against what is to be administered. This process, called "type and cross," makes sure that patients do not have a transfusion reaction to blood that does not match their own.

Plasma and plasma expanders come from whole blood that has been separated to remove the red, white, and clotting cells. Plasma does not have to be typed and crossmatched and can restore normal blood volume. Plasma is useful for replacing fluid (e.g., that lost through burns). Dextran and Plasma-Plex are examples of plasma expanders.

A *transfusion reaction* is a serious negative response to the administration of blood or blood products. Signs and symptoms of a reaction include a rapid change in vital signs, dyspnea, restlessness, fever, chills, blood in the urine (hematuria), and chest, back, or flank pain. To discontinue a blood

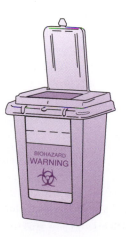

FIGURE 7.12. Biohazard container.

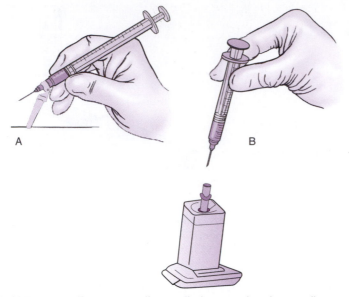

FIGURE 7.13. Recap a sterile needle by pressing the needle cap against a firm object (A) or placing it in a special recapping device to recap with the pressure of the device (B), not the hand.

transfusion, the health care worker first clamps the line infusing the blood and opens the line infusing the NSS, which is hung like a "Y" with the blood (Fig. 7.15) (see Fast Tip 7.5). You should closely watch the patient's vital signs, including pulse, temperature, respiratory rate, and blood pressure.

CRITICAL THINKING

Why do physicians prescribe different blood products instead of just giving whole blood?

IV setups

Most IV lines have the basic components illustrated in Figure 7.16. To set up an IV system, the health care worker *spikes* the IV bag or bottle and attaches it to the IV tubing. He or she does this by inserting the end of the tubing into the outlet port of the bag or bottle. The cap on the spike section of the IV tubing is removed just before it is inserted into the IV container to keep the spike sterile. An IV bottle may have an air vent located below the spike. The health care worker needs to remove a diaphragm to let air in and release the vacuum. The vent allows air to enter the bottle as fluid flows out.

Bags collapse as the solution flows out. Bottles maintain their shape as they empty. Calibration marks on the bag or bottle show how much IV solution has been administered and how much is left (see Fig. 7.16).

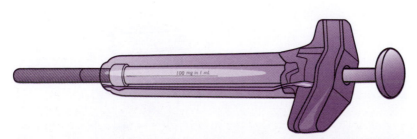
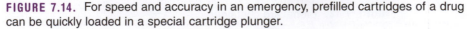

FIGURE 7.14. For speed and accuracy in an emergency, prefilled cartridges of a drug can be quickly loaded in a special cartridge plunger.

A CLOSER LOOK: Types of IV Administration

Medication can be given into a vein either by IV "push" or infusion. *IV push* refers to quick delivery of a small amount of medication in a syringe. IV push cannot be used for drugs that irritate the vein, those that can be deadly if given too quickly, or a large amount of medication. Only a licensed health care professional can give IV push medication.

Infusion is slow IV administration of a large volume of fluid. The solution can contain additives such as medications, electrolytes, or minerals. IV fluid is usually packaged in a 500- to 1000-mL bag or bottle. The health care worker hangs the bag on a pole that is raised higher than the patient's heart. The fluid then flows into the vein by gravity or via an infusion pump. Fluid may also be pushed into the patient's vein with a pump. *Patient-controlled analgesia* (PCA) allows patients to push a button and get medication (most often pain medication) on demand within parameters ordered by the prescriber. Usually licensed health professionals program these pumps.

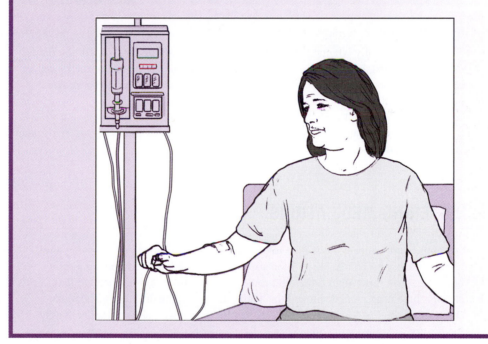

Below the spike is a *drip chamber* (see Fig. 7.16). The drip chamber allows the flow of fluid from the bag after it has been *primed* (emptied of air) by squeezing it. The purpose of the drip chamber is to encourage any air in the line to remain in the chamber while only the solution flows down to the patient. The flow rate is set by counting the drops going into the drip chamber.

On the IV tubing, the *flow regulator* adjusts the flow through the line (see Fig. 7.16). The *ports* in various places along the line allow IV medications to be infused through them. The *needle adapter*

⬤ *Fast Tip 7.4* Storage of IV Solutions

IV solutions are usually stored in cabinets away from light because they can deteriorate if exposed to light for long periods of time. IV solutions look similar, so it is important to check the label against the order three times.

enters the patient's vein but is usually removed, leaving a flexible cannula in the vein. A protective cap covers the needle until ready for use.

The length of the IV tubing varies from 6 to 120 inches, depending on need. The amount of fluid needed for priming the tubing varies depending on the length of the tubing, but the use of a final filtration device can reduce the need for flushing the line with a large amount of IV fluid before attaching it to the needle or catheter.

A CLOSER LOOK: Types of IV Lines

Peripheral lines are IV lines placed in veins in the arms or hands. *Central lines* are IV lines inserted in large veins such as the subclavian vein or internal jugular vein. These catheters terminate in the superior vena cava. That is, the tip of the catheter lies in the superior vena cava, just above the heart. Central lines are used to give additives that irritate small veins, such as lipids.

Intravenous sets are individually wrapped and sterilized, ensuring a sterile pathway for the fluids. Damaged packages are not used, because sterility may be compromised. Rigid parts of the IV set are made from plastic or polymerized chloride. Only plastic sets may be used for nitroglycerin, which interacts with polymerized chloride (see Fast Tip 7.6).

Needles used for IVs are usually 10–16 gauge and can be the winged "butterfly" type or a straight needle within a catheter, called an angiocath (Fig. 7.17). Table 7.2 compares the two types. A 20-gauge or smaller size needle is used in adults.

ADMINISTERING MEDICATIONS

Once the needed supplies are collected, it is time to administer the medication. When giving any medication, you must wash your hands, observe the six "rights" of medication administration— right patient, right drug, right dose, right time, right route, right documentation—compare the order to the container three times, and document the administration of the drug. Remember that the patient needs to know what is going to be done before proceeding with administration. Safely administering medications requires strict adherence to the protocols listed in this chapter or in your facility's manual.

Oral Medications

Unless a patient has trouble swallowing, most prefer the oral route to receiving injections with needles; hence, this is the most common way to deliver medication. Oral medications can be delivered by mouth or through a special tube in the stomach.

Medications by mouth

To give pills by mouth, you need to assemble supplies: medication, medication cup, order, and a cup of liquid to help the patient to swallow the medication. Box 7.1 provides a step-by-step procedure for administering solid oral medications.

The first part of the procedure for administering liquid medication is the same as for solid medication (Box 7.2). However, in this case you need a calibrated medicine cup. It is important to place the medicine cup on a flat surface and pour the liquid into the cup to ensure accurate dosing. The patient may need some water after swallowing a thick or bad-tasting medication; however, if the medication is used to coat the throat, do not offer water.

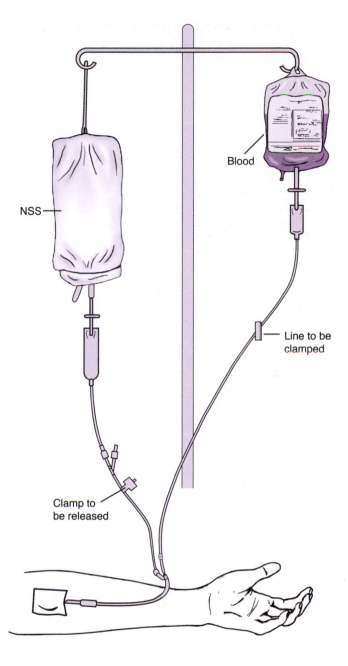

Blood

NSS

Line to be
clamped

Clamp to
be released

FIGURE 7.15. To discontinue a
blood transfusion, the health care
worker first clamps the line infusing blood and opens the line infusing NSS, which is hung like a "Y"
with the blood.

⊙ *Fast Tip 7.5* Dialysis: Not for Veins

A treatment option for patients with kidney problems that involves IV solutions, but
not veins, is dialysis. If you work at a dialysis clinic, you need to understand the
process. Dialysis refers to the passage of small particles through membranes.
Electrolytes and drugs move from areas of high concentration to areas of lower
concentration (osmosis). Normally, our kidneys perform this function, but when they
are not working correctly a machine must be used.

Dialysis solutions are never put directly into patients' veins but can be placed in
dialysis machines or across a membrane such as the peritoneum. If the patient
lacks the electrolyte needed, it crosses from the solution into the blood. If the patient
has too much of an electrolyte, it crosses from the blood into the dialysis solution.

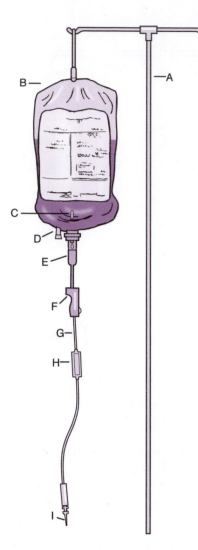

FIGURE 7.16. IV setup with: (A) pole; (B) IV solution bag; (C) spike; (D) injection port; (E) drip chamber; (F) flow regulator clamp; (G) tubing; (H) filter; (I) needle adapter with protective cap.

◯ *Fast Tip 7.6* IV Lumen
_____

The standard lumen of an IV set is usually 0.28 cm. The size of the lumen determines the flow rate. It is important to use a gentle flow rate with infants, as they may quickly build up too much fluid.

Nasogastric and gastric tube administration

Medications can be administered through a nasogastric (NG) tube, which leads from the nose to the stomach, or a gastric tube, which a surgeon places directly into the patient's stomach under sterile conditions (Box 7.3). These tubes are used for patients who have trouble swallowing.

Only liquids or tablets that have been crushed and mixed in water can be delivered through the tube. Before the drug is given, the NG tube must be checked to be sure it is in the proper place. Be sure to flush the tube with NSS before and after medications are administered (see Fast Tip 7.7).

Ophthalmic Administration

Many patients are anxious about having medicine dropped into their eyes, so it is especially necessary in this situation to keep the patient informed (Box 7.4). When placing medication in the eye, wear

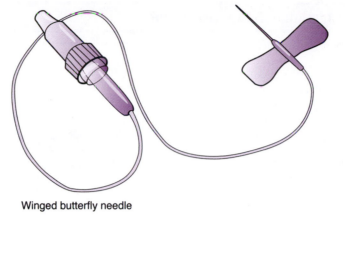

Winged butterfly needle

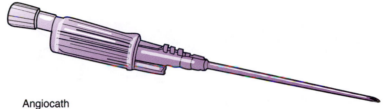

Angiocath

FIGURE 7.17. Needles used for IVs are usually 20 gauge or 16 gauge and can be a winged "butterfly" or a straight needle in a catheter, also called an angiocath.

TABLE 7.2 Comparison of Winged and Straight IV Needles	
WINGED	**STRAIGHT**
Short-term use	Long-term use
Easy to insert	More difficult to insert
More likely to lead to infiltration (leakage of fluid from the vein into the tissue)	Inadvertent vein puncture less likely
Uncomfortable	More comfortable once placed

gloves and be careful not to touch the dropper to the eye itself. Have the patient look upward as you drop in the exact number of drops ordered (Fig. 7.18). After instilling the drops, have the patient close his or her eyes. This helps prevent the medication from entering a tiny tube called the *nasolacrimal duct,* which runs from the inside corner of the eye to the nose. Light pressure with a finger on the inner part of the closed eyelid after administration of the medication also helps keep the drug from leaking into the nasolacrimal duct.

Some eye medications come in the form of ointment in a tube. Instead of dropping in the medicine, apply a thin layer of ointment into the bottom eyelid. Be sure not to touch the tube to the eye or lid.

⊙ *Fast Tip 7.7* Checking Tube Placement

You can check that the tube is in the stomach either by injecting air into the tube and listening with a stethoscope for the sound of air in the hollow stomach or by drawing back on a syringe attached to the tube and checking if stomach contents flow backward into the syringe.

BOX 7.1 Administration of Solid Medications

- Observe the six "rights" of medication administration.
- Read the medication order and compare with the medication container.
- Wash hands.
- Compare medication order with container a second time. Check expiration date.
- Assemble equipment needed: medication, medication cup, order, and cup of liquid to help swallow medication.
- Identify the patient and explain what you will be doing.
- Compare order and container a third time.
- Without touching the medication, gently tap the correct amount into the cap of the container.
- If the medication is scored and needs to be cut, place it (without touching it) into a scoring device and cut correctly.
- Place solid medication in a medicine cup.
- Give medication to patient with a glass of water.
- Instruct patient to swallow the medication completely.
- Assess patient for any negative response (e.g., choking).
- Wash hands.
- Document medication administration and patient response.

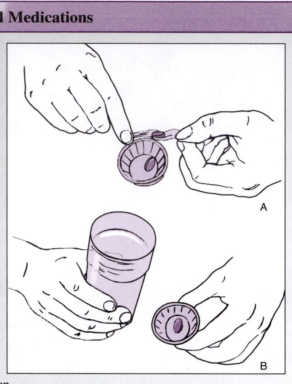

Otic Administration

Ear medications should be at room temperature before they are given. Instill the exact number of drops ordered (Box 7.5). Although ear medications do not leak out as easily as ophthalmic medicines, the patient needs to remain with the affected ear upright for a few minutes to allow maximum absorption of the medication.

Pull on the outer ear (pinna or auricle) to adjust the canal for best access. For adults, pull the pinna up and back, and for children pull the outer ear down and backward.

Nasal Administration

If a patient requires nasal drops, perhaps to clear out the nose or sinuses, you may need to help the patient administer these drops with a dropper or spray mist (Box 7.6). Instruct the patient to blow the nose before giving nasal drops, because this clears the mucosa for maximum absorption. Administer according to the order in the correct nostril or both nostrils. Instruct the patient to tilt the head backward to facilitate absorption. Be sure that the dropper is patent, and rinse the dropper afterward.

The same technique is used with a spray inhaler, but you press the spray container to spray mist into the nose. You do not rinse spray bottles, and you never use them for more than one patient.

Administration by Inhalation

Administering medications through inhalation into the respiratory system is a quick and effective way to access blood vessels. Techniques for administration include cannulas, masks, and a CPAP machine (discussed earlier in the chapter), as well as inhalers and nebulizers.

BOX 7.2 Administration of Liquid Medications

- Observe the six "rights" of medication administration.
- Read medication order and compare with the medication container.
- Wash hands.
- Compare medication order with container a second time. Check expiration date.
- Assemble equipment needed: medication, order, calibrated medication cup.
- Identify the patient and explain what you will be doing.
- Shake bottle if needed.
- Compare the order and the container a third time.

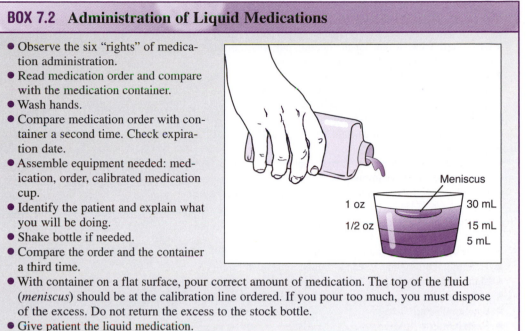

- With container on a flat surface, pour correct amount of medication. The top of the fluid (*meniscus*) should be at the calibration line ordered. If you pour too much, you must dispose of the excess. Do not return the excess to the stock bottle.
- Give patient the liquid medication.
- Instruct patient to completely swallow all the medication. If medicine is thick or tastes bad, offer patient water afterward.
- Assess patient for any negative response (e.g., choking).
- Wash hands.
- Document medication administration and patient response.

A CLOSER LOOK: Special Situations for Administering Medications by Mouth

Liquid medications. If the patient is a small child or has trouble swallowing a liquid medication, it can be drawn up into a syringe (without a needle) and injected gently into the mouth.

Crushing medications. Sometimes the prescriber orders a medication to be crushed for ease of swallowing or to insert it into a tube in the stomach. Be sure that the medication is not a timed-release or delayed-release drug. If it is a capsule that does not contain a timed-release medicine, it can be opened and mixed into food. If it is a tablet, you need a mortar and pestle to crush the medication. Then add it to a spoonful of soft, thick food, such as ice cream or applesauce, and give it to the patient. The patient needs to swallow all the food and medication on the spoon.

Metered-dose inhaler

Patients may have their own inhalers for administering a specific dose of medication. Be sure to instruct the patient to take the medication exactly as ordered. The prescribed medication should be inserted into the plastic inhaler, so the opening on the prescription is inserted into the hole in the bottom of the chamber (Box 7.7). Instruct the patient to put his or her mouth around the plastic inhalation device opening and depress the medication vial as he or she inhales for the number of puffs prescribed (see Fig. 7.19). Tell patients not to use other people's inhalers. Not only is it unsanitary to do so, but sometimes the prescription dosages are different. The plastic inhaler mouthpiece (not the prescription bottle) can be cleaned with soap and water after use to prevent infection.

BOX 7.3 **Administration of Medications by Nasogastric or Gastric Tube**

- Observe the six "rights" of medication administration.
- Compare the order to the medication container.
- Wash hands.
- Compare medication order with container a second time. Check expiration date.
- Assemble equipment needed: syringe, medication, flushing fluid, order.
- Compare order and container a third time.
- Identify the patient and explain what you will be doing.
- Elevate patient's head.
- Hold end of the tube up and remove clamp, plug, or adapter.
- Attach the syringe (without a needle) to the port.
- Make sure the tube is in the stomach (see Fast Tip 7.7).
- Use syringe to flush tube with NSS.
- Use syringe to administer medications and flush with NSS.
- Place more critical medications into the tubing first, so it is less likely that a crucial medication will be vomited out of the tube.
- After medications have been administered, flush tubing.
- Clamp tube with fingers by pinching it.
- While tube is closed, remove syringe and reattach securing device.
- Assess patient.
- Wash hands.
- Document medication administration and patient response.

Nebulizer

A nebulizer may be attached to an electric pump to force air into the patient's lungs (Fig. 7.20), or the patient may inhale from a whistle-like portable nebulizer. Place the liquid medication in the chamber on the nebulizer tubing or in the electric pump, as ordered by the prescriber. As the patient inhales the room air, the medication is added to the air and inhaled by the patient (Box 7.8).

Transdermal Administration

Most patches come prepared for administration. Wear gloves so medication from the patch does not enter your body. Remove the sticky backing on the patch, and apply the patch to an appropriate location on the body (Fig. 7.21). Be sure the area is free of tattoos, scarring, and redness. Teach the patient to rotate sites to prevent skin irritation.

BOX 7.4 **Administration of Ophthalmic Medication**

- Observe the six "rights" of medication administration.
- Read order and medication container.
- Make sure that the medication is at room temperature, not cold.
- Wash your hands.
- Compare the order with the medication container a second time. Check expiration date.
- Put gloves on.
- Identify the patient and explain what you will be doing.
- Check medication container with order a third time.
- Ask patient to look upward.
- Drop the medication with a dropper into the affected eye, or apply ointment, as ordered.
- For drops, provide gentle pressure on the corner of the eye.
- Assess patient.
- Remove gloves.
- Wash hands.
- Document dosage, site of placement, and patient response.

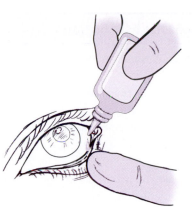

FIGURE 7.18. When placing medication in the eye, wear gloves and be careful not to touch the dropper or bottle to the eye itself. Have the patient look upward as you drop in the exact number of drops ordered.

To remove the patch, apply gloves to avoid getting any of the remaining medication on your own skin. Then fold the patch inward and dispose of it carefully.

Box 7.9 describes how to prepare a transdermal patch that is not already prepared. The most common patch you will need to make is nitroglycerin.

Vaginal Administration

The vaginal route is used for certain medications that prevent conception and soothe the vagina. Vaginal suppositories and foams are usually applied by the patient herself for the sake of modesty. The patient should wash her hands and lie on her left side to make is easer to insert the foam or opened suppository. If a patient is young or impaired, your help may be needed. If you need to administer a vaginal medication, do so according to the instructions in Box 7.10.

Rectal Administration

Rectal medications soften when warm, so they must be kept cool before administration. Insert a rectal suppository immediately after opening it, or it will melt in your hand. Wear a glove even though you are just using one finger for insertion. To administer a rectal suppository or enema, follow the instructions in Box 7.11.

Injections

Medications can be given by injection and thus bypass the gastrointestinal (GI) system. This is called parenteral administration and includes three types: intramuscular (IM), subcutaneous (SC), and intradermal (ID). An IM injection goes deep into muscle and its rich blood supply. The SC injection goes into the subcutaneous fatty tissue, where medications are absorbed more slowly. The ID site is just below the epidermis, in the dermis itself. The health care worker selects the proper needle length and adjusts the angle of injection to reach the appropriate tissue level (Fig. 7.22).

For all injections, the fluid must be drawn up from the ampule or vial into a syringe. (Check your organization's policy as to whether you are permitted to draw up and administer parenteral medication.) More viscous fluids need a lower gauge (larger lumen) needle. Choose a syringe with enough capacity to hold the medication and some extra space to draw the fluid into the syringe. Refer to Box 7.12 for a detailed description of how to draw a fluid into a syringe.

Intramuscular injections

The IM route is usually preferred for hormones, vaccinations, and pain medications. Most muscles provide a good blood supply for the medications to be absorbed. Be sure to select an appropriate needle length (usually $1-1^{1}/_{2}$ inches) and width (usually 21–23 gauge) and proper syringe capacity (up to 5 cc), depending on the patient, the viscosity (thickness) of the fluid, and the amount of medication.

BOX 7.5 Administration of Otic Medication

- Observe the six "rights" of medication administration.
- Read order and medication container.
- Make sure that the medication is at room temperature, not cold.
- Wash your hands.
- Compare the order with the medication container a second time. Check expiration date.
- Assess patency of the ear dropper.
- Put gloves on.
- Identify the patient, and explain what you will be doing.
- Check medication container with order a third time.
- Ask patient to place head on a counter or examining table, with the affected ear upward.
- Drop the medication with a dropper into the affected ear.
- Ask patient to remain still, or apply cotton ball to the ear.
- Assess patient.
- Remove gloves.
- Wash hands.
- Document dosage, site of placement, and patient response.

CRITICAL THINKING

Would you use a different length needle for a pediatric or very thin patient? Why or why not?

Sites for IM injections. Site selection depends on the viscosity of the liquid, the size and development of the muscle, and to a certain extent patient preference. Be sure not to inject into a scar or tattoo because the tissue under these areas may have an inadequate blood supply.

A common site for adults is the *deltoid* muscle, a triangular muscle on the upper arm that is usually well developed and easily accessed (Fig. 7.23).

If a larger amount of medication (2 mL or more) is needed or the patient has a very small deltoid muscle, the buttock is an alternative site. The sciatic nerve runs medially in (in the middle of) the buttock, so the safest area for injection is the upper, outer quadrant (Fig. 7.24). This is known as the *dorsogluteal* site. Usually, a patient removes clothing and leans over the examining table in a standing position.

The *ventrogluteal* site is used when the patient cannot stand and, instead, lies on his or her side (Fig. 7.25).

BOX 7.6 Nasal Administration

- Observe the six "rights" of medication administration.
- Read order and medication container.
- Wash your hands.
- Compare the order with the medication container. Check expiration date.
- Assess patency of the nose dropper.
- Put gloves on.
- Identify the patient and explain what you will be doing.
- Check medication container with order a third time.
- Ask patient to tilt head backward.
- Draw up medication into dropper, as ordered.
- Insert dropper with medication into nostril, as ordered.
- Squeeze dropper.
- Ask patient to maintain head tilt while you squeeze nostril—to prevent medication from leaking out.
- Rinse nose dropper with soap and water because it has entered the patient's body.
- Dry thoroughly.
- Assess patient.
- Remove gloves.
- Wash hands.
- Document medication dosage, site of placement, and patient response.

✳ CRITICAL THINKING

Are the dorsogluteal and ventrogluteal the same site? When would you use each method?

BOX 7.7 Administration of Medication by Inhaler

- Observe the six "rights" of medication administration.
- Read order and medication container.
- Wash your hands.
- Compare the order with the medication container. Check expiration date.
- Identify the patient and explain what you will be doing.
- Compare order and container a third time.
- Insert medication into inhaler.
- Ask patient to exhale.
- Insert inhaler into patient's mouth, and depress container when patient inhales for the number of times ordered.
- Assess patient.
- Wash hands.
- Document medication, dosage, and patient response.

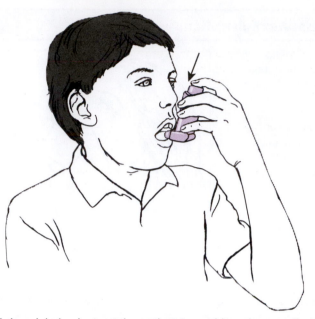

FIGURE 7.19. Metered-dose inhaler. Instruct the patient to put his or her mouth around the mouthpiece and depress the medication vial as he or she inhales for number of puffs prescribed.

The deltoid muscle is not well-developed in infants and small children, so a better site is a thigh muscle—the *vastus lateralis*. As the name suggests, it is the large muscle on the side of the thigh (Fig. 7.26).

The procedure for IM injections is described in Box 7.13. A different method is used for medications that might dye the skin surface, called the Z-track method. If a health care professional does not use the Z-track method with a medication such as Inferon, the patient may have permanent discoloration of the skin at the site. It is important to follow the directions for Z-tracking closely or the needle may break in the skin (Box 7.14).

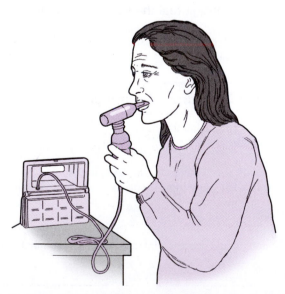

FIGURE 7.20. A nebulizer may be attached to an electric pump to force air into the patient's lungs.

BOX 7.8 Nebulizer Administration

- Observe the six "rights" of medication administration.
- Read order and medication container.
- Wash your hands.
- Compare the order with the medication container. Check expiration date.
- Identify the patient and explain what you will be doing.
- Compare order and container a third time.
- Insert medication into medication cup and add solution, as indicated.
- Apply nasal cannula or mask to patient.
- If electric, turn nebulizer on. If manual, have patient breathe deeply.
- Assess patient during treatment.
- After treatment, clean plastic parts in soap and water.
- Wash hands.
- Document medication administration and patient response.

Subcutaneous injections

Sometimes the prescriber wants the medication to be absorbed more slowly than what occurs with an IM injection. In this case, the prescriber may order the SC route, which places the medication into fat under the skin. Because fat does not have as generous a blood supply as muscle and there are fewer nerve endings, patients rarely complain of pain at the site and it rarely bleeds after injection.

Because SC injections are fairly easy, many patients give themselves injections at home. As an allied health professional, you may need to teach a diabetic patient how to self-administer insulin. Sometimes health care professionals also give SC injections of heparin or vaccinations.

Commonly used areas for a subcutaneous injection include the fleshy part of the upper arm, the abdomen, and the thigh. If the patient is to receive regular injections (e.g., insulin), the sites must be rotated so the medication does not accumulate in one area (Fig. 7.27). In the office or clinic setting, you might choose the back of the upper arms (not the deltoid muscle) (see Fast Tip 7.8).

Box 7.15 explains how to administer an SC injection. Note that the needle is injected at a 45° angle. You do not need to draw back on the syringe plunger to check for blood return because there are few blood vessels in subcutaneous tissue.

Intradermal injections

The usual sites for ID injections are the forearms and back (Fig. 7.28). After preparing the site with an alcohol swab, the health care professional holds the skin taut and inserts the needle just under the

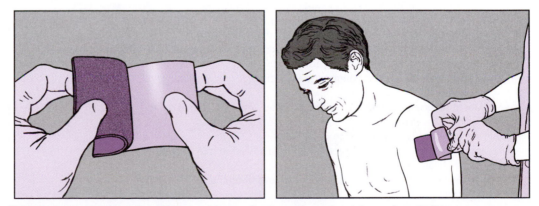

FIGURE 7.21. Remove the sticky backing on the transdermal patch, and apply it to an appropriate location on the body.

BOX 7.9   Transdermal Patch Administration

- Observe the six "rights" of medication administration.
- Read the order and medication container.
- Wash your hands.
- Compare order to medication container. Check expiration date.
- Put gloves on.
- Identify the patient and explain what you will be doing.
- Check medication container with order a third time.
- Apply the amount of ointment ordered to a patch template.
- Place patch on patient in area specified in order.
- Hold in place with tape.
- Assess patient.
- Remove gloves.
- Wash hands.
- Document dosage, site of placement, and patient response.

---

epidermis at a 10°–15° degree angle. Usually a short, high-gauge needle is used. ID injections are used for TB and allergy determination, so they need to be given right under the epidermis for easy evaluation.

Box 7.16 outlines how to perform an ID injection. Using a 10°–15° entry angle, be sure you gently push the needle just under the skin. Do not pull the plunger back for blood return. Instead, slowly inject the medication, forming a wheal. Gently remove the needle, and do not massage the site. If some of the medication leaks out, you will have to repeat the procedure.

CRITICAL THINKING

Can you think of a way to make it more pleasant for a child to receive an ID injection?

Table 7.3 summarizes the types of injections.

BOX 7.10   Vaginal Administration

- Observe the six "rights" of medication administration.
- Check order and medication container.
- Wash hands.
- Check order and medication container. Check expiration date.
- Identify patient and instruct patient on procedure. She must remove her underwear, so you need to be conscious of her need for modesty.
- Check order and medication container a third time.
- Put on gloves.
- Ask patient to assume a relaxed, supine position with legs spread apart.
- Drape patient for privacy.
- Remove suppository or foam from container.
- Use applicator (if needed) or fingers to insert medication into vagina.
- Remove applicator or fingers from vagina.
- Ask patient to close legs and remain still for several minutes.
- Assess patient.
- Remove gloves.
- Wash hands.
- Document medication administration and patient response.

BOX 7.11 Rectal Administration

This procedure can be used for a rectal suppository or an enema.
- Observe the six "rights" of medication administration.
- Compare order to medication container.
- Wash hands.
- Compare order to container a second time. Check expiration date.
- Identify the patient and explain what you will be doing.
- Compare order to container a third time.
- Have the patient remove underwear.
- Assist patient to left side.
- Place waterproof sheeting under patient.
- Drape patient for privacy.
- Put gloves on.
- Open suppository wrapping, or remove cover from enema bottle.
- Gently separate buttocks.
- Insert suppository with one finger into rectum, or insert tip of enema bottle and squeeze contents into the rectum.
- Remove finger or enema bottle from rectum.
- Assess patient.
- Ask patient to lie still for a few minutes.
- Clean patient and patient area.
- Remove gloves.
- Wash hands.
- Document medication administration and patient response.

INTRAVENOUS ADMINISTRATION

State and organization policies differ on which allied health professionals can start IV infusions, so you may not be asked to do this procedure. It is likely, however, that because so many patients are discharged from the hospital with IVs in place, and because so many are receiving infusion therapy over long periods of time, you may be asked to assess patients on IV therapy.

To ready the IV bag and tubing for administration, squeeze the drip chamber to begin the descent of fluid. Remove the cover from the end of the IV tubing and open the clamp. Prime the tubing by allowing some of the fluid to drip from the end of the IV tubing into a trash can. Clamp the IV tubing shut.

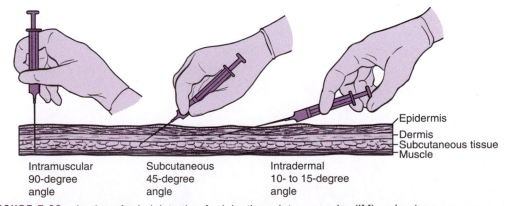

Intramuscular
90-degree
angle

Subcutaneous
45-degree
angle

Intradermal
10- to 15-degree
angle

Epidermis
Dermis
Subcutaneous tissue
Muscle

FIGURE 7.22. Angles of administration for injections: intramuscular (IM), subcutaneous (SC), and intradermal (ID).

BOX 7.12 Drawing Up Medication

- Observe the six "rights" of safe medication.
- Compare the order to the container.
- Wash hands.
- Calculate dosage correctly.
- Compare the order and the container a second time. Check expiration date.
- Select the correct equipment: syringe with correct needle length and gauge, disinfectant wipe, medication container, dressing, sharps container, and order.
- Identify the patient, and explain what you are going to do.
- Compare the order and container a third time.
- Remove cap from vial. If vial has been used before, wipe with a disinfectant wipe. If using an ampule, break it carefully. Use a piece of gauze to catch broken glass.
- Remove cover from needle by pulling straight off.
- If the drug is in an ampule, insert the needle into it and draw up the fluid into the syringe (see Fig. 7.5). Change the needle after drawing up the medication (see Fig. 7.5).
- If a vial is used, draw up an amount of air equal to the amount of fluid to be withdrawn. The air you inject will go above the medication and help to drive it downward. It will also break the vacuum that can exist in the vial. Insert the needle into the vial and inject the air (see Figure in this box).
- Turn the vial upside down, and remove the ordered amount of medication. If bubbles appear, tap the syringe with your fingernail or pull the plunger down farther and then push it back to the ordered calibration to push air above the medication and back into the vial.
- Leave needle in vial for support, and place vial back on surface.
- You are now ready to inject the medication into the patient.

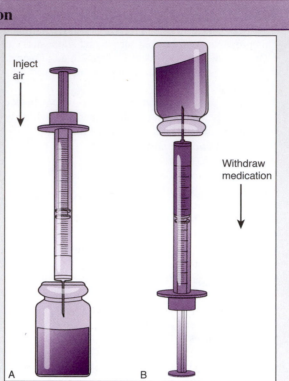

Inject air

Withdraw medication

A   B

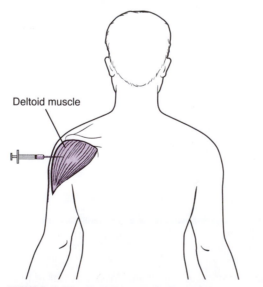

Deltoid muscle

FIGURE 7.23. Deltoid muscle insertion.

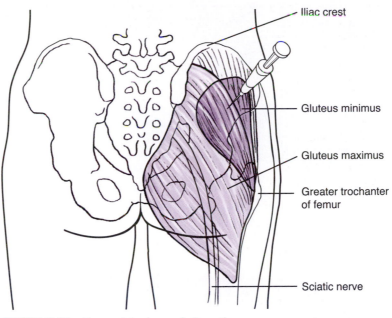

Iliac crest

Gluteus minimus

Gluteus maximus

Greater trochanter of femur

Sciatic nerve

FIGURE 7.24. Dorsogluteal muscle insertion.

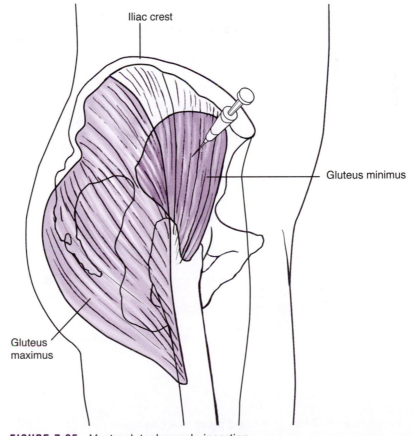

Iliac crest

Gluteus minimus

Gluteus maximus

FIGURE 7.25. Ventrogluteal muscle insertion.

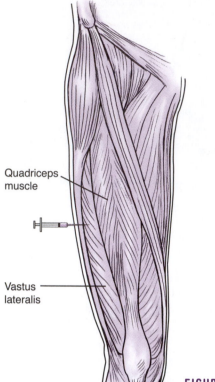

Quadriceps
muscle

Vastus
lateralis

FIGURE 7.26. Vastus lateralis insertion.

BOX 7.13   Administration of IM Injections

- Follow safety procedures described for oral medication.
- Assemble needed supplies (alcohol wipe, dressing, medication in syringe with needle)
- Identify patient and select site.
- Explain what you are going to do.
- Position patient comfortably.
- Put on gloves.
- Apply disinfectant wipe with circular motion to selected site.
- Allow to dry.
- Remove needle from vial.
- Hold skin taut.
- To reduce pain for the patient, use a dart-like motion to insert needle at a 90° angle completely to the hub.
- Release the skin.
- Check for blood return (accidental placement in a blood vessel) by pulling backward on plunger.
- If blood is noted, indicating that the needle is in a vein, remove the needle, and begin again with a new syringe and needle.
- If no blood is noted, gently and slowly inject all the medication.
- Remove needle and syringe quickly.
- Massage site if organization's policy suggests massage, or ask the patient to move the muscle.
- Dispose of needle and syringe. Do not recap.
- Assess patient.
- Cover wound if bleeding.
- Remove gloves.
- Wash hands.
- Document medication administration and patient response.

BOX 7.14 Z-Track Administration

- Before inserting needle, pull skin laterally $1\frac{1}{2}$ inches away from injection site (Figure, A).
- Insert needle at 90° angle, as for all IM injections.
- Pull plunger back to be sure you are not in a blood vessel.
- Gently inject medication.

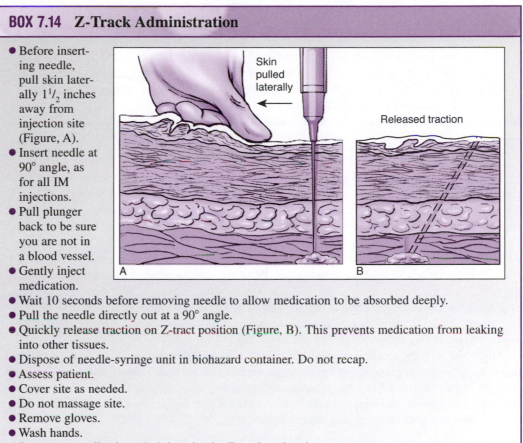

- Wait 10 seconds before removing needle to allow medication to be absorbed deeply.
- Pull the needle directly out at a 90° angle.
- Quickly release traction on Z-tract position (Figure, B). This prevents medication from leaking into other tissues.
- Dispose of needle-syringe unit in biohazard container. Do not recap.
- Assess patient.
- Cover site as needed.
- Do not massage site.
- Remove gloves.
- Wash hands.
- Document medication administration by Z-track and patient response.

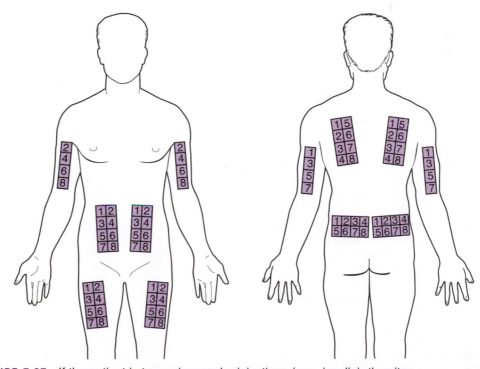

FIGURE 7.27. If the patient is to receive regular injections (e.g., insulin), the sites must be rotated.

> ◯ *Fast Tip 7.8* Rotating Sites for Regular SC Injections
>
> Be specific when you instruct the patient to rotate sites. For example, you could draw a chart: Sunday—above the navel; Monday—right thigh; Tuesday—below the navel; Wednesday—left thigh; Thursday—right side of navel; Friday—left side of navel; Saturday—back of left arm.

Generally, the best site for IV insertion is at the distal end of an arm. If a site infiltrates, the health care professional is then still able to use a more proximal site for reinserting the IV needle. Patient comfort should also be considered. Sites that bend, such as the elbow and wrist, are usually not good sites for insertion. The nondominant arm is most often used. Site selection depends on how long the IV line is expected to be in place and how mobile the patient needs to be.

To begin IV therapy, the health care worker assembles the necessary equipment, including a bag or bottle of the medication solution ordered, IV tubing, and a needle/cannula set to insert into the vein.

Placing the IV needle and cannula into the patient is similar to drawing blood, and only an indwelling cannula is left in the patient when the needle is removed (Box 7.17). Never insert an IV unless you are legally authorized to do so (see Fast Tip 7.9).

Allied health professionals are sometimes allowed to stop IV therapy. To do so, put on gloves and then loosen the securing tape. Gently pull out the needle or catheter and properly dispose of it. Apply pressure to the site with a 2 × 2 gauze pad until the bleeding stops. Be sure to assess the patient and document the removal, including the time and date. Follow your organization's policy for assessing the site, changing sites, flushing, and changing tubing.

Flushing Indwelling Devices

Health care professionals may be asked to flush an indwelling IV device that is not attached to a running IV line. Follow the organization's policy by flushing with heparin or normal saline as ordered and at the times specified. Clean the port with an antiseptic wipe, and enter the port with the needle and syringe drawn up with the ordered flush solution. If resistance is felt within the vein or the patient complains of a burning pain, stop and check whether the tip of the catheter is still in the vein. Pull back on the plunger, and check for blood return. If you see blood, remove the port device and notify a supervisor. If you don't see blood, gently flush again. Even if you are not allowed to flush a line, you should assess the patient with an indwelling port for signs and symptoms of infiltration, infection, and other problems.

BOX 7.15 Administration of SC Injections

- Grasp skin.
- Insert needle at a 45° angle with dart-like motion.
- It is not necessary to pull back for blood return because there are few blood vessels in fat.
- Slowly inject the medication.
- Quickly remove needle.
- Do not massage the site.
- Discard needle and syringe in a sharp biohazard container. Do not recap.
- Assess patient.
- Cover site if needed.
- Remove gloves.
- Wash hands.
- Document medication administration and patient response.

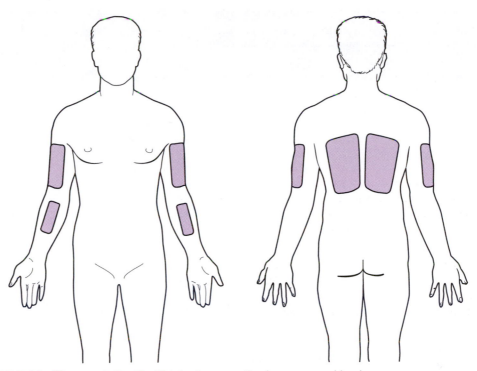

FIGURE 7.28. The usual sites for ID injections are the forearms and back.

Complications of IV Therapy

As an allied health professional, you must observe the IV site on a regular basis. If you see redness and swelling, feel unusual warmth at the site, hear the patient complain of tenderness or pain, or note that the site feels like a firm rope or that the cannula is no longer in a vein, notify your supervisor immediately. The supervisor may ask you to stop the IV quickly, although do not remove the IV line without permission. Specific complications include the following.

Thrombus (blood clot) or *phlebitis* (vein inflammation) can result from extremes in solution pH, needle or catheter trauma, particulate material, irritating drugs, or selecting a vein too small for the volume of solution infused. Check the vein for signs of inflammation (e.g., redness, swelling, warm to the touch) or pain.

BOX 7.16 Administration of ID Medications

- Pull the skin taut.
- Insert the needle gently at a 10°–15° angle, bevel up, for about $1/4$ inch. Do not aspirate, because it would traumatize tissue.
- Slowly inject the medication to produce a wheal (slight elevation under the skin).
- Remove needle steadily and gently.
- Dispose of needle and syringe in a sharps container. Do not recap.
- Do not massage.
- Assess patient.
- Cover site if needed.
- Remove gloves.
- Wash hands.
- Observe patient for reaction for 15 minutes, because allergic reactions are more likely with ID wheals than with other types of drug administration.
- Document medication administration and patient response.

TABLE 7.3   Parenteral Injections

TYPE	DEPTH	INJECTION VOLUME	USUAL NEEDLE SIZE	ANGLE
IM (deltoid)	Muscle	0.5–1 mL (maximum 2 mL)	23–25 gauge, $^5/_8$–1 inch	90°
IM (ventrogluteal)	Muscle	1–4 mL (maximum 5 mL)	18–23 gauge, $1^1/_4$–3 inches	Toward the iliac crest
IM (vastus lateralis in adult)	Muscle	1 mL (maximum 5 mL)	20–23 gauge, $1^1/_4$–$1^1/_2$ inches	90°
IM (vastus lateralis in child)	Muscle	0.5–1 mL (maximum 1 mL in infants and 2 mL in children)	22–25 gauge, $^1/_8$ inch	45°
IM (dorsogluteal)	Muscle	1–4 mL (maximum 5 mL)	18–23 gauge, $1^1/_4$–3 inches	90°
SC (various locations)	Subcutaneous tissue	Up to 1 mL	25–31 gauge	45°
ID (various locations)	Under the epidermis	Up to 1 mL, usually smaller	25–31 gauge	10°–15°

Note: This information addresses the typical patient. Make adjustments based on individual patient assessment.

CHECK UP

For all injections, it is important to document the name of the medication, dosage, site, and patient response. Practice documenting by completing the following exercises.

1. Document that you gave 1 mL of Depo-Provera in the left deltoid of a patient.

2. Document that you gave 0.1 mL of tuberculin in the right anterior forearm of a patient.

3. Document that you gave 7 units of insulin 1 inch to the right of the umbilicus.

4. How would you document that you observed a patient after giving an ID injection?

5. If that patient experienced a rash after a TB test, how would you document it?

BOX 7.17 Insertion of IV

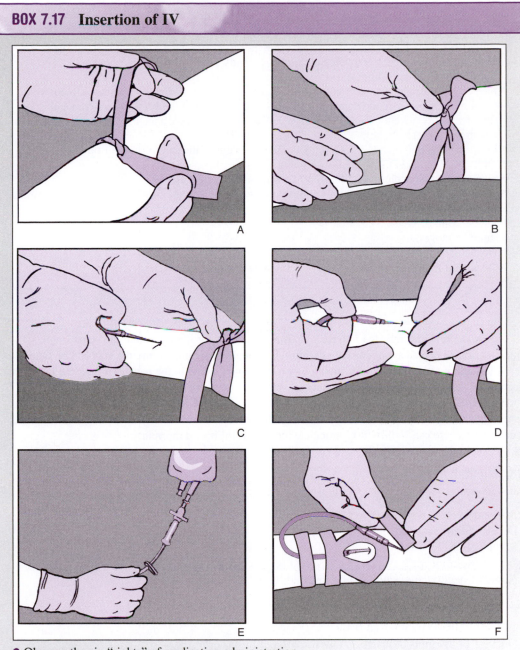

- Observe the six "rights" of medication administration.
- Assemble needed supplies (constricting band, needle/catheter or port, IV bag and tubing, disinfectant swab).
- Compare order to medication bag.
- Wash hands.
- Compare order to medication bag and check expiration date.
- Identify patient and explain what you will do.
- Compare order to medication bag a third time.
- Assess appropriate site.
- Put gloves on.
- Place constricting band (tourniquet) 6–8 inches proximal to site to be used (Figure, A).
- Ask patient to close fist 4–6 times. If necessary, gently tap the vein.
- Cleanse site with circular motion, using disinfecting swab, either povidone-iodine or alcohol (Figure, B).

(box continued on page 126)

BOX 7.17 Insertion of IV (continued)

- Administer a local anesthetic if ordered. Give the anesthetic ID at a 30° angle. Draw back to be sure that you are not in a vein, and massage gently after the injection.
- Stabilize vein by stretching skin 1 inch from the insertion site.
- Insert IV needle/catheter with bevel upward at a 30°–45° angle directly into the selected vein (or slightly adjacent to the vein and slip in through the side of the vein), then advance the catheter and remove the needle (Figure, C). *Note:* Advance the catheter (without a needle) into a vein at a 10°–15° angle.
- Connect IV tubing that has been primed (fluid runs out of the end to flush air out) (Figure, D).
- Turn on IV infusion using the flow regulator or slide clamp (Figure, E).
- Secure site with occlusive, waterproof dressing and tape (Figure, F).
- Some organizations require certain information be written on the dressing, such as your initials and the date and time.
- Assess patient.
- Remove gloves.
- Wash hands.
- Document medication administration and patient response.

Air emboli (bubbles released into the bloodstream) can occur if air gets into the vein. Small amounts of air in veins are not usually harmful, but rapidly injecting air into the vein can be fatal. Be careful to purge all air from the IV tubing before securing the line in the patient. Assess the patient's respiratory status and report and document any changes.

Particulate material (small particles) can cause vein irritation. Small pieces of glass can chip away from the vial or bottle. For this reason most IV tubing contains a final filter in the line. Swelling and redness at the site can signify that particulate matter has infiltrated the vein.

Documentation of IV Therapy

After inserting an IV, the following information needs to be documented.

- Size and type of device
- Date and time inserted
- Site location
- Type of solution
- Name of health care provider who inserted the IV or hung an IV bag
- Any additives added to the bag
- Flow rate
- Type of infusion pump used
- Number of attempts at insertion (successful and unsuccessful)
- Patient response (including the fact that the patient was observed for 15 minutes)
- Complications, if any, and your interventions
- Patient teaching

○ *Fast Tip 7.9* Tourniquets

Wrapping a constricting band (tourniquet) around the arm helps the vein become more visible. The tourniquet should never be placed on the patient for more than 2 minutes. If it takes longer to find a good site, release the tourniquet and begin elsewhere. Check your organization's policy, but usually you should call for assistance if you cannot insert the IV after three attempts.

A CLOSER LOOK: Advantages and Disadvantages of IV Therapy

Advantages

• Provides several options for medication and fluid delivery: direct injection or continuous or intermittent infusion.
• Avoids multiple injections for patients.
• An indwelling (in the vein) catheter with tubing or a port can be used. Ports are more comfortable for patients.

Disadvantages

• Incompatibility of medications. The health care provider should check compatibility before combining any drugs in an IV line.
• Risk of complications, such as infiltration and infection.
• Costs more than other types of parenteral administration.
• Clots can form in an IV catheter or port, making it useless.

After assessing an existing IV site, document:

• Date and time
• Condition of site
• Site care provided
• Dressing change
• Site change
• Tubing and solution change
• Patient teaching

SUMMARY

Safe medication administration requires familiarity with the routes and techniques of preparing and administering drugs. Always observe the six "rights" of safe medication administration (right patient, right drug, right dose, right time, right route, right documentation) and document the patient's response. Become familiar with which medications and routes you are allowed to administer according to your state's and organization's policies.

Activities

To make sure that you have learned the key points covered in this chapter, complete the following activities.

True or False

Write *true* if the statement is true. Beside the false statements, write *false* and correct the statement to make it true.

1. Signs and symptoms of infection are redness, heat, swelling, and pain. _____

2. IV tubing is clamped off with a filter. _____

3. IM injections are given at a 90° angle. _____

4. A mortar is a club used to pulverize drugs. _____

5. An ampule is usually broken open to remove the solution. _____

6. Vials come only in single-dose units. _____

7. A 27-gauge needle is wider than a 20-gauge needle. _____

8. IM injections usually use $3/8$ inch needles. _____

9. Drug viscosity determines needle length. _____

10. Tuberculin syringes are used to give insulin. _____

11. A U-100 insulin syringe holds 200 mL. _____

12. Cartridge plunger units are disposed of with the cartridge. _____

13. Otic medications go in the eye. _____

14. Always wash an ear dropper after use with soap and water. _____

15. Place used needles in biohazard sharps containers after use. _____

Multiple Choice

Choose the best answer for each question.

1. By which route is insulin usually given?
   a. ID
   b. SC
   c. IM
   d. Z-track

2. At which angle is a TB test given?
   a. 10°–15°
   b. 45°
   c. 90°
   d. 100°

3. Ophthalmic medications are given in the:
   a. Buttock
   b. Eye
   c. Ear
   d. Arm

4. Infants should get IM injections in which muscle?
   a. Deltoid
   b. Ventrogluteal
   c. Vastus lateralis
   d. Dorsogluteal

5. Which of the following is *not* true about Z-track injections?
   a. Enter the needle at a 90° angle.
   b. Inject medication slowly and completely.
   c. Release skin before removing needle.
   d. Do not massage site after injecting.

Short Answer Questions

Answer these questions on a separate sheet.
State which syringe would be used for the following procedures.

1. Insulin
2. Allergy testing
3. Flu shots
4. TB testing
5. IM injections

What length needles would you use for each of these procedures?

1. Insulin
2. Allergy testing
3. Flu shots
4. TB testing
5. IM injections

Application Exercises

Respond to the following scenarios on a separate sheet.

1. The physician orders you to give ID, IM, and SC injections. **Which supplies would you assemble (remember gauge and needle length) for each type?**
   a. ID
   b. IM
   c. SC

2. A patient is to receive an IV with lactated Ringer's solution. You have been asked to obtain the necessary supplies for a registered nurse to insert it. **What do you obtain?**
3. Dr. Mangrum asks you to go to the drug cabinet and get $D_{2.5}W/0.45$ NSS. **What is it?**
4. You are monitoring a patient receiving a blood transfusion who suddenly complains of chills and begins to have trouble breathing. **What do you do?**
5. You break an ampule and get glass in your finger. **What do you do? What might you have done to prevent this accident?**

Virtual Field Trips

1. Go to http://www.osha.gov and research the Occupational Safety and Health Administration regulation for needle safety.
2. Visit http://www.mooremedical.com and investigate the various safety devices offered for needles.
3. Go to http://www.pssd.com and find the price of IV sets.
4. Visit http://www.edruginfo.com or a similar site and print the instructions for IM and SC injections.
5. Go to http://www.ivprehospital.com or a similar site and print flash cards on IV therapy.

Calculations

Basic Review of Mathematics

*T*he next three chapters work slowly through dosage calculations. If you fear mathematics and do not work the problems included in the chapters, you will continue to struggle with mathematical concepts. The more you read these chapters and the more problems you work, the easier it will be to understand what you need to know to calculate dosages safely. If you enjoy mathematics, then get ready for some fun. This chapter reviews key mathematical concepts you must understand to calculate drug doses.

OBJECTIVES

At the end of this chapter, the student will be able to:

- Define all key terms.
- Discuss numerical relationships.
- Perform calculations involving whole numbers.
- Calculate problems using fractions.
- Find the lowest common denominator.
- Perform calculations involving decimals.
- Calculate percents, ratios, and proportions.
- Solve problems for an unknown quantity.

KEY TERMS

Addition	Divisor	Invert
Decimal	Equivalent	Lowest common
Denominator	Extremes	denominator
Dividend	Fraction	Means
Division	Improper	Mixed

Multiplication	Proper	Subtraction
Numerator	Proportion	Sum
Percent	Quotient	Whole numbers
Prime	Ratio	

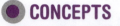 CONCEPTS

It is easier to learn math concepts by breaking them down: whole numbers, fractions, decimals, percentages, and ratios.

Whole Numbers

Sometimes dosage calculations involve *whole numbers* (not fractions, decimals, or percentages). Whole numbers have no subdivisions to them. They are simply a whole amount of an entity (1, 2, 3. . .). Many times a situation requires that you add, subtract, multiply, or divide whole numbers.

Addition calculations

Frank Lachance is on a fluid restriction of 30 oz. To calculate what he has consumed, simply add the amounts together.

He drinks:

A 12-oz Mountain Dew	12 oz
An 8-oz glass of water	8 oz
And 6 oz of a 12-oz Dr. Pepper	6 oz
Total	26 oz

Did he exceed his fluid restriction? His total fluids were 26 oz, which is less than ($<$) 30 oz, so the answer is no.

Here is one for you to try. Cory Gagne is on a 1800-calorie diet. He eats cereal with one-half cup of milk (150 calories) for breakfast and an apple (90 calories), a soft drink (170 calories), and a cupcake (250 calories) for lunch. How much has he consumed so far today?

$$
\begin{array}{r}
150 \\
90 \\
170 \\
+\ 250 \\
\hline
\end{array}
$$

Write total here ☐

The answer is 660. Because 660 is less than 1800, he has not exceeded his restriction. However, Cory needs to look at the quality of his food as well as the quantity.

CHECK UP

Now, you try a few addition problems.

250	3	1000	5	150
+150	+ 4	+ 480	+ 6	+25

Subtraction calculations

In the above example of calories, Cory consumed (ate and drank) 660 calories. If he is on a 1800-calorie restriction, how many calories can he consume the rest of the day? To find out, you need to subtract the 660 he has already consumed from the maximum of 1800.

$$
\begin{array}{r}
1800 \\
-660 \\
\hline
1140
\end{array}
$$

In this case, you answered the question, "What number is left when I subtract this amount from the larger amount?" Other times, you can use subtraction to answer another question, "Which number needs to be added to this number to get the larger one?"

$$660 + ? = 1800$$
$$1800 - 660 = 1140$$

CHECK UP

Now, you try a few subtraction problems.

250	500	21	35	90
− 175	− 300	− 7	− 8	− 60

Multiplication calculations

Multiplication is simply repeated addition.

3×4	is	$4 + 4 + 4$ (adding 4 three times)
5×6	is	$6 + 6 + 6 + 6 + 6$ (adding 6 five times)

If Sally Monnes takes 3 pills per day for 7 days, how many does she need to take in a week?

Sunday		Monday		Tuesday		Wednesday		Thursday		Friday		Saturday
3	+	3	+	3	+	3	+	3	+	3	+	3

Or $7 \times 3 = 21$

Is it not easier to multiply 3×7 to get 21 than to add? It usually is. However, you can always use addition to check your multiplication: $3 + 3 + 3 + 3 + 3 + 3 + 3 = 21$. Table 8.1 provides more examples of when multiplication is used.

CHECK UP

Try a few multiplication calculations.

4	2	3	30	100
× 10	× 90	× 7	× 7	× 3

Division calculations

Division is multiplication in reverse. You learned in an earlier example that Corey is allowed 1140 calories for the rest of his day. How can we split this amount throughout his day more evenly? A possible solution is to divide the remaining calories into two meals.

$$1140 \div 2 = 570 \text{ calories during each of the two meals}$$

TABLE 8.1 Examples of the Practical Use of Multiplication

If Alex Boles drinks six 12-oz sodas per day, how much does he consume in 1 week?
$$6 \times 7 = ? \text{ sodas per week}$$
$$6 \times 7 = 42 \text{ sodas per week}$$

If each soda is 12 oz, how many ounces of soda does he consume in 1 week?
$$42 \text{ sodas} \times 12 \text{ oz each} = 504 \text{ oz}$$

If each soda has 150 calories, how many calories does he consume from soda in 1 week?
$$42 \text{ sodas} \times 150 \text{ calories} = 6300 \text{ calories from soda per week}$$

CHECK UP

Here are a few division calculations for you to try.

500	6	18	21	90
÷250	÷3	÷ 6	÷ 7	÷10

Or you could divide by 2.5 and allow 500 calories at each meal and two 70-calorie snacks at bedtime and when he comes home from school.

Fractions

A fraction is simply part of a whole. It is important to understand fractions because sometimes a dose may not be a whole number.

Let us say that you have a whole pie and want to give some to your friends. You can divide the pie in many ways to get smaller pieces (Fig. 8.1). For example, you can divide the pie into three pieces or four pieces; a slice of pie from the three-piece division is larger than a slice of pie from the four-piece division. In other words:

$$\frac{1}{3} \text{ is greater than } \frac{1}{4}$$
$$\frac{1}{4} \text{ is smaller than } \frac{1}{3}$$

The number on the top of the fraction is called the *numerator.* It is part of the whole being divided. The *denominator* is the number on the bottom. It represents the total number of equal parts in the problem.

If the numerator is smaller than the denominator, it is called a *proper* fraction (Fig. 8.2). In the pie example, you would have some pie left over after some of the numerator was carved out. If the pie is divided into 4 pieces and each of your 3 friends gets a piece, that leaves $\frac{1}{4}$ for you. That is proper, or polite.

CRITICAL THINKING

What happens to the pie slices when a numerator becomes larger? A denominator becomes larger? If you have trouble remembering this concept, ask yourself, what would happen if you and your siblings were inheriting some money? The more brothers and sisters you have, the less your share would be.

As the numerator gets larger, the number itself is larger because there are more pieces available. As the denominator gets larger, however, the amount gets smaller because you are dividing the pie into smaller sections.

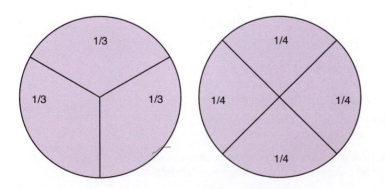

FIGURE 8.1. Slices of a pie (represented as this circle) divided into three sections are larger than one divided into four sections: $\frac{1}{3}$ is larger than $\frac{1}{4}$.

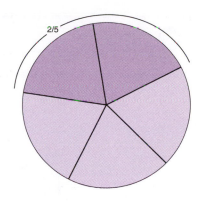

FIGURE 8.2. Proper fraction. This figure shows the proper fraction $2/5$. It is a proper fraction because the numerator (top number) is smaller than the denominator (bottom number).

An *improper* fraction is against etiquette. For example, you divide a pie into four pieces but have five friends. You will need to find another pie, be "improper," or cut smaller pieces (Fig. 8.3). You can write $5/4$ or $1\frac{1}{4}$. It means the same thing because $5/4 = 4/4$ (or 1) $+ 1/4$.

🔵 CHECK UP

Circle the fraction with the largest value in each listing. Then, using the same numbers, underline the lowest value in each listing.

- 4/25, 5/25, 10/25
- 1/300, 1/200, 1/100
- 5/3, 2/3, 4/3
- 1/75, 1/100, 1/125
- 4/8, 1/8, 2/8

Circle the fraction with the lowest value and underline the highest.

- 1/10, 1/8, 1/6
- 3/6, 2/6, 5/6
- 1/25, 1/75, 1/50
- 2/16, 1/16, 4/16
- 2/12, 1/12, 6/12

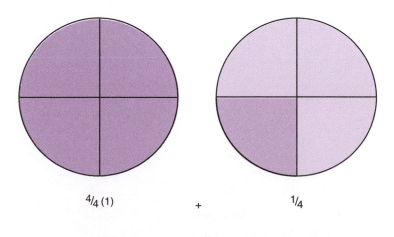

$$4/4 \ (1) \qquad + \qquad 1/4$$

$$= 5/4 \text{ or } 1\tfrac{1}{4}$$

FIGURE 8.3. Improper fraction. If you divide a pie into four pieces but have five friends, you need to find another pie, be "improper," or cut smaller pieces. This shows the improper fraction of 5/4. You can also write $1\frac{1}{4}$ because $5/4 = 4/4$ (or 1) $+ 1/4$.

✏️ CHECK UP

1. Shade the circles to represent the improper fraction 16/5.

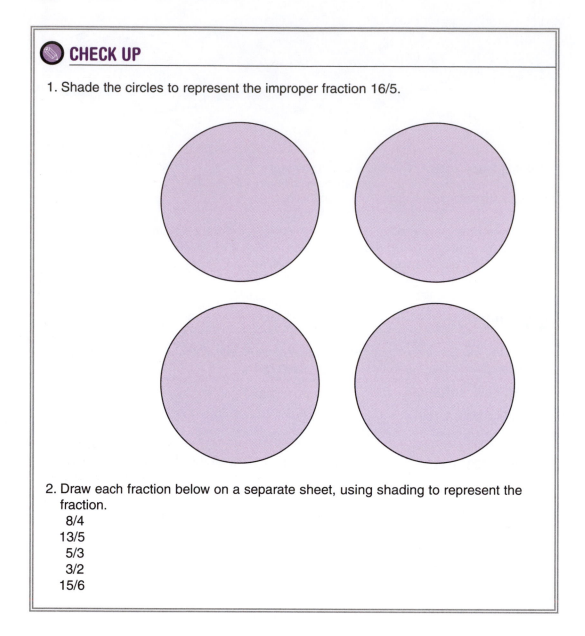

2. Draw each fraction below on a separate sheet, using shading to represent the fraction.
   8/4
   13/5
   5/3
   3/2
   15/6

Figure 8.4 lets you practice creating fractions.

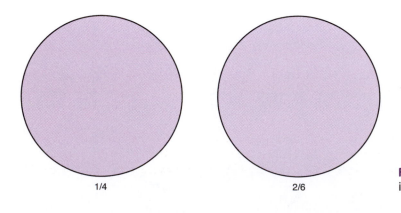

1/4   2/6

FIGURE 8.4. In each of the circles, divide the pie into the denominator and shade the numerator.

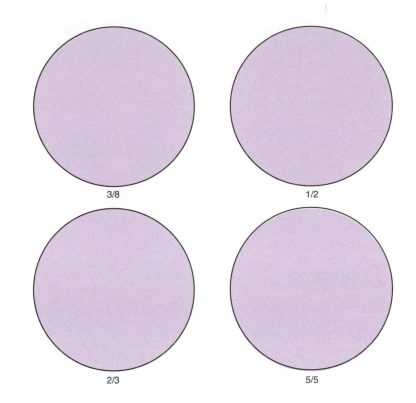

FIGURE 8.4. (continued)

Least common denominators

A common denominator is a number that is a common multiple of two (or more) denominators. Finding the least number into which both denominators can be divided to keep the fraction small makes it easier to work with. To find the least common denominator (LCD) of two or more fractions:

• List the multiples of each denominator.
• Compare the lists. Any numbers that appear on all lists are common denominators.
• The smallest number that appears on all the lists is the LCD.

Example: 1/9 + 1/6

Write the multiples of each number:

$$
\begin{array}{ccc}
9 & \rightarrow & 9\ldots\mathbf{18}\ldots27\ldots36 \\
6 & \rightarrow & 6\ldots12\ldots\mathbf{18}\ldots24\ldots36
\end{array}
$$

Once you have the LCD, it becomes the denominator of each fraction. You multiply the numerator by the number that you need to multiply the denominator by to get the least common denominator. For the fraction with the denominator of 9

$$9 \times \mathbf{2} = 18$$

So you would multiply the numerator 1 by 2 and place it over 18. For the fraction with the denominator of 6, you would multiply by 3 to get to 18, so you would multiply the 1 in the numerator by 3 and place it over 18. Thus, 1/9 + 1/6 = 2/18 + 3/18 = 5/18. Although 36 appears on both lists, 18 is the least (lowest) common denominator.

Equivalent is a fancy word for equal. When doing dosage calculations, it is good to use equivalents. For example, you may want to give a fluid dose equivalent to the powder dose that a prescriber orders, using what is written on a label as a standard. Equivalencies are more fully explained in Chapter 10.

If a numerator and denominator are multiplied by the same number, an equivalent fraction is made. Multiplying the entire fraction by the same number over itself is like multiplying by 1.

Example:

$$\frac{1}{3} \times \frac{2}{2} = \frac{2}{6}$$

$$\frac{1}{3} \times \frac{3}{3} = \frac{3}{9}$$

$$\frac{1}{3} \times \frac{4}{4} = \frac{4}{12}$$

$$\frac{1}{3} \times \frac{5}{5} = \frac{5}{15}$$

All are 1/3.

✎ CHECK UP

Find the LCD, then work out the problem on a separate sheet.

• 1/15 + 1/45 = _____

• 1/3 + 3/8 = _____

• 5/12 + 1/10 = _____

• 1/4 + 1/5 = _____

• 3/8 + 1/6 = _____

• 4/5 + 5/12 = _____

• 5/6 + 3/5 = _____

• 1/2 + 1/19 = _____

• 3/25 + 4/75 = _____

• 1/4 + 3/16 = _____

✎ CHECK UP

Examine the fraction 3/4.

1. What are the total equal parts in one whole? _____

2. What is the size of each part? _____

3. How many parts are being talked about? _____

4. The numerator is: _____

5. The denominator is: _____

6. Give three fractions equivalent to 3/4.

(box continued on page 139)

Based on what you have learned, write an equivalent for each of the following:

• 5/25 = _____

• 3/4 = _____

• 160/40 = _____

• 25/75 = _____

• 5/6 = _____

Mixed numbers and improper fractions

Sometimes you must convert a *mixed number*, which is a whole number plus a fraction, into an improper fraction. To do this:

• Multiply the denominator by the whole number.
• Add the result from the first step to the numerator.
• Keep the denominator.

$$Example: 5\tfrac{1}{2}$$
$$2 \times 5 = 10$$
$$10 + 1 = 11/2$$

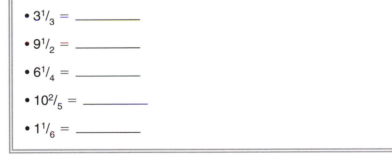

CHECK UP

Convert these mixed numbers into improper fractions.

• $3\tfrac{1}{3}$ = _____

• $9\tfrac{1}{2}$ = _____

• $6\tfrac{1}{4}$ = _____

• $10\tfrac{2}{5}$ = _____

• $1\tfrac{1}{6}$ = _____

CRITICAL THINKING

Sometimes we need to teach the patient how to break certain pills. For example, if Haley Watkins takes $1\tfrac{1}{2}$ pills per dose, how long will 30 pills last?

On the other hand, sometimes you need to convert improper fractions to mixed numbers. The process for this is:

• Divide the numerator by the denominator.
• The remainder becomes the numerator.
• The denominator stays the same.

$$Example: 29/5 =$$
$$29 \div 5 = 5 \text{ remainder } 4$$
$$29/5 = 5\tfrac{4}{5}$$

CHECK UP

Convert these improper fractions to mixed numbers.

• 28/5 = _____

• 42/5 = _____

• 30/7 = _____

• 52/10 = _____

• 7/6 = _____

? CRITICAL THINKING

If you give ⅓ tablespoon of a medication four times daily, how much of the medication do you need per day?

Reducing to lowest terms

Sometimes you start with numbers that are large. It is easier to work with smaller numbers, so you should reduce the numbers to the lowest terms.

To reduce a large fraction:

• Determine the largest common divisor (the number by which a dividend is divided) of the two numbers.
• Divide the numerator and denominator by this number to reduce to lowest terms.

Example: 6/10 is 6/10 ÷ 2/2 = 3/5

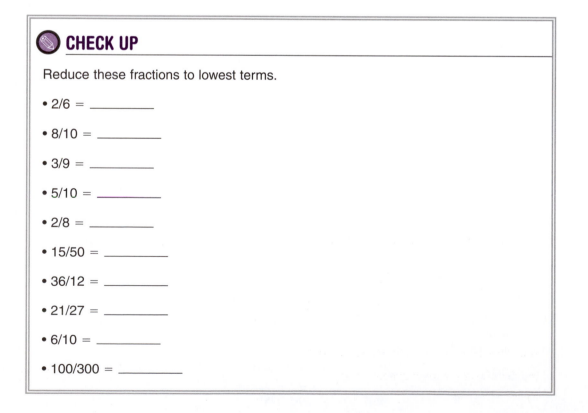 **CHECK UP**

Reduce these fractions to lowest terms.

• 2/6 = _____

• 8/10 = _____

• 3/9 = _____

• 5/10 = _____

• 2/8 = _____

• 15/50 = _____

• 36/12 = _____

• 21/27 = _____

• 6/10 = _____

• 100/300 = _____

Adding fractions

Adding fractions is easy when they have the same denominator.

- Add the numerators.
- Place the *sum* (what you get when you add) over the denominator.
- Reduce to lowest terms.

$$\textit{Example:} \quad \frac{1}{4} + \frac{2}{4} = \frac{3}{4}$$

To add fractions with different denominators:

- Change fractions to an equal fraction with the least common denominator:
- Add the numerators.
- Place the sum over the denominator.
- Reduce to lowest terms.

$$\textit{Example:} \quad \frac{1}{3} + \frac{1}{4} = \frac{4}{12} + \frac{3}{12} = \frac{7}{12}$$

$$\textit{Example:} \quad \frac{1}{4} + \frac{1}{5} = \frac{5}{20} + \frac{4}{20} = \frac{9}{20}$$

CHECK UP

Add these fractions.

- 1/2 + 1/3 = _____
- 1/10 + 2/5 = _____
- 5/8 + 3/7 = _____
- 1/4 + 1/6 = _____
- 1/9 + 2/3 = _____

Subtracting fractions

To subtract fractions with the same denominators:

- Subtract the numerator.
- Preserve the same denominator.
- Reduce if necessary.

$$\textit{Example:} \quad \frac{5}{6} - \frac{1}{6} = \frac{4}{6} = \frac{2}{3}$$

If the denominators are different, you must:

- Find the lowest common denominator.
- Change to equivalent fractions.

- Subtract the numerators.
- Place the sum over a common denominator.
- Reduce if necessary.

$$\textit{Examples}: \quad \frac{12}{5} - \frac{1}{2}$$

$$\frac{12}{5} \times \frac{2}{2} = \frac{24}{10}$$

$$\frac{1}{2} \times \frac{5}{5} = \frac{5}{10}$$

$$\frac{24}{10} - \frac{5}{10} = \frac{19}{10}$$

✏ CHECK UP

Subtract these fractions.

- 2/3 − 1/3 = _____

- 5/6 − 5/12 = _____

- 250/500 − 50/500 = _____

- 10/6 − 2/3 = _____

- 15 − 7¹/₂ = _____

Multiplying fractions

Multiplying fractions is also easy. You do not have to worry about common denominators. Simply:

- Multiply the numerators.
- Multiply the denominators.
- Reduce if necessary.

$$\frac{2}{5} \times \frac{3}{4} = \frac{2 \times 3}{5 \times 4} = \frac{6}{20} = \frac{3}{10}$$

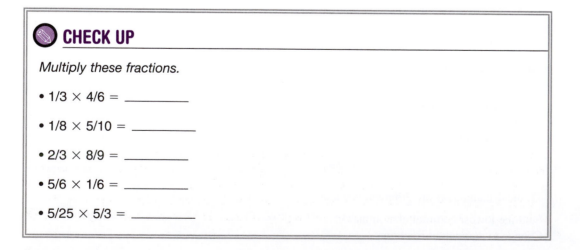

✏ CHECK UP

Multiply these fractions.

- 1/3 × 4/6 = _____

- 1/8 × 5/10 = _____

- 2/3 × 8/9 = _____

- 5/6 × 1/6 = _____

- 5/25 × 5/3 = _____

Dividing fractions

Remember that division is multiplication in reverse. When you multiply 1/5 × 2/3, you get 2/15.

Suppose you divide 2/15 by 1/5? You should get 2/3.

To reverse multiplication, *invert* the fraction you are dividing by (flip the numerator and denominator over) and change the process to multiplication instead of division.

$$2/15 \div 1/5 \rightarrow 2/15 \times 5/1 = 10/15 = 2/3$$

So to divide, simply:

• Invert the second fraction.
• Multiply the two fractions.
• Reduce if needed.

🖉 CHECK UP

Divide these fractions.

• 4/6 ÷ 1/2 = _____

• 15/30 ÷ 5 = _____

• 2/3 ÷ 3/2 = _____

• 6/2 ÷ 3/4 = _____

• 2/3 ÷ 6/8 = _____

Decimals

A *decimal* is similar to a fraction, but it is a fraction with 10, 100, 1000, and so on in the denominator. Instead of writing it as a fraction, you can use a decimal point. It is not unusual for drug doses to contain decimal points, so it is important to understand decimals and how they work. Figure 8.5 shows how to identify units in a number that has a decimal.

Rounding decimals

Tablets are not usually dispensed in parts unless they are specifically scored (cut) to do so. Capsules cannot be broken apart and separated evenly. Thus, you would usually round up or down if a dosage calculation does not produce a whole number. With fluids, you can give an exact decimal (e.g., 1.3 mL), but you may need to round up or down between 1.3 and 1.4 if the decimal is between those marks on the syringe or a measuring cup.

If a tablet is not scored, and you must round the amount off:

For 0.01 to 1.49 → give 1 tablet
For 1.50 to 1.99 → give 2 tablets

For dosage calculations, it is rarely necessary to go past the hundredths place.

Larger/smaller

You must understand whether a decimal is larger or smaller to check your dosage calculations. When decimal numbers contain whole numbers, the whole numbers must be compared to determine which is larger. For example, 5.8 is larger than 2.9, and 7.37 is larger than 6.39.

If the whole numbers are the same or zero and the numbers in the tenths place are the same, the decimal with the higher number in the hundredths place is larger. For example, 0.66 is larger than 0.64, and 2.17 is larger than 2.15.

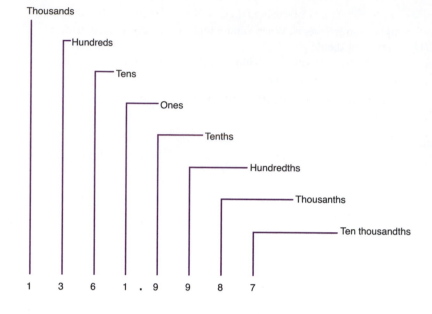

FIGURE 8.5. Decimal system. The decimal system is based on units of 10. Each numerical place in the number 1361.9987 has a specific unit name. Note that the first number in front of a decimal point is a whole number, in this case 1. The next numbers are based on units of 10 (tens, hundreds, thousands). The numbers behind the decimal point are also based on 10, but because they are less than a whole number the unit names are tenths, hundredths, thousandths, ten thousandths, and so on.

✏ CHECK UP

If you had a scored tablet, what would you give for each of the following dosages?

• 1.1 = _____

• 1.5 = _____

• 1.0 = _____

• 2.1 = _____

• 2.49 = _____

If you had an unscored tablet, what would you give?

• 1.1 = _____

• 1.5 = _____

• 1.9 = _____

• 2.1 = _____

• 2.59 = _____

The addition of zeros to the right of the end of a decimal does not alter its value, so they are usually deleted. The zero to the left of the decimal point, however, is very important; it shows that the dosage is very small.

CRITICAL THINKING

Why is it important when writing a prescription to write the leading "0" (e.g., 0.25 instead of .25)?

CHECK UP

Circle the larger number, if there is one.

• 0.25 or 0.52

• 0.24 or 0.355

• 0.322 or 0.321

• 0.5 or 0.05

• 4.4 or 4.4

Adding decimals

Adding decimals is easy. Just line up the decimal points and add each column—carrying over a number, as necessary.

$$
\begin{array}{r}
1.25 \\
+ \ 2.56 \\
\hline
3.81
\end{array}
$$

CHECK UP

Add the following. *Hint:* You may want to rewrite them on top of each other, as above.

• 0.3 + 0.07 = _____

• 219.8 + 14.02 = _____

• 9.07 + 19.1 = _____

• 5.44 + 60.66 = _____

• 8.774 + 0.26 = _____

Subtracting decimals

To subtract decimals, line up the decimal points and subtract.

$$
\begin{array}{r}
4.3000 \\
-\ 1.7942 \\
\hline
2.5058
\end{array}
$$

Note: To make the problem easier to work, you may have to add zeros to the right of the decimal.

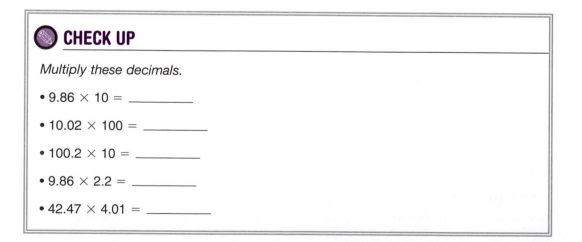

CHECK UP

Subtract these decimals. *Hint*: You may want to rewrite them on top of each other, as above.

- 13.2 − 6.82 = _____

- 3.005 − 1.882 = _____

- 29 − 10.03 = _____

- 64.1 − 1.999 = _____

- 25.4 − 3.9 = _____

Multiplying decimals

To multiply decimals, multiply as you do for whole numbers, and insert the decimal point into the product so that the number of places to the right is equal to the sum of the decimal places in the factors.

$$
\begin{array}{r}
21.4 \rightarrow 1 \text{ place to the right of the decimal point} \\
\times\ 0.36 \rightarrow 2 \text{ places to the right of the decimal point} \\
\hline
1284 \\
642 \\
\hline
7.704 \rightarrow 3 \text{ places to the right of the decimal}
\end{array}
$$

To multiply a decimal by a power of 10 (10, 100, 1000 . . .), move the decimal point to the right the same number of places as there are zeros in the power of 10. This is important to know in case the prescriber orders a medication in a different unit of measure than what is on the label (see Fast Tip 8.1). Chapter 10 discusses this in more detail.

CHECK UP

Multiply these decimals.

- 9.86 × 10 = _____

- 10.02 × 100 = _____

- 100.2 × 10 = _____

- 9.86 × 2.2 = _____

- 42.47 × 4.01 = _____

⬤ *Fast Tip 8.1* Power of 10

Notice that, as a zero is added to the number 1 (i.e., 10, 100, 1000), the decimal point moves to the right the same number of places as the number of zeros. When two zeros are added you get 100, and when three zeros are added you get 1000. You add the number of zeros that correspond with the power of 10 involved. For example, 100 is 10 to the power of two, so it has two zeros. The number 1000 is 10 to the power of three and has three zeros.

$$3.9825 \times 10^{1} = 39.825$$

$$3.9825 \times 100^{2} = 398.25$$

$$3.9825 \times 1000^{3} = 3982.5$$

Dividing decimals

To divide decimals, follow these steps.

1. Move the decimal in the *divisor* (number doing the dividing) to the right of the decimal place to make the divisor a whole number. If you were dividing 100 by 0.5, 0.5 would become 5.0.
2. Move the decimal the same number of places in the *dividend* (number being divided). In the above example, 100 would become 1000.
3. Then do the long division. In this case, 1000 ÷ 5 = 200.

  This does not change the *quotient* (answer we get) because this process is the same as multiplying the numerator and denominator of a fraction by the same number.

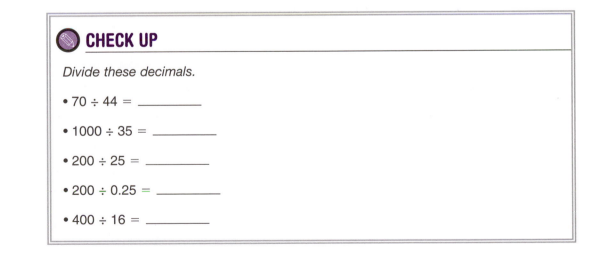

⬤ **CHECK UP**

Divide these decimals.

• 70 ÷ 44 = _____

• 1000 ÷ 35 = _____

• 200 ÷ 25 = _____

• 200 ÷ 0.25 = _____

• 400 ÷ 16 = _____

Decimal and fractional forms

Have you noticed that decimals are really fractions? For example, 0.3 is simply 3/10 and 0.95 is 95/100.

  To convert a decimal to a fraction, place it over the number of the place it signifies. For example:

  0.4 = 4/10 (four tenths)
 0.04 = 4/100 (four hundredths)
0.004 = 4/1000 (four thousandths)

Another way to do this is to count the number of places to the right of the decimal point, add that number of zeroes to "1," and use it as the denominator. For example:

0.3   = 3/10 (Use one zero because there is one place after the decimal point.)
0.95 = 95/100 (Use two zeroes because there are two places after the decimal point.)
0.002 = 2/1000 (Use three zeroes because there are three places after the decimal point.)

To convert a fraction to a decimal, simply put the decimal point one place to the left of the decimal for each 0 in the denominator. For example:

3/10 = 0.3 (The decimal point is one place to the left of the number because there is one zero in the denominator.)

95/100 = 0.95 (The decimal point is two places to the left of the number because there are two zeroes in the denominator.)

2/1000 = 0.002 (The decimal point is three places to the left of the number because there are three zeroes in the denominator.)

Of course, if the fraction is not over a number divisible by 10, you just have to perform long division.

CHECK UP

Convert each of the fractions below to a decimal. Use a separate sheet.

• 4/10 = _____

• 6/100 = _____

• 71/100 = _____

• 192/1000 = _____

• 20/1000 = _____

• 3/10 = _____

• 43/100 = _____

• 5/1000 = _____

• 5/12 = _____

• 55/1000 = _____

Percentages

Percents, quite simply, are numbers "over" 100.

A quarter = 25 cents = 0.25 = 25/100, or 25%
A penny = 1 cent = 0.01 or 1/100, or 1%

If you are asked to leave a 15% tip on a $15.00 dinner:

$$15\% = 0.15$$

$$
\begin{array}{r}
\$15.00 \\
\times\,0.15 \\
\hline
7500 \\
1500 \\
\hline
\$2.2500
\end{array}
$$

The tip would be $2.25. In this case, you have converted the percentage to a decimal.

CHECK UP

Convert each number below to a percentage.

- 20/100 = _____

- 2/100 = _____

- 0.2 = _____

- 0.20 = _____

- 0.02 = _____

Ratios and Proportions

Ratios and proportions are ways to compare items. (Colons indicate ratios.) For example:

100 syringes : (*relates to*) 1 box :: (*as*) 200 syringes : 2 boxes

This can also be written as:

$$\underset{1\ box}{\underset{(is\ to)\rule{3cm}{0.4pt}}{100\ syringes}} \underset{(as)}{=} \underset{2\ boxes}{\underset{(is\ to)\rule{3cm}{0.4pt}}{200\ syringes}}$$

Both sides of the equal sign must relate to each other in the same way. For example:

$$\frac{1}{1} = \frac{2}{2} = \frac{3}{3} = \frac{4}{4} = \frac{5}{5} = \frac{6}{6} = \frac{7}{7}$$

All these relate to each other in the same way because they all are equal to 1. They might instead be equal to 1/2.

$$\frac{1}{2} = \frac{2}{4} = \frac{3}{6} = \frac{4}{8} = \frac{5}{10} = \frac{6}{12} = \frac{7}{14}$$

To get from 1/2 to 2/4, you multiply the numerator and denominator by 2. They are still equal. To get from 1/2 to 3/6, you multiply the numerator and denominator by 3. As you multiply the numerator and denominator by the same number, you are basically multiplying by 1 and thus not changing the relationship of the numbers.

CRITICAL THINKING

By what numbers did we multiply them to get to the equivalents?

Ratios and proportions expressed as fractions

Ratios and proportions are also expressed as fractions. If we are asked to make a 1:10 bleach solution, it is a 10% or 10/100 bleach solution.

1:10 → 1/10 = one tenth is bleach, nine tenths are water

Ratios as decimals

Ratios also relate to decimals. To convert a ratio to a decimal, write it as a fraction over a number divisible by 10 and convert it to a decimal.

1:10 = 1/10 = 0.1

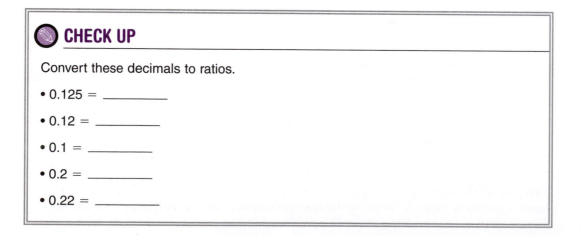

🖋 **CHECK UP**

What number makes each ratio correct?

• 1:10 :: 4: _____

• 3:6 :: 5: _____

• 6:3 :: _____:4

• 10:100 :: 1: _____

• 250:500 :: _____:2

🖋 **CHECK UP**

Write each ratio as a decimal.

• 1:8 = _____

• 1:5 = _____

• 1:10 = _____

• 1:100 = _____

• 1:1000 = _____

If the number is not divisible by 10, you will need to perform long division. For example,

$$1:9 = 1/9 = 1 \div 9 = 0.11$$

Converting decimals to ratios

To convert a decimal to a ratio, write the decimal as a fraction in lowest terms. Restate the fraction as a ratio. For example:

$$0.14 = 14/100 \text{ (need to reduce this fraction)} = 7/50 = 7:50$$

🖋 **CHECK UP**

Convert these decimals to ratios.

• 0.125 = _____

• 0.12 = _____

• 0.1 = _____

• 0.2 = _____

• 0.22 = _____

Converting ratios to percents

To convert a ratio to a percentage, change it to a decimal first and then multiply the decimal by 100 and add the % sign.

$$1:50 = 1/50 = 0.02$$
$$0.02 \times 100 \ = 2\%$$
$$1:50 = 1/50 = 0.02 = 2\%$$

✏ CHECK UP

Convert each ratio to a percentage.

• 2:3 = _____

• 1:2 = _____

• 100:200 = _____

• 1:10 = _____

• 1:3 = _____

Converting percents to ratios

To convert a percentage to a ratio, write it as a fraction in lowest terms. Write the fraction as a ratio.

$$25\% = 25/100 = \frac{1}{4} = 1:4$$

✏ CHECK UP

Convert these percentages to ratios.

• 50% = _____

• 10% = _____

• 75% = _____

• 67% = _____

• 33% = _____

Checking ratio and proportions

If you are not sure you calculated a ratio correctly, there is an easy way to check yourself.

Consider: 1:3 :: 100:?

Suppose in this problem you thought the correct answer was 300. To check yourself, you could multiply the *means* (middle numbers) by the *extremes* (outer numbers). If you have calculated correctly, the means and extremes should be equal (Fig. 8.6).

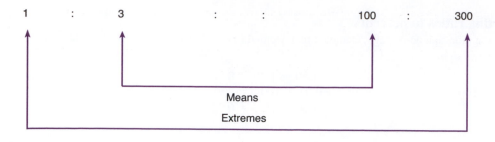

Means
3 X 100 = 300

Extremes
3 X 100 = 300
300 = 300 correct

FIGURE 8.6. Means and extremes check for proportions. To verify that your answer for a proportion is correct, multiply the means and the extremes. The two results should be equal.

Here are two examples to illustrate this point.

Problem: 1: 2 :: 3:?
Proposed answer: 1:2 :: 3:6
Means: 2 × 3 = 6
Extremes: 1 × 6 = 6
6 = 6, so the answer is correct

Problem: 2:3 :: 4:?
Proposed answer: 2:3 :: 4:7
Means: 3 × 4 = 12
Extremes: 2 × 7 = 14
12 does not equal 14, so the answer is incorrect

CHECK UP

Check if these ratios are proportional. Write true or false.

• 1:4 :: 100:200 _____

• 1:2 :: 50:100 _____

• 1:3 :: 3:6 _____

• 1:5 :: 20:100 _____

• 1:6 :: 2:7 _____

You can also use the means and extremes method to check your work when you get an answer.

◉ CHECK UP

Check if these ratios are equal. Write true or false.

• 1:2 :: 2:5 _____

• 2:3 :: 4:6 _____

• 10:100 :: 2:20 _____

• 200:150 :: 1:2 _____

• 250:200 :: 5:4 _____

Solving for an Unknown

You must solve for an unknown number when you calculate some drug doses, so it is important that you know how to do it.

If you are given a ratio or fraction, you need to find an unknown. For example:

$$\frac{100}{200} = \frac{1}{?}$$

This might also be written 100 : 200 :: 1 : ?

There are several ways to solve for ? (the unknown). You can use WORDS.

> 100 relates to 200 as 1 relates to an unknown number.
> 100 is 100 times greater than 1.
> Therefore, 200 is 100 greater than the unknown number, which is 2.

You can use MEANS AND EXTREMES.

$$100 \times ?$$
$$100 : 200 :: 1 : ?$$
$$200$$

$$100 \times ? = 200$$

$$? = \frac{200}{100}$$

$$? = 2$$

You can use fractions and CROSS MULTIPLY.

$$100 \times ? = 1 \times 200$$
$$100? = 200$$
$$\frac{100?}{200} = \frac{200}{100}$$
$$? = 2$$

✳ CRITICAL THINKING

Did you notice how similar the last two methods are? Why does cross-multiplying work?

CHECK UP

Solve for the ? (unknown).

• 100 : 200 :: ? : 2 _____

• 2 : 1 :: 400 : ? _____

• 300 : ? :: 100 : 1 _____

• 50 : 150 :: ? : 3 _____

• 250 : 1 :: 500 : ? _____

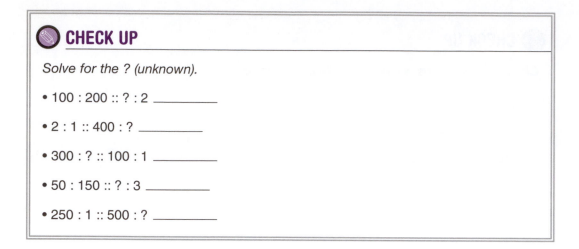

CRITICAL THINKING

Sometimes it is easier to leave a calculation in a fractional form, and sometimes it is better to work with a decimal. When would you use a decimal rather than a fraction? When would it be easier to write a numeric equation as a fraction, and when as a ratio?

SUMMARY

If you are competent with whole numbers, fractions, decimals, percents, ratios and proportions, and solving for unknowns, you can safely calculate dosages. If you are still uncomfortable with any of these problems, review the exercises in this chapter and ask your instructor for help.

You should also use the *Calculating Drug Dosages* CD-ROM packaged with this book. This interactive tutorial contains many dosage calculation problems and takes you step-by-step through solving them. It's a great tool when first learning dosage calculations, and you should use it frequently to become comfortable with this important part of health care.

In addition, many websites provide tutorials on dosage calculations. See the Virtual Field Trips activity at the end of this chapter.

Activities

To make sure that you have learned the key points covered in this chapter, complete the following activities.

Calculations
Find the answer to each equation below.

1. $90 \div 3 =$ _____

2. $3 \times 7 =$ _____

3. $28 \div 4 =$ _____

4. $4 + 3 + 2 =$ _____

5. $30 - 28 =$ _____

Find the least common denominator.

1. 1/3 and 1/4 _____

2. 1/8 and 1/6 _____

3. 1/2 and 1/3 _____

4. 1/5 and 1/15 _____

5. 1/15 and 1/90 _____

6. 1/7 and 1/9 _____

7. 1/4 and 1/9 _____

8. 1/10 and 1/4 _____

9. 1/100 and 1/25 _____

10. 1/2 and 1/10 _____

Add the following:

1. $3/4 + 1/4 =$ _____

2. $1/5 + 2/5 =$ _____

3. $1/6 + 2/3 =$ _____

4. $1\ 1/3 + 1/3 =$ _____

5. $1\ 1/3 + 2/3 =$ _____

6. $8/17 + 6/17 + 2/17 =$ _____

7. $2/3 + 3/8 =$ _____

8. $2/5 + 1/3 =$ _____

9. 1/4 + 1/6 = _____

10. 1 1/3 + 1/2 = _____

Subtract the following:

1. 1 1/2 − 1/2 = _____

2. 15/7 − 8/7 = _____

3. 150/50 − 75/50 = _____

4. 21/1 − 3/1 = _____

5. 5/6 − 3/6 = _____

6. 3/4 − 2/4 = _____

7. 6/3 − 1 1/2 = _____

8. 3/4 − 1/4 = _____

9. 7/18 − 3/24 = _____

10. 4/6 − 1/6 = _____

Multiply the following:

1. 1/3 × 1/4 = _____

2. 250/1 × 1/500 = _____

3. 200/400 × 1/2 = _____

4. 5/1 × 1/4 = _____

5. 3/1 × 10/1 = _____

6. 1/2 × 90 = _____

7. 4/1 × 2 1/2 = _____

8. 3/7 × 3/9 = _____

9. 300/600 × 1 = _____

10. 150/450 × 2 = _____

Divide the following:

1. 4/4 ÷ 5/9 = _____

2. 5/10 ÷ 2/4 = _____

3. 1/6 ÷ 1/6 = _____

4. 9/10 ÷ 3/5 = _____

5. 6/9 ÷ 9/10 = _____

6. 6 ÷ 1/6 = _____

7. 1 2/3 ÷ 2/4 = _____

8. 3/5 ÷ 5/9 = _____

9. 100 ÷ 4 = _____

10. 6 ÷ 6/8 = _____

Reduce the following fractions.

1. 500/250 = _____

2. 600/3 = _____

3. 1000/10 = _____

4. 100/4 = _____

5. 75/150 = _____

6. 240/3 = _____

7. 250/25 = _____

8. 50/500 = _____

9. 100/150 = _____

10. 15/150 = _____

Calculate these decimal problems.

1. 0.04 ÷ 0.2 = _____

2. 10.87 − 0.345 = _____

3. 100 × 9.8 = _____

4. Arrange from smallest to largest: 0.135, 0.13, 0.03 _____

5. Write fifty-two thousandths as a decimal. _____

6. Divide 17.25 by 0.85. Round to the nearest tenth. _____

7. Round to the nearest tenth: 18.75 _____

8. Convert to a decimal: $6^1/_4$ _____

9. Write as a decimal: $7^1/_5$ _____

10. 1.054 + 3.15 = _____

11. Add: 0.05 + 0.005 _____

12. Subtract: 250.98 − 5.55 _____

13. Multiply: 250 × 0.2 _____

14. Divide: 250 ÷ 500 _____

15. Divide: 250 ÷ 0.5 _____

Which is greater?

1. 0.12 or 0.012 _____

2. 4.4 or 0.44 _____

3. 0.15 or 0.16 _____

4. 1.6 or 0.16 _____

5. 0.05 or 0.50 _____

Answer the following questions.

1. What is 10% as a fraction? _____

2. What is 5/100 as a percentage? _____

3. What is 50% of 60? _____

4. What is 0.25 as a percentage? _____

5. What is 75% as a decimal? _____

Convert these ratios to decimals.

1. 1:4 _____

2. 1:10 _____

3. 2:3 _____

4. 1:3 _____

5. 1:2 _____

Convert these decimals to ratios.

1. 0.33 _____

2. 0.50 _____

3. 0.67 _____

4. 0.75 _____

5. 0.90 _____

Convert these ratios to percentages.

1. 1:2 _____

2. 2:3 _____

3. 1:4 _____

4. 2:5 _____

5. 4:6 _____

Convert these percentages to ratios.

1. 50% _____

2. 67% _____

3. 80% _____

4. 99% _____

5. 60% _____

Check if the following ratios are correct. Write true or false.

1. 1 : 10 :: 4 : 50 _____

2. 250 : 500 :: 1 : 2 _____

3. 100 : 400 :: 3 : 5 _____

4. 1 : 2 :: 200 : 400 _____

5. 50 : 150 :: 1 : 2 _____

Solve for the ? (unknown).

1. 1 : 10 :: 3 : ? _____

2. 100 : 1 :: 400 : ? _____

3. 200 : 400 :: 2 : ? _____

4. 2 : 3 :: 4 : ? _____

5. 1 : 2 :: ? : 8 _____

6. 100 : 300 :: ? : 3 _____

7. 100 : 300 :: ? : 6 _____

8. 100 : 200 :: ? : 4 _____

9. 200 : 1 :: 400 : ? _____

10. 1 : 200 :: ? : 400 _____

11. 100 : 1 :: 200 : ? _____

12. 1 : 3 :: 2 : ? _____

13. 0.5 : 1 :: ? : 2 _____

14. 0.25 : 1 :: 25 : ? _____

15. 75 : 150 :: 1 : ? _____

Application Exercises

Respond to the following scenarios on a separate sheet.

1. If one slice of bread contains 100 calories. **How many calories do you reduce if you omit a slice of bread per day for 30 days?**

2. One serving of crisp bread is 60 calories. If you eat three servings, **how many calories did you eat**?

3. A banana split has 550 calories. If you burn 350 calories, **how many more calories do you still have to burn to work off the banana split calories?**

4. Jamie Miller received 21 sample pills from her physician. **If she has to take three per day, how many days will the pills last before she needs to fill the written prescription her physician gave her?**

5. James Critz weighed 102 lb at the end of January. He gained 4 lb in February and 2 lb in March. **How much does he weigh at the end of March?**

6. Joyce Powell gives her daughter $^1/_2$ T at each of three meals each day. **How much does she give in 1 day?**

7. Diana Swink drank $2^1/_2$ cups of water, $1^1/_4$ cups of milk, and 1 cup of orange juice. **How many cups did she drink?**

8. At the beginning of the day, you have a 30-oz bottle of medication. If each dose is $^1/_2$ oz, **how many doses in total do you have?**

9. Jasmine Waddy weighed 100 lb at the last visit. She has lost $4^1/_2$ lb this month. **How much does she now weigh?**

10. Annabelle Fenton is receiving 500 mL of fluid IV. A total of 250 mL has been used in 1 hour. **How much is left?**

11. Peter Hubbard, CMA, makes $10.50 per hour. If he works for 32 hours, **how much does he make?**

12. Colleen Walsh is feeling very drowsy on 50 mg of Zoloft. The nurse practitioner says to cut the prescription by 50%. **How much should she take?**

13. Donnie Wiggins, a pharmacist, made sales totaling the following this hour: $15.28, $77.42, $35.00, $10.00, $35.00, $98.99, and $17.44. **How much in total did he make this hour?**

14. Kathy Thomas owes a medical office $498.43 and pays $35.00. **How much does she now owe?**

15. Gary Gledhill sees the physician four times this month. Each time he pays $35.50. **How much does he pay in total?**

16. Dr. Binderwald has allotted $240.60 in bonuses to be split equally among his six staff members. **How much should each person receive?**

17. In this medical office, the ratio of allied health professionals to patients is 1:3. If there are 60 patients, **how many allied health professionals are needed at this time?**

18. If there are 50 vials of flu vaccine in a box and you need 200 vials, **how many boxes do you need?**

19. If 3 grams of a drug are contained in 50 mL of solution, write the ratio.

20. Describe a 10% bleach solution as a ratio.

21. **How much bleach is in the solution mentioned in question 20? How much water?**

22. David Burrows weighs 50 lb. He is about one third of an adult's weight. **How much of an adult dose should he get?**

23. Ian Metcalfe weighs 300 lb. If an adult dose is based on 150 lb and he is twice that size, **how much should he get of a medication whose dosage is based on weight?**

24. Judith Beyrant is slicing a pie. She sliced six pieces for her three children. If the children get equal shares, **how many slices does each get?**

25. Sheri Yamada is adding up her paychecks for this month. She received $355.60, $320.00, $440.00, and $350.40. **How much did she make this month?**

Virtual Field Trips

Go to the following websites to find the information. If a website is not available, try to find the information through another source.

1. Go to http://www.ebig.com and search for a website to help you with whole numbers. Print a copy of the website information.

2. Surf the web to http://www.excite.com and go to a website with a tutorial about decimals. Print a copy of the information.

3. Visit http://www.lycos.com and search for a website with information about cooking equivalencies. Print the equivalencies.

4. Surf the web to http://www.dogpile.com and use the search engines to find a tutorial on fractions. Print the information.

5. Go to http://www.hotbot.com and search for information on ratios. Print that information.

Measurement Systems

You have reviewed the basic mathematics necessary to calculate dosage calculations, and the next step is to examine the four systems of measurement used for drug dispensing: avoirdupois, apothecary, household, and metric.

OBJECTIVES

At the end of this chapter, the student will be able to:

- Define all key terms.
- Compare three systems of measurement used for drug dosages.
- State the basic units of measurement in the metric system.
- Correctly convert between the systems of measurement.

KEY TERMS

Apothecary	Deci-
Avoirdupois	Household
cc	Kilo-
Centi-	Metric
Compound	Micro-
Conversion triangle	Milli-

● MEASURING SYSTEMS

Years ago, before the metric system was developed, pharmacists mixed (compounded) and dispensed drugs. Patients often measured drugs with handy utensils such as teaspoons and tablespoons. Now drugs are usually ordered using the metric system, although some of the older systems are still used for different purposes. The four systems of measurement discussed here are avoirdupois, apothecary, household, and metric.

Avoirdupois and Apothecary Systems

The *avoirdupois* system is used both for drugs and general purposes. All units of measures in this system are based on the pound. You often use the avoirdupois system when you weigh a patient because most scales give weight in pounds and ounces. You must learn to weigh the patient in pounds and convert that number into kilograms to calculate some drug dosages.

$$1 \text{ kg} = 2.2 \text{ lb}$$
$$1 \text{ lb} = 0.45 \text{ kg}$$

For example, it might not be appropriate to give the same dose of drug to someone who weighs 100 pounds and someone who weighs 300 pounds.

⁕ CRITICAL THINKING

Would you rather be weighed in kilograms or pounds? Why?

The *apothecary* system is one of the oldest systems of measurement. Pharmacists used it for compounding drugs. Whereas the metric system uses decimals, the apothecary system uses fractions. Because it is complicated and less accurate (rounding of numbers is necessary), you do not often see it. However, some prescribers continue to use it, and some patients continue to use nonmetric measuring utensils, so you must be familiar with it.

Household System

At home, a patient may use available teaspoons, tablespoons, cups, glasses, teacups, or other utensils. Unfortunately, they are not standardized, so this practice is unsafe. Encourage your patients to use the metric system or standardized measuring tools. Box 9.1 provides key equivalents of household measures.

A CLOSER LOOK: Apothecary Symbols and Abbreviations

Although not recommended, some prescribers still use symbols and abbreviations for some apothecary measurements, so you should be familiar with them.

UNIT	ABBREVIATION	SYMBOL
Grain	gr	None Used
Minim	—	♏

UNIT	ABBREVIATION	SYMBOL
Dram	dr	ℨ
Ounce	oz	℥

Box 9.1   Household Measures

3 teaspoons (t) = 1 tablespoon (T)
2 T = 1 fluid ounce (oz)
8 oz = 1 cup
2 cups = 1 pint (pt)
2 pints = 1 quart (qt)
4 quarts = 1 gallon (gal)
1 juice glass = 4 ounces
1 teacup = 6 ounces
1 glass = 8 ounces

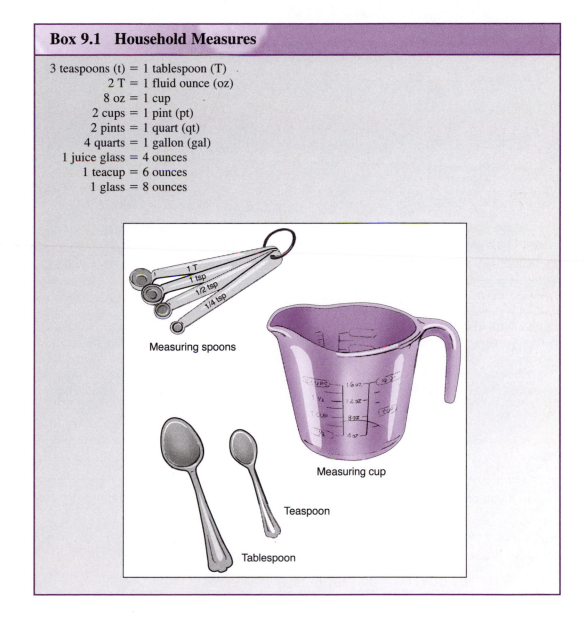

Measuring spoons

Measuring cup

Teaspoon

Tablespoon

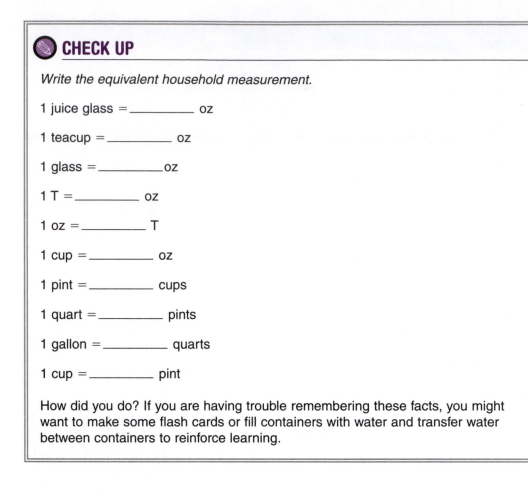

CHECK UP

Write the equivalent household measurement.

1 juice glass = _____ oz

1 teacup = _____ oz

1 glass = _____ oz

1 T = _____ oz

1 oz = _____ T

1 cup = _____ oz

1 pint = _____ cups

1 quart = _____ pints

1 gallon = _____ quarts

1 cup = _____ pint

How did you do? If you are having trouble remembering these facts, you might want to make some flash cards or fill containers with water and transfer water between containers to reinforce learning.

Equivalents in Systems

Before discussing the metric system, it is important to understand the equivalents between the apothecary and household measuring systems. To start, think about the number of minutes your favorite television drama lasts. Most likely, it is 60 minutes. This association may help you remember that 1 dram (a measurement used for fluids) = 60 minims. You also need to know that 8 drams (dr) = 1 ounce (oz).

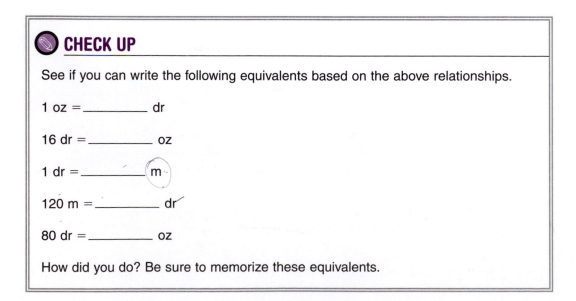

CHECK UP

See if you can write the following equivalents based on the above relationships.

1 oz = _____ dr

16 dr = _____ oz

1 dr = _____ m

120 m = _____ dr

80 dr = _____ oz

How did you do? Be sure to memorize these equivalents.

Larger fluid measurements are pints, quarts, and gallons. Here are some equivalents that you might already know.

1 pint   = 16 fluid ounces
2 pints = 1 quart
4 quarts = 1 gallon

CHECK UP

Fill in the blanks with equivalents.

1 quart = _____ gallon

1 pint = _____ fluid ounces

4 pints = _____ quarts

8 fluid ounces = _____ pint

1 gallon = _____ quarts

How did you do? If you did not know some of these equivalents, you may need to make flashcards to review them.

Some equivalents are tiny—so tiny that there can be a large variable in the number of tiny amounts in a larger amount—similar to grains of sand in a cup.
One drop (gtt) is so small that 360–480 gtt = 1 oz.
There are 360–480 grains or minims in an ounce.
Did you notice that 1 drop (gtt) = 1 grain = 1 minim because they are all about the same size?

CHECK UP

Fill in the blanks with equivalents.

360 gtts = _____ oz

1 oz = _____ grain

1 gtt = _____ oz

CRITICAL THINKING

Does it bother you that 1 oz = something between 360 and 480 gtts, minims, or grains? What does this say about the accuracy of this system?

Sometimes Roman numerals are used when ordering grains. For example, V grains (gr) = 5 grains. Table 9.1 provides a list of ways Roman numerals are used.

TABLE 9.1 Values of Roman Numerals

Roman numerals can be written one of three ways, with the first two the most common. Sometimes these numerals are difficult to read. Be sure to check with the prescriber if you are ever in doubt about an order.

VALUE	ROMAN	NUMERAL	OPTIONS
1	i	I	$\frac{1}{i}$
2	ii	II	$\frac{1}{ii}$
3	iii	III	$\frac{1}{iii}$
4	iv	IV	$\frac{1}{iv}$
5	v	V	$\frac{1}{v}$
6	vi	VI	$\frac{1}{vi}$
7	vii	VII	$\frac{1}{vii}$
8	viii	VIII	$\frac{1}{viii}$
9	ix	IX	$\frac{1}{ix}$
10	x	X	$\frac{1}{x}$

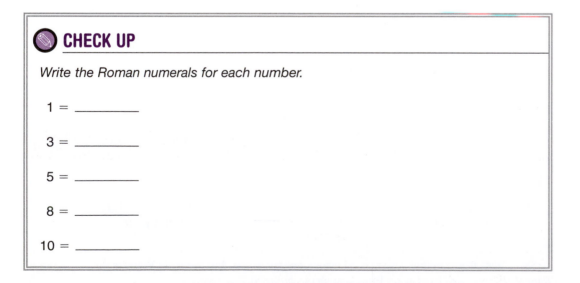

CHECK UP

Write the Roman numerals for each number.

1 = _____

3 = _____

5 = _____

8 = _____

10 = _____

Metric System

The metric system is based on the decimal system of places of 10 (100, 100, 1000). The metric system is used by many countries and most researchers, so it is the most popular system for calculating drugs. The basic units of measurement in this system are as follows.

$$Mass \text{ or weight} = gram$$
$$Length = meter$$
$$Volume/fluids = liter$$

For dosage calculations, you do not usually have to deal with very large or very small numbers. The units of measures typically used are listed in Table 9.2. The prefixes in the table are added to the unit to make the measurement. For example, the term "kilo" means thousands of units; when it is added to "grams," the result is "kilograms." When the term "deci," which means 1/10 of a unit, is added to "liter," the result is "deciliter." When the term "centi," which means 1/100 of a unit, is added to "meter," the result is centimeter. When "milli," which means 1/1000 of a unit, is added to "gram," the result is milligram. When "micro," which means 1/1,000,000 of a unit, is added to "gram," the result is microgram.

🔵 CHECK UP

Define these prefixes.

kilo-

micro-

milli-

centi-

deci-

Write them in order from smallest to largest: _____

Write them in order from largest to smallest: _____

Dosage calculations predominantly use liters and grams. When you use a syringe, the syringe is calibrated so 1 cubic centimeter (cc) of space holds 1 mL of fluid.

If a syringe is thin, more length is needed to form 1 cc of length, depth, and width. If a syringe is wide, you do not pull the plunger back as far to fill the syringe with 1 cc.

TABLE 9.2 Common Metric Units of Measures

PREFIX	LEVEL OF MEASUREMENT
Deci-	Tenths
Centi-	Hundredths
Milli-	Thousandths
Micro-	Millionths

CHECK UP

Shade the syringes to show the amount of fluid indicated.

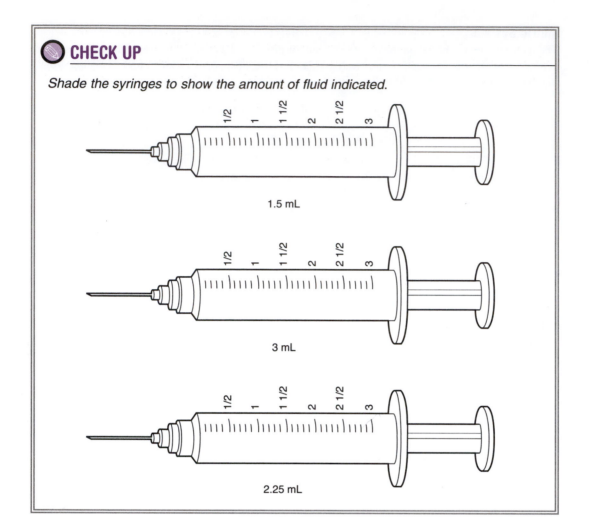

1.5 mL

3 mL

2.25 mL

CHECK UP

A prescriber orders 100 mg of a drug; according to the label, there are 200 mg in each 1 mL of fluid. How many cubic centimeters would you give?

CHECK UP

Converting units within the metric system

Suppose a prescriber orders a drug in grams. Could you convert to milligrams, which is how the label usually states the drug amount? This is how you would do it.

A prescriber orders 0.2 gram; you can think of this as 0.200.

Milligrams are 1/1000 gram, so multiply 0.200 by 1000.

0.200 × 1000 = 200 mg

The prescriber may order a drug in grams or milligrams of weight, but this number must be converted into fluid, or milliliters, so the correct amount can be injected. That conversion information is found on the label of the drug bottle. Once you have calculated the milliliters to administer, remember that 1 cc of space in the syringe is equal to 1 mL of fluid, so you do not need to convert to cubic centimeters.

For example, a prescriber orders 100 mg of drug. According to the label on the drug, 100 mg of drug is dispersed in 1 mL of fluid. To draw up 100 mg of the drug, you would need to fill the syringe with 1 mL of the fluid, so you would pull back the syringe to 1 cc.

Sometimes it is helpful to use fractions or ratios to convert.

$$\frac{0.500 \text{ gram}}{? \text{ mg}} = \frac{1 \text{ gram}}{1000 \text{ mg}}$$

You can cross-multiply to find that the answer.

$$1 \times ? = 0.500 \times 1000$$
$$? = 500/1$$
$$? = 500$$

🔵 CHECK UP

Would you multiply or divide to solve the following problems?

0.200 gram to milligrams _____

200 mg to grams _____

2 grams to kilograms _____

0.5 L to mL _____

1 kg to grams _____

How did you do? If you have trouble with this, it might help to create a chart. One is started for you in Box 9.2.

❋ CRITICAL THINKING

Do you have trouble seeing the decimal point? Do you think pharmacists ever do? How can you be sure that a patient is given 0.5 gram instead of 5 grams?

Box 9.2   Converting from One Unit to Another

Kilo-	×1000 to get to unit → 1 km = 1000 meters
Centi-	÷ 100 to get to unit → 100 cm = 1 meter
Milli-	÷ 1000 to get to unit → 1000 mm = 1 meter
Micro-	÷ 1,000,000 to get to unit → 1,000,000 mcm = 1 meter

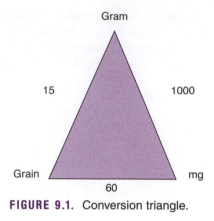

FIGURE 9.1. Conversion triangle.

If you prefer to use words to visualize concepts, you may find this story helpful. There was once a king named Gram. He had 1000 servants called milligrams. He owned 15 grain fields (apothecary). In each grain field, 60 milligrams worked.

Repeat this story, and learn to draw the picture (conversion triangle) in Figure 9.1. The words in the story can help you understand whether to use 1/15 or 15 in the triangle. You can also just memorize these equivalents:

1 gram = 1000 mg
1 gram = 15 grains
1 grain = 60 mg

⬤ CHECK UP

Using the above story and triangle or memorization tables, answer the following.

1. How many servants did King Gram have? _____

2. How many milligrams are in a gram? _____

3. How many grain fields did King Gram have? _____

4. How many grains are in a gram? _____

5. How many milligrams worked in each field? _____

6. How many milligrams are in a grain? _____

Keeping in mind the story and triangle, let us tackle more difficult questions.

Example: King Gram has 1000 milligram servants. Each milligram is 1/1000 of his workforce. If a milligram is sick one day, 1/60 of the workforce in the field is missing. If King Gram gives his child a grain field as a wedding gift, he gave 1/15 of his fields away. Refer to Figure 9.2 as a guide.

Of course, you can just memorize the conversions.

1 mg   = 1/1000 gram   1 g   = 1000 mg
1 grain = 1/15 gram   1 g   = 15 grains
1 mg   = 1/60 grain   1 grain = 60 mg

You must know these conversions to calculate drug dosages safely.

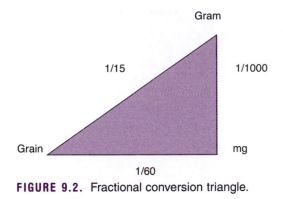

FIGURE 9.2. Fractional conversion triangle.

CHECK UP

Using the above story and triangle, answer the following questions.

1. If King Gram gives away 1 grain field, what fraction of his wealth has he given away? _____

2. A grain is _____ of a gram.

3. Each milligram is what fraction of his workforce?

4. A milligram is _____ of a gram.

5. A milligram is sick today. What fraction of the workers in the field is out sick?

6. A milligram is _____ of a grain.

Table 9.3 summarizes whether you need to multiply or divide when converting from one type of unit to another.

Are you feeling like there is much to memorize? Fast Tip 9.1 may be helpful to you.

TABLE 9.3   How to Convert from One Unit to Another

Grams to kilograms	Divide by 1000
Grams to milligrams	Multiply by 1000
Kilograms to grams	Multiply by 1000
Milligrams to grams	Divide by 1000
Liters to milliliters	Multiply by 1000
Milliliters to liters	Divide by 1000

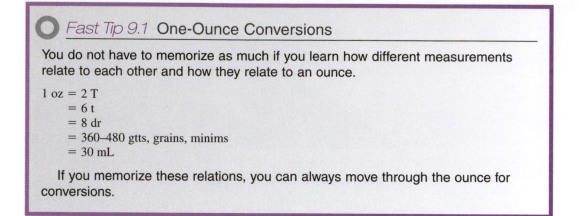

Fast Tip 9.1 One-Ounce Conversions

You do not have to memorize as much if you learn how different measurements relate to each other and how they relate to an ounce.

1 oz = 2 T
    = 6 t
    = 8 dr
    = 360–480 gtts, grains, minims
    = 30 mL

    If you memorize these relations, you can always move through the ounce for conversions.

CHECK UP

Fill in the blanks with equivalents.

1 oz = _____ mL

1 oz = _____ dr

1 oz = _____ T

1 oz = _____ t

1 oz = _____ gtts, minims, or grains

CHECK UP

Fill in the blanks with equivalents.

8 oz   =   _____ mL

2 T   =   _____ dr

1000 mL =   _____ oz

12 oz   =   _____ mL

1 pint   =   _____ oz

Be sure to know these conversions before proceeding to the next chapter.

● ● ● S U M M A R Y

There are four measurement systems: avoirdupois, apothecary, household, and metric. If you are familiar with these measurement systems and can convert between them, you will do well in the next chapter, where we apply these conversions to dosage calculations. If you are not confident, ask your instructor for more problems to work on or refer to your *Calculating Drug Dosages* CD-ROM.

Activities

To make sure that you have learned the key points covered in this chapter, complete the following activities.

Exercises

Fill in the blanks to show what you have memorized.

1. 1 juice glass = _____ oz

2. 1 teacup = _____ oz

3. 1 cc = _____ mL

4. 1 kg = _____ lb

5. 1 lb = _____ kg

6. 1 dr = _____ m

7. 1 oz = _____ dr

8. 1 pint = _____ oz

9. 1 quart = _____ pints

10. 1 gallon = _____ quarts

11. 1 oz = _____ gtts

12. 1 T = _____ t

13. 1 cup = _____ oz

14. 1 kg = _____ gram

15. 1 gram = _____ mg

16. 1 grain = _____ mg

17. 1 gram = _____ grain

18. 1 glass = _____ oz

19. 1 oz = _____ gtts

20. 1 oz = _____ grain

Write Roman numerals three ways for numbers 1 through 5.

1.
2.
3.
4.
5.

Define the following terms on a separate sheet.

1. kilo-
2. micro-

3. deci-
4. milli-
5. centi-

Application Exercises

Respond to the following scenarios on a separate sheet.

1. Faith Ramer calls the medical office. The over-the-counter cough syrup she is using requires that 30 mL be given. She wants to know how many teaspoons to take. **What would you say?**
2. Charlie Armstrong weighs 110 lb. **How many kilograms is that?**
3. Doug Curtis is on a fluid restriction of 1000 mL/day. He has drunk 40 oz today. **Has he exceeded his restriction? Show your calculations**.
4. Nancy Acosta is calculating a drug dosage. The doctor ordered 0.500 gram. **She calculates that as 500 mg. Is she correct?**
5. Jaquan Hulick calls from the pharmacy. The physician ordered 1/15 gram, and he was given 2 grains. He wants to know if he received the correct dosage. **Did he? Show your work.**

Virtual Field Trips

Go to the following websites to find the information. If a website is not available, try to find the information through another source.

1. Go to http://www.factmonster.com/ and download cooking equivalents.
2. Visit http://www.history.org/Almanack/life/trades/tradeapo.cfm and print information about what it was like to work in an apothecary in Williamsburg.
3. Surf to http://www.colostate.edu and type 'lamar' into the site's search window. Write down one interesting fact about the metric system. Try some other site that has information about the United States Metric Association as well.

Dosage Calculations

Having learned the mathematical principles necessary to calculate dosages safely and the systems of measurement, this chapter shows you five ways to calculate dosages. You might want to work problems different ways and then select one method as your preferred working method and another to check your work. Depending on how you were originally taught mathematics as a child, some methods will seem clearer to you than others. This chapter also discusses dosage calculations you may need to know for special circumstances in your career, such as dosage based on weight and administration of an intravenous (IV) solution. It also covers issues surrounding reconstituting solutions and how to help your patients calculate their intake and output.

OBJECTIVES

At the end of this chapter, the student will be able to:

- Define key terms.
- Use dimensional analysis to calculate dosages for administering drugs accurately.
- Use the formula method to calculate dosages accurately.
- Use fractions to solve dosage calculations accurately.
- Use ratios and proportions to solve dosage calculation problems by cross-multiplying to calculate or check a dosage given.
- Correctly solve word problems.
- Accurately calculate dosages ordered by weight.
- Use a child's weight to calculate the desired dosage correctly.
- Use a body surface area nomogram to calculate pediatric dosages.
- Discuss how pediatric patients differ from adults.
- Correctly reconstitute powdered medication and calculate desired dosage.
- Use dimensional analysis to calculate IV drip rates accurately.
- Calculate fluid intake accurately.

KEY TERMS

Body surface area (BSA)
Conversion factor
Desired dose
Dimensional analysis
Formula

Geriatric
Ordered dose
Pediatric
Reconstitute

⬤ METHODS FOR CALCULATING DRUG DOSAGES

Correctly calculating dosages is critical for safe administration of drugs. When approaching mathematics problems, you may use multiple methods to find the correct answer. For this reason, five ways to calculate dosages are illustrated: dimensional analysis, formula, fractions, ratio and proportions, and word problems. You may want to choose one as your preferred method of calculation and use another to check the accuracy of your results. No matter which method you choose, you must first read the label correctly.

Reading Drug Labels

Figure 10.1 shows a sample drug label. Note that sometimes the quantity is in tablets, capsules, milliliters, or another unit. Also note that each label has its own equivalents. The manufacturer, lot number, and expiration dates are included on the label as well as the name, dosage, form, and route of the drug. Now you are ready to learn the five ways to calculate dosages.

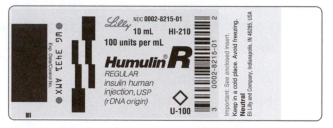

FIGURE 10.1. Sample drug label. (© Copyright Eli Lilly and Company. All rights reserved. Used with permission. ® Humulin is a registered trademark of Eli Lilly and Company.)

Dimensional Analysis

The prescriber includes both a quantity and a *dimension* (or unit of measurement) in each medication order. If you focus on the dimension, not the numbers, you can create a template to use for every problem.

Dimensions or units vary depending on the circumstance. They may be tablets, capsules, bottles, milliliters (mL), ounces (oz), tablespoons (T), milligrams (mg), grams, grains, or something else.

Dimensional analysis uses the ordered amount of a drug to multiply with two equal quantities in different dimensions (units of measurement) to derive the answer. This method is a basis for calculating IV drip dosages (discussed later in the chapter) and also to calculate dosages when a conversion between units is necessary or if the units ordered are not the same as those found on the drug label. You can do this in four easy steps.

Step one

Write the unit of the dose ordered. If the prescriber orders a dose in milligrams, write "mg" in the first position. If the order is in grams, write "grams." This is the *ordered dose*. For example, if the order is for 500 mg, you would write "mg."

Step two

Write the *units* that are on the label and the *unit* that you plan to give to the patient. For instance, a label shows that a drug is available in milligrams, and you want to give the drug in milliliters.

Place the unit of the ordered dose on the bottom of the *conversion factor* (found on the label) to cancel with the ordered unit. The *desired* unit is the unit that you want to give. The desired unit is used on the top of the conversion factor.

$$\text{mg} \times \frac{\text{mL}}{\text{mg from label}} = \text{mL}$$

The conversion factor effectively multiplies the other units by 1/1 because the two values are equal but in different units. The answer to this equation is the *desired dose*. The example below shows that one equivalent over another equals one.

$$\frac{1}{1} = \frac{2}{2} = \frac{3}{3} = \frac{4}{4} \qquad \text{Finish the rest: } \frac{}{5} = \frac{}{6} = \frac{}{7}$$

Therefore, if 250 mg = 1 mL (from the label), then

$$\frac{250 \text{ mg}}{1 \text{ mL}} = \frac{1}{1}$$

Can you find equivalents?

$$\frac{1 \text{ oz}}{? \text{ mL}} = \frac{1}{1} \qquad \frac{1 \text{ gram}}{? \text{ mg}} = \frac{1}{1}$$

Step three

Now fill in the numbers for each unit and cancel the ordered units.

$$500 \text{ mg} \times \frac{1 \text{ mL}}{250 \text{ mg (from label)}} = 2 \text{ mL}$$

Note: 1 mL = 250 mg (from label), so it is a conversion that equals 1/1.

Check each label carefully; different vials may have different equivalents. Sometimes a label may not have a conversion of 1 mL. It may read 250 mg = 2 mL. You can reduce this fraction to be 125 mg = 1 mL or leave it as 250 mg = 2 mL for calculations. Both are equivalents.

Step four

Check the work for reasonableness.

Would you inject 2 mL? Yes, OK.

What if your calculations resulted in an answer of 20 mL? Would you inject that much fluid? No. You would go back and check your calculations again.

Are these values equivalents?

$$\frac{500 \text{ mg}}{2 \text{ mL}} = \frac{250 \text{ mg}}{1 \text{ mL}}$$

OK.

🖉 CHECK UP

You try it.

Using the information in the box, calculate the amount of drug you would give according to the orders below.

100 mg

200 mg

50 mg

300 mg

250 mg

> Generic cough syrup
>
> 100 mg/1 mL
>
> For oral use only.

BOX 10.1	**Household Measures**

1 oz	= 30 mL
1 juice glass	= 4 oz
1 teacup	= 6 oz
1 cup	= 8 oz
1 glass	= 8 oz

Dimensional analysis is particularly useful when converting between apothecary and household systems (Box 10.1).

You can use dimensional analysis for other purposes too, including converting between measurement systems. For example, the nurse practitioner orders 1000 mL fluid restriction for Clark Castillo. Clark drinks 50 oz of fluid today. Did he exceed the restriction?

Step 1: mL (units in which the fluid restriction is ordered)

Step 2:
$$mL \times \frac{}{mL} \ oz = oz \ \text{(units for the fluid he drank)}$$

Step 3:
$$1000 \ mL \times \frac{1 \ oz}{30 \ mL} = 33.3 \ oz$$

Thus, 33.3 oz is less than 50 oz.

If he drank 50 oz, he exceeded the 33.3 oz restriction.

Step 4: Check for reasonableness. Think of a liter (1000 mL) as about a quart. Fifty ounces is larger than a quart. You may need to teach Clark not to drink more than a quart a day because he may not know what a liter looks like.

Dimensional analysis can also be used when dosages are not in the unit on the label—if equivalent conversion units are used. For example, the physician orders $\frac{1}{2}$ gram of medication. The label says 250 mg = 1 capsule.

Step 1:
$$\frac{1}{2} \ \text{gram} = 0.5 \ \text{gram}$$

Step 2:
$$\text{grams} \times \frac{mg}{grams} = \text{capsule}$$

⬤ CHECK UP

A mother calls your office from home, saying that she does not know how many teaspoons to give her child because the directions on the medication bottle read "Give 15 mL."

Step 1: Write the units ordered.

Step 2: Write the known equivalent (*hint*: teaspoons to mL).

Step 3: Do the math.

Step 4: Is the answer reasonable?

If you worked out the answer like this, congratulations!

$$15 \ mL \ \times \ \frac{6 \ \text{teaspoons}}{30 \ mL} = 3 \ \text{teaspoons}$$

Suggestion: Make sure your patient uses a properly calibrated teaspoon because kitchen teaspoons can vary in size.

Step 3:
$$0.5 \text{ gram} \times \frac{1000 \text{ mg}}{1 \text{ gram}} = 500 \text{ mg}$$

$$500 \text{ mg} \times \frac{1 \text{ capsule}}{250 \text{ mg}} = 2 \text{ capsules}$$

Step 4: Is an answer of two capsules reasonable? Yes.

Try another: Suppose you weighed a patient in pounds but needed to know the weight in kilograms to do a dosage calculation. Could you use dimensional analysis? The patient weighs 70 lb. What is that in kilograms?

Step 1: lb

Step 2:
$$\text{lb} \times \frac{\text{kg}}{\text{lb}} = \text{kg}$$

Step 3:
$$70 \text{ lb} \times \frac{0.45 \text{ kg}}{1 \text{ lb}} = 31.5 \text{ kg}$$

Step 4: If a pound is approximately $\frac{1}{2}$ kg, the amount of kilograms should be approximately one half of the number of pounds.

$$7 \text{ lb} \times \frac{1}{2} = 35 \text{ lb}$$

Is 31.5 approximately 35 lb? Yes.

Formula Method

If you prefer, you can use a *formula* instead of dimensional analysis. With the formula method, you stack the units that are the same and multiply by the unit requested. Note that the desired dose equals the dosage that has been ordered. It *must* be in the same units as the dosage on hand. If the prescriber orders 200 mg, and the label reads 200 mg = 1 tablet, you would give 1 tablet when following this formula, where D = the desired dose, H = the on-hand amount in ordered units, and Q = quantity in the unit given.

$$\frac{D}{H} \times Q = \frac{200 \text{ mg}}{200 \text{ mg}} \times 1 \text{ tablet} = 1 \text{ tablet}$$

CHECK UP

Calculate these dosages.

1. Physician's order: 400 mg
   Label: 200 mg/mL
   What would you give in mL? _____

2. Nurse practitioner's order: 100 mg
   Label: 200 mg/scored tablet
   What would you give in tablets? _____

3. Physician's order: 500 mg
   Label: 500 mg/capsule
   What would you give in capsules? _____

4. Physician assistant's order: 200 mg
   Label: 1 oz = 100 mg
   What would you give in oz? _____

5. The patient weighs 100 lb. How many kilograms is that? _____

Ordered units do not always match the units on the drug's label. Here is how you can proceed if they do not.

Example: The prescriber orders 0.25 gram, but the label says 250 mg/mL.

Step 1. Convert grams to milligrams.

$$0.25 \text{ grams} \times 1000 \text{ mg (the number of milligrams in 1 gram)} = 250 \text{ mg}$$

Step 2. Set up the D/H × Q formula:

$$\frac{250 \text{ mg (order)}}{250 \text{ mg (label)}} \times 1 \text{ mL} = 1 \text{ mL}$$

Step 3. Solve the formula.

Note that the D/H × Q formula is a slight variation on dimensional analysis (Fig. 10.2).

CHECK UP

Using the D/H × Q formula, calculate the following.

1. D = 700 mg   H = 350 mg   Q = 1 tablet

2. D = 250 mg   H = 500 mg   Q = 2 mL

3. D = 200 mg   H = 400 mg   Q = 1 tablet

4. D = 1000 mg   H = 1 gram   Q = 2 bottles

5. D = 1000 units   H = 10,000 units   Q = 10 mL

Fractions

To use the fraction method for calculating dosages, the ordered dose and units given must be in the same proportion as the amount on the label. This method uses two equivalent proportions (the label and the desired dose) to find the missing number.

$$\frac{\text{Dosage on hand}}{\text{Dosage unit}} = \frac{\text{Desired dose}}{\text{Dose given}}$$

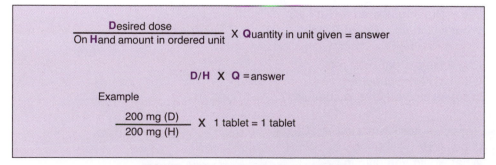

$$\frac{\text{Desired dose}}{\text{On Hand amount in ordered unit}} \times \text{Quantity in unit given} = \text{answer}$$

$$\text{D/H} \times \text{Q} = \text{answer}$$

Example

$$\frac{200 \text{ mg (D)}}{200 \text{ mg (H)}} \times 1 \text{ tablet} = 1 \text{ tablet}$$

FIGURE 10.2. Sliding formula example.

For example, if the label reads that 200 mg of a drug is in 1 mL of fluid, the correct dosage must maintain that proportion.

$$\frac{100 \text{ mg}}{0.5 \text{ mL}} = \frac{200 \text{ mg}}{1 \text{ mL}} = \frac{300 \text{ mg}}{1.5 \text{ mL}} = \frac{400 \text{ mg}}{2 \text{ mL}} = \frac{500 \text{ mg}}{2.5 \text{ mL}} = \frac{600 \text{ mg}}{3 \text{ mL}} = \frac{700 \text{ mg}}{3.5 \text{ mL}}$$

All these proportions are the same. Sometimes you can even cancel down into lower numbers—so long as you maintain the same proportion.

Here is how this method would be used. If the label reads 100 mg/tablet, what would be given if 200 mg is ordered?

Step 1: To find the desired proportion, write the label ratio on one side and the same units on the other:

$$\overset{\text{On hand}}{\frac{\text{mg}}{\text{tablets}}} = \frac{\text{mg}}{\text{tablets}} \quad or \quad \overset{\text{Desired}}{\frac{\text{mg desired}}{\text{mg on label}}} = \frac{\text{tablets desired}}{\text{tablets on label}}$$

Step 2: Write the same units on the other side of the equal sign.

$$\frac{\text{mg}}{\text{tablets}} = \frac{\text{mg}}{\text{tablets}}$$

Step 3: Insert the numbers.

$$\frac{100 \text{ mg}}{1 \text{ tablet}} = \frac{200 \text{ mg}}{? \text{ tablets}}$$

Step 4: Perform the calculation.

$$\frac{100 \text{ mg}}{1 \text{ tablet}} = \frac{200 \text{ mg}}{2 \text{ tablets}}$$

Step 5: Check for reasonableness. Would you reasonably give 2 tablets? Yes.

🔵 CHECK UP

Solve the problems using fractions.

1. $\dfrac{1 \text{ mL}}{200 \text{ mg}} = \dfrac{? \text{ mL}}{100 \text{ mg}}$

2. $\dfrac{1 \text{ tablet}}{250 \text{ mg}} = \dfrac{? \text{ tablets}}{500 \text{ mg}}$

3. $\dfrac{1 \text{ oz}}{300 \text{ mg}} = \dfrac{? \text{ oz}}{150 \text{ mg}}$

4. $\dfrac{1 \text{ capsule}}{200 \text{ mg}} = \dfrac{? \text{ capsules}}{400 \text{ mg}}$

5. $\dfrac{1 \text{ bottle}}{1000 \text{ mL}} = \dfrac{? \text{ bottles}}{500 \text{ mL}}$

If it is easier for you, you can also align the like dosage units on each side so long as you are careful.

Does $\dfrac{Label: \ 1 \text{ mL}}{Desired: \ ? \text{ mL}} = \dfrac{200 \text{ mg}}{100 \text{ mg}}$ get the same result as $\dfrac{? \text{ mL}}{100 \text{ mg}} = \dfrac{1 \text{ mL}}{200 \text{ mg}}$?

Yes, but you must be sure that the numerators are the ordered quantity and the given information becomes the denominators. Or reverse them, with the given quantities being the numerators and the desired quantities the denominators. For example,

$$\frac{Desired}{On \ label} = \frac{2 \text{ mL}}{1 \text{ mL}} = \frac{200 \text{ mg}}{100 \text{ mg}}$$

✳ CRITICAL THINKING

Does it make any difference if you align like units on one side and desired units on the other? Explain.

 CHECK UP

Calculate the correct dosages.

1. $\dfrac{250 \text{ mg}}{1000 \text{ mg}} = \dfrac{? \text{ mL}}{4 \text{ mL}}$

2. $\dfrac{100 \text{ mg}}{200 \text{ mg}} = \dfrac{? \text{ scored tablets}}{1 \text{ scored tablet}}$

3. $\dfrac{0.250 \text{ gram}}{0.750 \text{ gram}} = \dfrac{1 \text{ mL}}{? \text{ mL}}$

4. $\dfrac{1 \text{ oz}}{2 \text{ oz}} = \dfrac{30 \text{ mL}}{? \text{ mL}}$

5. $\dfrac{100 \text{ mg}}{50 \text{ mg}} = \dfrac{? \text{ T}}{1 \text{ T}}$

✳ CRITICAL THINKING

Can you use the fraction method to check the accuracy of other methods?

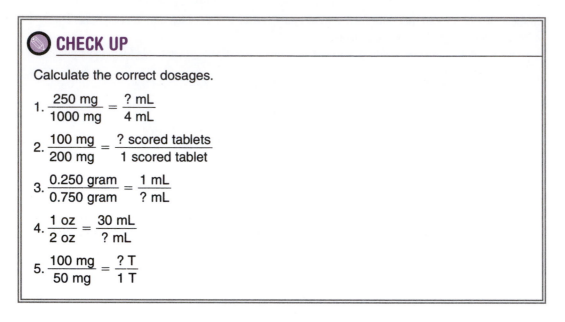 **CHECK UP**

Using the fractions, check to see if these dosage calculations are correct. You may reduce or cross-multiply. Write *true* or *false* next to each calculation.

1. $\dfrac{250 \text{ mg}}{1000 \text{ mg}} = \dfrac{1 \text{ mL}}{3 \text{ mL}}$

2. $\dfrac{100 \text{ mg}}{200 \text{ mg}} = \dfrac{1 \text{ mL}}{2 \text{ mL}}$

3. $\dfrac{500 \text{ mg}}{250 \text{ mg}} = \dfrac{2 \text{ mL}}{1 \text{ mL}}$

4. $\dfrac{700 \text{ mg}}{350 \text{ mg}} = \dfrac{1 \text{ mL}}{2 \text{ mL}}$

5. $\dfrac{300 \text{ mg}}{100 \text{ mg}} = \dfrac{3 \text{ mL}}{1 \text{ mL}}$

Ratio and Proportions

You can use the means and extremes method discussed in Chapter 8 as a shorthand to solve problems. If, for example, the order is 100 mg, but the label says 200 mg/mL, Figure 10.3 shows how you would solve it.

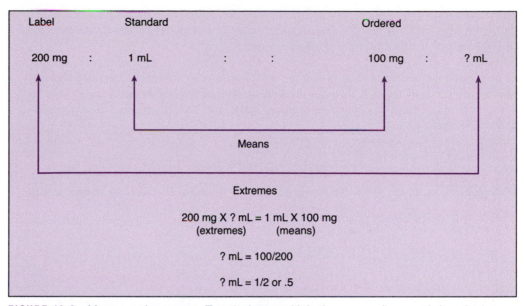

FIGURE 10.3. Means and extremes. To calculate, multiply the means (inner units) and relate them to the extremes (outer units).

First, write what is on the label:

$$\frac{200\ mg}{1\ mL}\quad 200\ mg : 1\ mL$$

Then multiply as shown in Figure 10.3. Note that each unit relates to another in a ratio. Remember that both sides of the equation should have the same units (e.g., mg-mL or mg-tablets).

$$200\ mg : 1\ mL :: 200\ mg : ?\ mL$$
$$mL \times mg\ (means)$$
$$mg \times mL\ (extremes)$$

Setting it up in this way should help you set up ratios correctly.

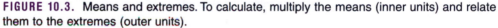 **CHECK UP**

Using ratios and proportions, calculate what amount you would give.

1. 400 mg : 1 mL :: 200 mg : ? mL _____

2. 250 mg : 1 mL :: 750 mg : ? mL _____

3. 200 mg : 2 mL :: 100 mg : ? mL _____

4. 50 units : 1 mL :: 150 units: ? mL _____

5. 100 mg : 1 tablet :: 200 mg : ? tablets _____

Word Problems

Some people understand words better than numbers because different parts of the brain perform these different functions.

It may be helpful for you to create a word template such as one of these:

If the prescriber orders _____ *mg, multiply the order by the amount of tablets, caplets, milliliters, etc. on the label and divide by the number of milligrams on the label.*

OR

If the prescriber orders _____ *mg, divide that number by the milligrams on the label and multiply by the unit per milligram.*

OR

If the prescriber orders _____ mg, place it over the milligrams on the label. Place the quantity of units on the label and write it as the denominator of a fraction on the other side of the equals sign. Then find what numerator makes the two fractions equal.

OR

Express the label quantities as a ratio of mg:units. On the other side of the two colons, place the prescriber's order in milligrams. Solve for the units that you should give by multiplying the extreme (far right and left) amounts together and the mean (inside right and left) amounts together—solving for what you need to give.

In mathematics, that would be:

$$\frac{?\ mg}{\text{label mg}} \times \text{no. of tablets, capsules, mL, etc.} = \text{answer in tablets, capsules, mL, etc.}$$

Which seems easier to you—words or numbers? Write words for the following in the space to the right:

$$\text{Rx in mg} \times \frac{\text{units from label}}{\text{mg from label}} = \text{answer}$$

$$\frac{\text{Order in mg}}{\text{Desired mL}} = \frac{\text{mg on label}}{\text{mL on label}}$$

$$\frac{\text{Order in mg}}{\text{Label in mg}} = \frac{\text{desired mL}}{\text{label in mL}}$$

Order in mg: desired mL :: label mg : label mL

Because it is your brain that translates the words into calculations, it is important for you to select your own words for your template. If you have had trouble with mathematics in the past, it may be because someone else (a textbook writer, for example) did not use words your brain likes to use to process mathematics (see Fast Tip 10.1.).

🖊 CHECK UP

Using the word templates you made, calculate the following dosages.

1. $\dfrac{200\ mg}{400\ mg} = \dfrac{?\ mL}{2\ mL}$

2. $\dfrac{?\ tablets}{500\ mg} = \dfrac{1\ tablet}{250\ mg}$

3. D = 50 mg, H = 150 mg, Q = 1 mL

4. 400 mg : ? mL :: 200 mg : 1 mL

5. Rx = 125 mg. Label reads 250 mg/1 oz.

⭘ *Fast Tip 10.1* Critical Thinking Symbols

Some English phrases translate into symbols that can help you create templates more easily.

×	times
=	equals, is, was, has, has the value, costs, weighs
>	greater than
<	less than
÷	divided by
3×	three times
2×	two times

● SPECIAL CIRCUMSTANCES

Sometimes prescribers order medications based on a patient's weight. For example, an order might be for a drug in milligrams per kilogram per day (mg/kg/day). Weight is frequently used to calculate children's dosages because children are usually smaller than adults and cannot tolerate a full adult dosage. Similarly, small, thin adults may also benefit from calculating dosages based on weight. If you are caring for infants, children, adolescents, or small adults, you must know how to calculate dosages by weight.

Weight-Based Calculations in Adults and Children

You can use the methods already discussed to calculate the dosage when a drug is ordered based on weight. Children are especially sensitive to variations in medication dosages. A dosage appropriate for an adult might harm a child. Although calculating dosages correctly is important, it is even more critical with pediatric (child-age) patients. Most drug references list a pediatric dosage for drugs used in children. When a dose is not listed, the drug may not be indicated for children. Consult with the prescriber and a pharmacist.

Here's an example. The prescriber orders a drug that has a recommended dosage of 30 mg/kg/*day*. How much would you give a 100-lb child each *day*?

$$100 \text{ lb} \times \frac{0.45 \text{ kg}}{1 \text{ lb}} = 45 \text{ kg}$$

$$45 \text{ kg} \times \frac{30 \text{ mg}/\textbf{\textit{day}}}{1 \text{ kg}} = 1350 \text{ mg}/\textbf{\textit{day}}$$

If the drug is given bid (twice daily), you would divide the *daily* dose by 2.

$$\frac{1350 \text{ mg}}{\text{Day}} \div 2 = \frac{675}{\text{Dose}}$$

How would you calculate the dose if it is labeled bid? Would you multiply or divide? What if it is tid? These situations require *dividing* the daily dose by 2 or 3.

❋? CRITICAL THINKING

You may find it bothersome that dosages sometimes come out to be odd numbers relative to the usual dosages—for example, when the dose is 337.5 mg/dose. If the medication comes in 200 mg tablets, what would you do?

Sometimes the order is given in milligrams per kilogram per *dose* (mg/kg/dose). To determine the total *daily dose*, multiply by the times per day the dosage is given.

For example, the patient weighs 100 lb. What is the total *daily dose* of a drug ordered as 20 mg/kg/*dose* bid?

$$100 \text{ lb} \times \frac{0.45 \text{ kg}}{1 \text{ lb}} = 45 \text{ kg}$$

$$45 \text{ kg} \times 20 \text{ mg}/\textbf{\textit{dose}} = 900 \text{ mg}/\textbf{\textit{dose}}$$

bid: 900 mg × 2 = 1800 mg/*day*
tid: 900 mg × 3 = 2700 mg/*day*
qid: 900 mg × 4 = 3600 mg/*day*
If the drug was dosed in 500-mg tablets, what would you give for each dose?

Calculation Using Body Surface Area

Dosages can be ordered according to the patient's *body surface area* (BSA), a ratio of height to weight. The following formula shows the figures for calculating BSA.

$$\text{BSA} = (\text{W}^{0.425} \times \text{H}^{0.725}) \times 0.007184$$

where the weight is in kilograms, and the height is in centimeters.

CHECK UP

Answer these questions.

1. If a drug is ordered at 10 mg/kg/day, how much would a 20-lb patient need each day? _____

2. If the drug in question 1 is given tid, what would be the mg/dose? _____

3. If a different drug is ordered at 20 mg/kg/day for the same patient, how much would he or she need each day? _____

4. If the 20 mg/kg/day drug is to be given qid, what would be the mg/dose? _____

5. If a drug is ordered bid, how many doses do you give per day? _____

6. If the drug is ordered at 10 mg/kg/dose for a 50-lb patient, how much is given per dose? _____

7. If the drug in question 6 is given tid, how much is given per day? _____

8. If the drug is ordered at 20 mg/kg/dose for a 50-lb patient, how much is given per dose? _____

9. If the drug in question 8 is given qid, how much is given per day? _____

10. Write a word template to explain when you divide and when you multiply to solve these problems. _____

To find the BSA:

Fortunately, you do not need to use this formula but can use the chart in Figure 10.4 instead.

1. Find the child's height on the left side of the chart, and put a ruler or piece of paper at that point.
2. Find the child's weight on the right side (be sure to find it in kilograms or pounds—depending on how it was measured), and place the other side of the ruler or piece of paper at that point.
3. Note that the ruler or paper cuts across the chart. The intersection point indicates the child's BSA.

● RECONSTITUTING POWDERS

Sometimes powdered medication needs to be turned into liquid so it can be given. This process is called *reconstituting*. After adding a specified amount of sterile water or saline solution, use the conversion ratio on the label to calculate the dosage. Remember that the amount of fluid (diluent) used to reconstitute adds to the powder's volume, so the final solution (powder and fluid) may be greater than the volume of the diluent.

Consider this situation. A drug label indicates that you should mix 9 mL sterile water with 500 mg powder, which makes a total of 10 mL. To calculate the dosage after reconstituting, just use the ratio 500 mg/10 mL.

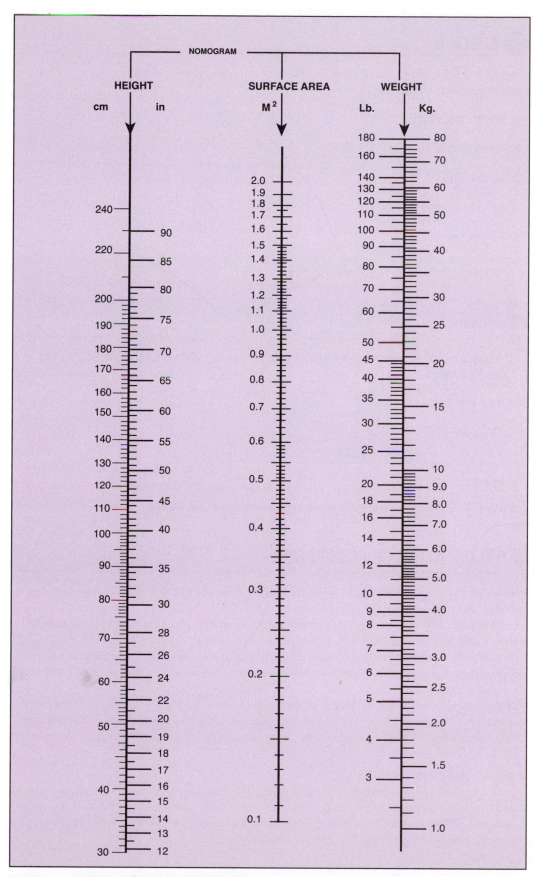

FIGURE 10.4. Body surface area (BSA) chart.

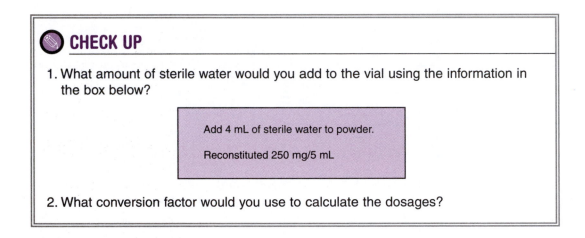

CHECK UP

Using the BSA chart, determine the BSA of the patient. Be sure to note the dimensions (cm, kg, inches, lb):

1. 50 cm and 6 kg

2. 45 inches and 36 lb

3. 80 cm and 25 lb

4. 14 inches and 7.5 lb

5. 58 cm and 9 kg

CHECK UP

1. What amount of sterile water would you add to the vial using the information in the box below?

> Add 4 mL of sterile water to powder.
>
> Reconstituted 250 mg/5 mL

2. What conversion factor would you use to calculate the dosages?

CALCULATION OF IV DOSAGES

Many patients who might have been hospitalized for IV therapy at one time are now coming to outpatient facilities or receiving IV therapy at home.

Laws related to IV therapy vary from state to state. Check with your state Board of Medicine to determine your legal responsibilities.

IV therapy policies also vary from organization to organization. No matter what the scope of your responsibilities, you should know how IV dosages are calculated so you can double-check other health care workers' calculations.

IV drip calculations are not as difficult as they might seem—so long as you understand the equipment and the therapy (see Chapter 7). Dimensional analysis is the best way to calculate the drip rate. Calculations are needed whether an electronic pump or a manual setup is used to regulate the infusion.

Electronic Regulator Pumps

Electronic regulator pumps make our job much easier. The prescriber gives an order in milliliters to be infused over a certain period of time (e.g., 1000 mL over 2 hours or 400 mL over 8 hours). The IV tubing, which is specific to the type of pump, is run through an electronic regulator; someone needs to program the rate for the regulator. The rate is expressed as:

$$\frac{\text{Total mL ordered}}{\text{Total time ordered in hours}} = \text{mL/hour (rounded to a whole number)}$$

Example: If the physician ordered 1000 mL over 2 hours:

$$\frac{1000 \text{ mL}}{2 \text{ hours}} = \frac{500 \text{ mL}}{1 \text{ hour}}$$

Does this seem reasonable? Cross-multiply to double-check.

CHECK UP

What is the electronic mL/hr for the following:

1. 1000 mL over 3 hours _____

2. 500 mL over 2 hours _____

3. 1000 mL over 4 hours _____

4. 250 mL over 1 hour _____

5. 150 mL over 3 hours _____

Sometimes patients want to know when their infusion will be finished. If the prescriber orders an amount over a certain number of hours, it is easy to calculate the completion time.

For example, a patient arrives at 10 a.m., and the physician orders 1000 mL of IV fluid to be given over 3 hours:

10:00 plus 3 hours = 13:00, or 1 p.m. (13:00−12:00 = 1 p.m.)

At noon, the patient asks if the infusion will be done on time. You see there is still 500 mL to be infused. The physician ordered 500 mL/hour. There is 500 mL left.

$$\frac{500 \text{ mL}}{500 \text{ mL}} \times 1 \text{ hour} = 1 \text{ hour}$$

You can tell the patient that the infusion will be finished in 1 hour. Noon + 1 hour is 1 p.m.

Suppose you looked up at noon and there was 750 mL left? When will the patient be finished?

$$\frac{750 \text{ mL}}{500 \text{ mL}} \times 1 \text{ hour} = 1.5 \text{ hours}$$

Noon + 1.5 hours is 1:30.

Not only will your patient be disappointed, but something might have malfunctioned. If the flow rate is not constant and correct, report it to your supervisor. Do not just change the flow rate, because the change may cause the fluid or medication to be infused too quickly or the patient's IV may be infiltrated. In either case you could cause damage by increasing the flow rate.

CRITICAL THINKING

In the above case, where the flow rate has not been consistent, you see that the IV insertion site is swollen. Would you increase the flow rate to make up the difference? What would you do?

Manual IV Sets

Manual IV sets use gravity to infuse a solution at a set rate, which means you need to know the drop factor. The drop factor = gtt/mL and is stated on the package of the IV tubing. (The drop factor is built

A CLOSER LOOK: Military Time

Some facilities use military time, which is based on a 24-hour clock. The hours pass from 0100 to 1200, and then continue the next sweep from 1300 (1 p.m.) to 2400 (12 midnight). To return to the 12-hour clock, simply subtract 1200 from the number: 1300−1200 = 1.

*Complete the following
for 24-hour times.*
Noon =
 1 p.m. =
 2 p.m. =
 3 p.m. =
 4 p.m. =
 5 p.m. =
 6 p.m. =
 7 p.m. =
 8 p.m. =
 9 p.m. =
10 p.m. =
11 p.m. =
12 p.m. =

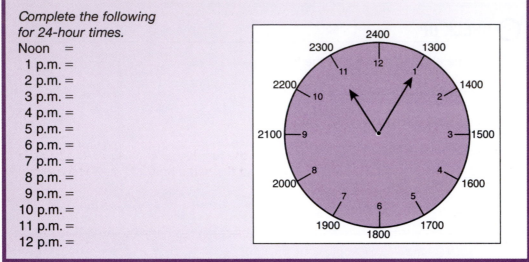

CHECK UP

1. It is 1 p.m. There is 500 mL of solution in an IV bag infusing at 250 mL/hr. When will the infusion be finished?

2. The patient needs an IV infusion in the medical office. The physician has ordered 1000 mL at 250 mL/hour. How much time should you allow for this patient?

3. It is noon. The patient wants to know if the infusion will be completed by 3 o'clock, when a favorite TV show airs. The infusion has 500 mL left at 250 mL/hr. Will the infusion be finished in time, for the patient to see the show?

4. The infusion is supposed to be 250 mL/hr. There is 1 hour left, and 325 mL is in the bag. Is this correct? If not, what would you do to correct it?

into electronic pumps because the tubing matches the pump.) IV tubing has either a micro or a macro drip chamber. The micro drip is usually 60 gtt/mL, and the macro is usually 10 or 15 gtt/mL.

The health care professional who starts the IV establishes the rate by hanging the bag or bottle at a certain height and adjusting the number of drops per minute with the roller clamp. The IV set must not be moved or adjusted; doing so might change the drip rate.

The formula for the IV flow rate is:

$$\frac{\text{Total volume (V) to be infused (mL)}}{\text{Total time in minutes}} \times \frac{\text{drop factor (D) (gtts)}}{\text{mL}} = \frac{\text{rate of flow (R) (gtts)}}{\text{min}}$$

or, more simply

$$\frac{V \times D}{T} = R$$

If you prefer the formula method, just assemble the information and solve the problem.

Example: $$\frac{250 \text{ mL}}{60 \text{ min}} \times \frac{60 \text{ gtts}}{1 \text{ mL}} = 250 \text{ gtts/min}$$

This is dimensional analysis, with an additional conversion factor.
Use this format if you prefer fractions:

$$\frac{V}{T} = \frac{R}{D}$$

Example: $$\frac{250}{60} = \frac{?}{60} = 250$$

CRITICAL THINKING

Because the actual order is the same, the real factor in these calculations is the drip rate. Which would drip faster at the same hourly rate, a macrodrip or a microdrip?

CHECK UP

For using a manual IV setup, calculate the following in drops per minute.

1. 1000 mL NS over 24 hours. Tubing: 20 gtts/mL.

2. 250 mL D$_5$W over 3 hours. Tubing: 10 gtts/mL.

3. 50 mL penicillin IV over 1 hour. Tubing: 60 gtts/mL.

4. 750 mL RL over 8 hours. Tubing: 15 gtts/mL.

5. 40 mEq KCl in 100 mL NS over 40 minutes. Tubing: 20 gtts/mL.

FLUID BALANCE

Fluid balance is vital for life. Pediatric and *geriatric* (older) patients can easily suffer from dehydration, overhydration, or electrolyte imbalances. Sometimes you need to calculate a patient's input and output of fluids as a measurement of fluid status.

Fluid output is determined by measuring urine (usually in milliters) caught in a special container placed on a toilet. If the patient vomits, the fluid (emesis) should also be measured. Calculating *fluid intake* presents more of a challenge. Patients may comply easily with urinating into a plastic container on their toilet, allowing correct calculation of output. However, patients may not remember to write down a complete log of ingested fluids, especially if they are cognitively impaired. Instruct patients on the importance of keeping an accurate log of both intake and output.

The prescriber usually orders fluid intake restrictions or goals in milliliters, so you may need to teach the patient how to convert household measurements into milliliters or to use metric equipment to measure input and output. Some patients forget how to do conversions, so you need to be able to convert household measurements to metric measurements. Box 10.2 is a reminder of some of these conversions.

BOX 10.2 Common Conversion

Remember:

1 oz	= 8 drams
	= 30 mL
	= 2 T
	= 6 t
	= 360–480 gtts, minims
1 kg	= 2.2 lb
1 lb	= 0.45 kg

For example, a dehydrated child, Nita Page, is required to drink 1500 mL/day. She drank:

> 1 20-oz soda
> 1 8-oz glass of water
> 1 4-oz juice glass of orange juice
> <u>1 8-oz cup of milk</u>
> 40 oz

Did she achieve 1500 mL?

$$40 \text{ oz} \times \frac{30 \text{ mL}}{1 \text{ oz}} = 1200 \text{ mL}$$

$$1200 \text{ mL} < 1500 \text{ mL}$$

No, she did not achieve 1500 mL.

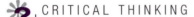 CRITICAL THINKING

What instructions do you need to give this child's parents?

Here is another example: Jeremy Jones has heart failure and is on 1000 mL fluid restriction. Did he achieve it if he drank:

2 6-oz cups of tea	$2 \times 6 = 12$
1 8-oz glass of water	$1 \times 8 = 8$
1 8-oz bowl of milk in cereal	$1 \times 8 = 8$
1 4-oz glass of prune juice	$1 \times 4 = 4$
	32 oz

$$32 \text{ oz} \times \frac{30 \text{ mL}}{1 \text{ oz}} = 960 \text{ mL}$$

$$960 \text{ mL} < 1000 \text{ mL}$$

Yes. Jeremy should be praised!

🔵 CHECK UP

Solve these problems.

1. John Elliott is on 1000 mL fluid restriction. He drank two 10-oz sodas, one 8-oz glass of milk, and one 8-oz cup of coffee. Did he exceed his restriction? Show your work.

2. Kathy Thomas is dehydrated. Her physician ordered her to drink at least 1200 mL/day. Did she achieve this goal if she drank two 12-oz sodas, one 8-oz cup of coffee, and one 8-oz glass of water? Show your work.

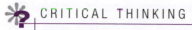

CRITICAL THINKING

Coffee, caffeinated sodas, and beer have a diuretic effect on the kidneys, meaning that they increase urination. Although consumption of these fluids does count as hydration, what would be better choices for dehydrated patients?

SUMMARY

It does not matter whether you calculate by dimensional analysis, formula method, fractions, ratio and proportion, or word problems. You should use the technique that is easiest for you and gives you the correct answer. You can use one of the other methods to double-check your mathematics. Always check your answer to be sure it is accurate and reasonable. That extra precaution can save a patient's life.

Activities

To make sure that you have learned the key points covered in this chapter, complete the following activities.

Calculate the following using dimensional analysis.

1. Order: 100 mg   Label: 50 mg/mL

2. Order: 2 oz   Label: 1 oz/30 mL

3. Order: 10,000 units   Label: 1000 units/mL

4. Order: 500 mg   Label: 250 mg/tablet

5. Order: 300 mg   Label: 100 mg/capsule

6. Order: 125 mg   Label: 250 mg/mL

7. Order: 125 mg   Label: 75 mg/mL

8. Order: 250 mg   Label: 1000 mg/bottle

9. Order: 250 mg   Label: 125 mg/mL

10. Order: 1 gram   Label: 500 mg/capsule

Use the formula method to calculate the following.

D	H/Q
1. 1.5 grams	500 mg/capsule
2. 90 mL	30 mL/oz
3. 200 mg	100 mg/tablet
4. 0.5 gram	1000 mg/bottle
5. 160 mg	80 mg/tablet
6. 600 mg	300 mg/capsule
7. 200 mg	100 mg/tablet
8. 750 mg	250 mg/tablet
9. 125 mg	250 mg/mL
10. 25 mg	100 mg/mL

Calculate the following using fractions.

Order	Label

1. 200 mg   100 mg/2 mL

2. 250 mg   500 mg/tablet

3. 160 mg   80 mg/capsule

4. 350 mg   70 mg/mL

5. 75 mg   150 mg/mL

6. 1000 units   500 units/mL

7. 250 mg   125 mg/mL

8. 25 mg   50 mg/tablet

9. 0.5 gram   500 mg/mL

10. 1 gram   500 mg/tablet

Using ratio and proportion, calculate the following.

1. 100 mg : 1 tablet :: 200 mg : ? tablets

2. 1000 units : 1 mL :: 10,000 units : ? mL

3. 1 gram : 1000 mL :: 500 mg : ? mL

4. 1 oz : 30 mL :: ? oz : 90 mL

5. 2 T : 1 oz :: ? T : 4 oz

6. 1 oz : 8 drams :: 3 oz : ? drams

7. 4 oz : 1 oz :: ? mL : 30 mL

8. 250 mg : 500 mg :: ? mL : 1 mL

9. 1000 units : 10,000 units :: ? mL : 1 mL

10. 500 mg : 250 mg :: ? mL : 1 mL

In your own words, create word problems for solving the following using a separate sheet.

1. 100 mg : 200 mg :: 1 tablet : ? tablets

2. 250 mg : 500 mg :: 1 capsule : ? capsules

3. D = 50 mg, H = 100 mg, Q = 1 mL

4. Rx = 100 mg. Label: 5 mg/mL

5. Rx = 1,000,000 units. Label: 1000 units/mL

Use the BSA nomogram in this chapter to determine the BSA for each of these patients.

Patient	Weight	Height
1	15 lb	24 inches
2	18 kg	35 inches
3	100 lb	60 inches
4	50 kg	62 inches
5	86 lb	58 inches

Give the flow rate for an IV solution that is being infused through an electronic pump.

1. 50 mL over 2 hours

2. 2500 mL over 4 hours

3. 1000 mL over 8 hours

4. 500 mL over 3 hours

5. 1000 mL over 2 hours

Give flow rates in gtts/min for a solution that is being infused through a manual IV setup.

1. 1000 mL D_5RL over 8 hours set at 20 gtts/mL

2. 500 mL NSS over 4 hours set at 10 gtts/mL

3. 1500 mL RL over 6 hours set at 60 gtts/mL

4. 2500 mL NS over 10 hours set at 20 gtts/mL

5. 1000 mL D_5 and $^1/_2$ NS over 6 hours set at 20 gtts/mL

6. 90 mL NS over 1 hour set at 15 gtts/mL

7. 50 mL over 40 minutes set at 10 gtts/mL

8. 200 mL NS over 2 hours set at 10 gtts/mL

9. Kefzol 0.5 gram in 50 mL D_5W over 30 minutes set at 60 gtts/mL

10. 250 mL $^1/_2$ NSS over 5 hours set at 20 gtts/mL

Application Exercises
Respond to the following scenarios on a separate sheet.

1. Dr. McCauley orders 400 mg. The label reads 100 mg is found in 1 mL. **How many cubic centimeters (cc) do you inject?**
2. Dr. Palmer orders 10,000 units of a drug. On hand you have 1000 units. The quantity is 1 mL. **How many mL do you give?**
3. Dr. Seiler orders 500 mg. The label says 250 mg/mL. **What do you give?**

4. The examination question says:
   100 mg : 1 mL :: 250 mg : ? mL. **What do you answer?**

5. You are asked to make a large quantity of 10% bleach solution. **If you need 20 mL of solution, how much bleach do you need?**

6. Emily Jane weighs 44 lb. If the doctor orders a medication for 10 mg/kg/day, **how much should she get per day?**

7. If the above patient was ordered a drug for 20 mg/kg/dose with two doses per day, **how much does she get per day?**

8. When Martia Shapiro goes to the drug cabinet, she notes that there is 1 gram of a medication in a bottle. She adds 4 mL of sterile water. This yields 250 mg/mL. **If the ordered dose is 500 mg, what should she give?**

9. Mr. Belcher calls to try to understand how to compute his child's fluid intake. All he has at home are regular cups, glasses, and mugs. **What would you suggest he do?**

10. Matthew Murphy-Moore is on 1000 mL fluid restriction. **Does he exceed it if he drinks two 20-oz. sodas, one 8 oz glass of milk, and one 4 oz juice glass of orange juice? Show your work.**

11. You notice that a nurse has not set the correct IV drip dose for an electronic pump. **What would you do or say?**

12. Kathy Helbert is having an infusion. She needs to pick up her children by 4:30 p.m. at the day care center. If the infusion begins at 10 a.m. at 125 mL/hr and she needs 750 mL, **will she be able to pick up her children on time?**

13. Gloria Loving is having an IV infusion. She is supposed to be finished in 2 hours at 150 mL/hr, and there is 450 mL left in the bag. **Is it infusing correctly? Show your work.**

Virtual Field Trips

Go to the following websites to find the information. If a website is not available, try to find the information through another source.

1. Visit http://www.discoveryschool.com and work on some of the above ratio and proportions problems. Print your work.
2. Surf to http://www.chemistrycoach.com and take the tutorial on dimensional analysis. Print your information.
3. Go to http://www.purplemath.com and gather information on how to translate word problems.
4. Visit http://school.discovery.com and work some fraction problems. Print your work.

   Note: If these websites are unavailable, go to http://dogpile.com and search for similar websites that can help you learn about ratio and proportion, dimensional analysis, and translating word problems.

5. Go to http://www.dogpile.com and search for a site to instruct patients on pediatric dosages. Print a teaching tool.
6. Visit your favorite search engine. Search for the key word "Body Surface Area," and print your own copy of the BSA nomogram.
7. Find three sites that manufacture IV tubing, and see what is used as a drop factor.

Classifications of Drugs

Nervous System Medications

The remaining chapters of this book discuss common medication classifications. (See Appendix A at the back of this text for a list of drug classifications and their general effects.) You need to recall your knowledge of physiology so you can understand how drugs work and how to administer them safely. Each chapter covers categories under the main classification and contains Master the Essentials tables, which contain key examples of side effects, contraindications (conditions under which a drug should not be given), precautions, and interactions.

Medications that affect the neurological system include psychotropic drugs, which influence the mind, emotions, and behaviors. Other medications include drugs to treat pain and fever, anesthetics, drugs for seizure control, and more. Neuropharmacology is the most complex branch of pharmacology because it involves the most complex system in the body—the nervous system.

OBJECTIVES

At the end of this chapter, the student will be able to:

- Define all key terms.
- List characteristics of neurological drugs.
- Discuss the side effects of each classification of nervous system medications: adrenergics, sympathomimetics, adrenergic blockers, cholinergics, parasympathomimetics, anticholinergics/cholinergic blockers, analgesics, anxiolytics, barbiturates, central nervous system (CNS) stimulants, antimanics, neuroleptics, antiparkinsonian agents, anesthetics, alcohol, and antidepressants.
- Describe safety precautions necessary when patients are anesthetized.

KEY TERMS

Adrenergic	GABA	Peripheral
Aura	Hallucination	Psychotropic
Autonomic	Hydantoins	Somatic
Cholinergic	Mania	SSRIs
Contraindications	MAO inhibitors	Status epilepticus
Delusion	Migraine headache	Succinimides
Dementia	Neurotransmitters	Sympathetic
Depression	Paranoia	Synapse
EEG	Parasympathetic	Tension headache

● NEUROLOGICAL MEDICATIONS

The nervous system is divided into the central nervous system (CNS), the peripheral nervous system, and the autonomic nervous system. The CNS includes the brain and spinal cord. The brain acts on information from inside and outside the body. It processes the information and tells the body how to respond. For example, the brain senses you are cold and tells the body to shiver to raise the temperature. Another example is when your body is not getting enough glucose because you skipped lunch; the brain then stimulates a headache, reminding you to eat.

A dysfunctional brain or one that is under the influence of mind-altering drugs can create information not consistent with reality. The body acts on that information as though it is real. For example, patients may be frightened because they believe people are out to get them. Psychotropic drugs can change the way patients behave and experiences the environment, so they can respond appropriately.

Nervous system medications are used to treat pain, anxiety, depression, mania, insomnia, convulsions, and schizophrenia. They act on the CNS and the peripheral nervous system (outside the spinal cord throughout the body) (Fig. 11.1). Because the peripheral nervous system extends throughout the body, these drugs can affect other body systems. For example, a drug meant to ease uterine pain may relieve leg pain too.

Most of these drugs act at the synapse (gap) between nerves and can adjust the transmission of messages by neurotransmitters (chemicals that facilitate the movement of messages across the synapses). These medications might excite the CNS or depress it. Because these drugs are powerful enough to cross the blood–brain barrier (a barrier in the brain that prevents toxic substances and some medications from entering the brain), they frequently have serious side effects. (See the Master the Essentials table for descriptions of the most common nervous system drugs.)

Medications of the Autonomic Nervous System

The peripheral nervous system consists of the somatic (voluntary) and autonomic (involuntary) systems (Fig. 11.2), which sense the environment and, usually after consulting the brain, respond to it. Drugs in this section include those that affect the autonomic system.

The autonomic system consists of two parts: the sympathetic system, which controls the body's "fight or flight" response, and the parasympathetic system, which helps the body rest and relax. Acetylcholine and norepinephrine are the two main neurotransmitters that affect the autonomic nervous system. A nerve cell that releases acetylcholine is referred to as being cholinergic. One that releases epinephrine or norepinephrine is referred to as being adrenergic.

Autonomic drugs that act on the sympathetic system (also called sympathomimetics or adrenergic agonists) stimulate the nervous system. Drugs that act on the parasympathetic system (also called parasympathomimetics or cholinergic agonists) calm the nervous system.

Adrenergics

Adrenergic drugs are called sympathomimetics because they mimic the sympathetic nervous system, exciting the fight or flight impulse. They stimulate the heart, increase blood flow to the skeletal

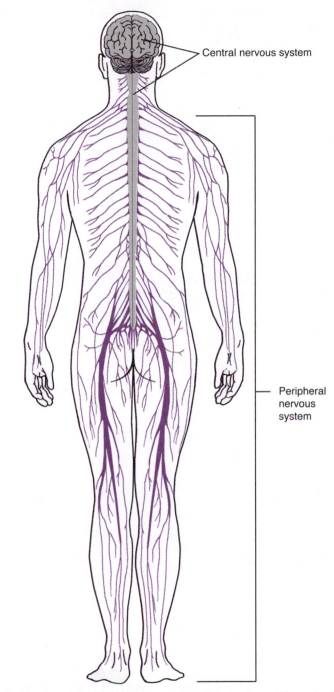

Central nervous system

Peripheral nervous system

FIGURE 11.1. Central and peripheral nervous systems. The brain and the spinal cord make up the central nervous system. The peripheral nervous system contains nerves outside of the brain and spinal cord that go to the arms, legs, hands, and feet.

muscles, and constrict peripheral blood vessels, which in turn leads to dilation of parts of the body, such as the bronchi and pupils.

Adrenergics are used to restore heart rhythm during cardiac arrest. They also increase blood pressure in cases of shock. They constrict capillaries if the patient is bleeding—for example, if the patient has a nosebleed. Adrenergics can dilate the bronchioles of the patient with asthma or the pupils for patients having eye procedures.

Adrenergic blockers. As the name suggests, adrenergic blockers block the action of adrenergics and thus have a parasympathetic effect. They shut off what the adrenergics do. Thus, they are useful for treating cardiac arrhythmias (heart rhythm problems), high blood pressure, migraine headaches, and chest pain.

Alpha blockers work on vascular smooth muscle. Beta blockers affect the heart, where beta-1 receptors are found.

Cholinergics. Cholinergics mimic the action of the parasympathetic system. Releasing acetylcholine relaxes the body's fight or flight mechanism. Cholinergics are rarely used because they severely slow the body systems (including the heart rate) and constrict respiratory passages. Nerve gases are an example of this class.

Anticholinergics or cholinergic blockers. Anticholinergics or cholinergic blockers inhibit the parasympathetic branch of the autonomic nervous system and thus promote fight or flight symptoms. These drugs dry secretions, including those in the respiratory tract. They can therefore be used for asthma and motion sickness. They are used for preoperative relaxation, neuromuscular blocking of spasms, antidotes for insect stings, and cholinergic crises. In an emergency, they can be used to treat a slow heart rate, heart block, or bronchospasm.

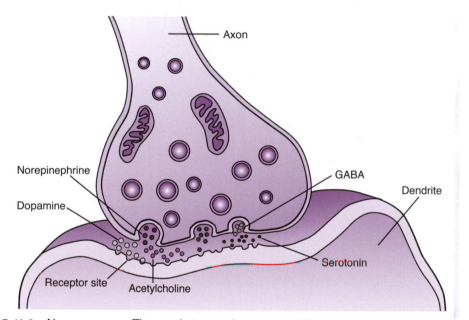

FIGURE 11.2. Nerve synapse. The gap between the axon and the dendrite of a nerve is called the synapse. Neurotransmitters such as gaba, serotonin, dopamine, norepinephrine, and acetylcholine help transmit the electrical impulse from the axon to the dendrite. The neurotransmitters fit into receptors on the dendrites. Some psychotropic drugs act by inhibiting the work of the neurotransmitters, thereby slowing the electrical impulses; others act by stimulating neurotransmitters, thereby promoting electrical impulses.

Master the Essentials: Nervous System Medications

This table shows the various classes of nervous system medications and key side effects, contraindications and precautions, and interactions for each class.

CLASS	SIDE EFFECTS	CONTRAINDICATIONS/PRECAUTIONS	INTERACTIONS
Adrenergics	Chest pain, fast heart rate, headache, increased blood glucose, nervousness, tissue death, tremors	Brain damage, cardiovascular and heart problems, glaucoma, hyperthyroidism	Adrenergic blockers, CNS drugs
Adrenergic blockers	Confusion; decreased blood pressure, blood glucose, energy, heart rate	Asthma, atrioventricular block (heart block), chronic heart failure, diabetes, low blood pressure	Alcohol, digitalis, epinephrine, insulin, MAO inhibitors (drugs that inhibit the action of monoamine oxidase), theophylline, tricyclic antidepressants
Cholinergics	Bronchospasm; decreased heart rate, respirations, blood pressure; increased salivation, tears, and sweating; muscle cramps and weakness	Asthma, benign prostatic hypertension, cardiac disease, gastrointestinal (GI) disorders, hyperthyroidism	Quinidine, procainamide
Anticholinergics	Blurred vision, confusion, decreased GI and genitourinary (GU) motility, dilation of pupils, drying of secretions, fever, flushing, headache, increased heart rate	Asthma, cardiac arrhythmias, chronic obstructive pulmonary disease (COPD), GI or GU obstruction, glaucoma, high blood pressure	Digoxin, nitroglycerin, tricyclic antidepressants
Salicylates	Coma, depression, dizziness, headache, drowsiness, increased bleeding time, bruising, GI bleeding, headache, liver and kidney disorders, tinnitus, rash	Asthma, bleeding disorders, lactation, pregnancy, vitamin K deficiency	Alcohol, antacids, anticoagulants, heparin, NSAIDs, insulin
Acetaminophen	Rash, urticaria (High dosages can cause kidney and liver failure.)	Alcohol abuse, hypersensitivity, liver disease, malnutrition	Alcohol, oral contraceptives, phenytoin, loop diuretics
NSAIDs	Blurred vision, constipation, dizziness, drowsiness, dyspepsia, edema, GI bleeding, headache, hepatitis, irregular heart rate, kidney disorders, prolonged bleeding, psychic disturbances, rash, tinnitus	Active GI bleeding, cardiovascular (CV) disease, hypersensitivity, liver disease, pregnancy, renal disease, ulcer	Corticosteroids, salicylates, cyclosporine, anticoagulants, beta blockers, digoxin

(table continued on page 208)

Master the Essentials: Nervous System Medications (continued)

CLASS	SIDE EFFECTS	CONTRAINDICATIONS/PRECAUTIONS	INTERACTIONS
Narcotics	Decreased blood pressure, heart rate, and respirations; agitation, blurred vision, confusion, constipation, flushing, headache, oversedation, rash, restlessness, seizures, urinary retention	Lactation and pregnancy. Patients with head injury, CNS depression, COPD, hypothyroidism, liver or kidney disease. Use with caution in addicted patients, children, elderly patients, hypersensitive patients, suicidal patients.	Alcohol, antiemetics, antihistamines, antihypertensives, antiarrhythmics, muscle relaxers, psychotropics, sedative-hypnotics
Anxiolytics	Agitation, amnesia, bizarre behaviors, confusion, decreased white blood cell count, depression, drowsiness, hallucinations, headache, lack of coordination, lethargy, oversedation, sensitivity to light, tremors	Children, decreased vital signs, depression, lactation, pregnancy, thoughts of suicide. Observe for addiction and for evidence that the patient is considering suicide.	Alcohol, antiemetics, antihistamines, analgesics, CNS depressants, digoxin, grapefruit juice, muscle relaxants, phenytoin, psychotropics
Barbiturates	Lethargy, dizziness, irritability, constipation, vessel swelling, confusion, decreased respirations and heart rate, bone softening, coma, fatal overdose, unsteady balance, liver inflammation, bone marrow suppression, vision disorders, anorexia, inflammation of the gums	Pregnancy, hypersensitivity, hepatitis, cardiac and renal disease, hemolytic disorders, decreased heart rate	Alcohol, analgesics, antacids, antineoplastics, CNS depressants, corticosteroids, folic acid, grapefruit juice, MAO inhibitors, oral anticoagulants, oral contraceptives, theophylline, sedatives
CNS Stimulants	Nervousness, insomnia, irritability, seizures or psychosis; increased heart rate, blood pressure, and irregularity of heart rhythm; dizziness, headache, blurred vision, GI disorders, dependence	Nervousness, insomnia, irritability, seizures or psychosis; increased heart rate, blood pressure, and irregularity of heart rhythm; dizziness, headache, blurred vision, GI disorders, dependence	Antacids, anticoagulants, anticonvulsants, clonidine, tricyclic antidepressants
MAO Inhibitors	Nervousness, headache, stiff neck, increased heart rate and blood pressure, diarrhea, blurred vision	Known hypersensitivity, heart disease, hepatic or renal impairment, headaches, cerebrovascular disease, pregnancy, lactation	Adrenergics, diuretics, antidepressants, CNS depressants, insulin, levodopa, foods containing tyramine, herbs such as St. John's wort

CLASS	SIDE EFFECTS	CONTRAINDICATIONS/PRECAUTIONS	INTERACTIONS
TCAs	Dry mouth, increased appetite, weight gain, blurred vision, drowsiness, dizziness, constipation, urinary retention, postural low blood pressure, irregular heart rhythms, confusion	Pregnancy and lactation; cardiac, kidney, liver, and GI disorders; glaucoma; obesity; seizures	Alcohol, CNS drugs, MAO inhibitors
SSRIs	Sexual dysfunction, anorexia, diarrhea, sweating, insomnia, anxiety, nervousness, tremor, fatigue, dizziness, drowsiness, headache	Pregnancy and lactation, patients with thoughts of suicide, diabetes, bipolar disorders, eating disorders	CNS drugs, MAO inhibitors, anticoagulants, beta blockers, antiarrhythmics
Lithium	GI distress, decreased blood pressure, cardiac irregularities, increased urination, tremors, thyroid problems	Seizure disorders, Parkinson's disease; CV, kidney, and thyroid diseases; dehydration, pregnancy, lactation	NSAIDs, diuretics, ACE inhibitors, sodium salts
Antipsychotics	ECG changes, hypotension, agitation, dizziness, sedation, drowsiness, dystonia, headache, constipation, dry mouth, photosensitivity, nausea	Known hypersensitivity, cardiac arrhythmias, seizure disorder, thyroid disease, renal or hepatic impairment	Anticholinergics, CNS depressants, alcohol, beta blockers, caffeine, antidepressants, lithium
Antiparkinsonian drugs	Involuntary movements, loss of appetite, anxiety, confusion, depression, psychosis, decreased blood pressure, dizziness, fainting	Pregnancy and lactation, asthma and emphysema, cardiac disease, decreased blood pressure, peptic ulcer, diabetes, glaucoma	Benzodiazepines, pyridoxine, phenothiazines, haloperidol, antihypertensives, phenytoin, vitamin B_6, MAO inhibitors
Local anesthetics	Heart block, hypotension, bradycardia, arrhythmias, restlessness, anxiety, dizziness, headache, nausea, vomiting	Known hypersensitivity, severe hypertension, shock, hematologic disorders, psychosis	Sedatives, sulfonamides
General anesthetics	Cardiopulmonary depression, confusion, sedation, nausea, vomiting, hypothermia, malignant hyperthermia	Known hypersensitivity, hepatic disorder, malignant hyperthermia, pregnancy, lactation	CNS depressants, neuromuscular blockers, catecholamines

● MEDICATIONS FOR CONTROL OF PAIN AND FEVER

Pain is an unpleasant sensory and emotional experience arising from actual or potential tissue damage. The perception of pain varies greatly among patients, but it is important to treat each person's pain based on his or her description of it. Pain management is based on a thorough patient assessment that includes the location and intensity of the pain.

A CLOSER LOOK: Headaches

There are two main types of headache. *Tension headaches* occur when the head and neck area become tight because of tension and stress. This causes a steady throbbing pain. These headaches can usually be treated with NSAIDs or mild narcotics.

Migraine headaches are more painful. They are usually preceded by a sensory cue known as an *aura.* The aura may include the perception of flashing lights, smelling bizarre odors, tasting food in the mouth when none exists, and hearing sounds that do not exist. The pain is often localized behind the eye, and patients often have nausea and vomiting. Mild analgesics may help with tension headaches, but migraines need special medications, such as sumatriptan (Imitrex), to prevent or stop the pain.

Triggers for migraines

Environmental
    Changes in barometric pressure and weather
    Bright colors
    Unusual odors
    Sun glare
    Tobacco smoke
Emotional/hormonal
    Stress and anxiety
    Fatigue
    Pregnancy
    Menstruation
    Decreased blood
      glucose
    Physical/sexual stress
Food
    Alcohol
    Aged cheese
    Aspertame
      (NutraSweet)
    Caffeine
    Chocolate
    Monosodium
      glutamate (MSG)
Medications
    Tagamet
    Nifedipine
    Theophylline

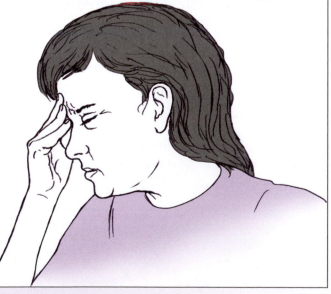

Analgesics reduce pain without eliminating feeling or sensation, which occurs with anesthetics. Choices include salicylates, acetaminophen, nonsteroidal antiinflammatory drugs (NSAIDs), and narcotics. Some of these drugs are also antipyretic, which means they reduce fever.

Salicylates

Salicylates, such as aspirin (acetylsalicylic acid), relieve mild to moderate pain and reduce inflammation and fever. Salicylates are also used to decrease inflammation in blood vessels, thus improving cardiovascular flow. Aspirin has the disadvantage of causing gastrointestinal (GI) distress and should not be used in children with viral infections.

Methylsalicylate is a topical antiinflammatory medication used to irritate the surface of the skin. This irritation increases blood flow to the area where it was applied, which decreases pain by increasing blood flow. An example of this classification is Bengay.

CRITICAL THINKING

Why would buccal powders (aspirin in a powder form you put in your cheek) work faster than aspirin tablets?

Acetaminophen

Acetaminophen (Tylenol) decreases pain but does not have an antiinflammatory effect. This drug is frequently an ingredient in combination products used to relieve pain, colds, or the flu. Because it typically does not produce severe side effects, acetaminophen is frequently combined with narcotics to treat moderate to severe pain.

NSAIDs

Salicylates are NSAIDs, but this term usually refers to other drugs in this category such as ibuprofen (Motrin). These drugs reduce both pain and swelling caused by inflammation.

Narcotics

Although most pain can be reduced without narcotics, they are excellent choices for pain not relieved by weaker drugs. Narcotics are generally made from opium, extracted from the poppy plant.

Narcotics are strong painkillers, but they are also CNS depressants. Too much narcotic can slow a patient's respirations to dangerous levels.

Opioid analgesics are the strongest. They are not routinely prescribed because of their addictive potential and the severe side effects they can produce, particularly in large doses. Because narcotics produce euphoria, or happy feelings, they can also cause physiological or psychological dependence. However, if a patient has pain that does not respond to other medications, he or she should not be denied adequate pain relief out of concern for addiction or dependence. Narcotics are rarely addictive in patients taking them for relief of acute pain. Narcotics can also be used for general anesthesia during surgery.

Sometimes combining analgesics with alternative methods of pain relief, such as meditation, can reduce pain effectively.

CRITICAL THINKING

What methods, other than drugs, can be used to decrease pain?

DRUGS FOR ANXIETY, INSOMNIA, SEDATION, AND SEIZURES

Medications can help relieve anxiety, promote sleep, reduce alertness, or help stop seizures.

Anxiolytic Medications

Anxiety is apprehension, tension, or uneasiness that stems from the anticipation of danger, the source of which is often unknown or unrecognized. In summary, it is an inappropriate fear. Some fears are exaggerations of normal anxieties (heights, animals), and others are based on previous experiences (such as being trapped on an elevator). Below is a list of phobias (fears). Use a medical dictionary to define them on a separate sheet.

- Acrophobia
- Agoraphobia
- Ailurophobia
- Arachnophobia
- Claustrophobia
- Mysophobia
- Panophobia
- Xenophobia
- Zoophobia

Examples of anxiety disorders are generalized anxiety disorder and panic disorder.

Anxiolytics reduce anxiety. They can be taken routinely or only when the patient feels anxiety building. These drugs work in the limbic system of the brain. CNS depressants treat anxiety and restlessness. Benzodiazepines are used for anxiety, seizures, alcohol withdrawal symptoms, and muscle relaxation. They can also be used to reduce anxiety before general anesthesia.

Barbiturates

Insomnia (having trouble sleeping) is a common complaint from patients. Sometimes barbiturates are used to induce sleep. They are also used to help the patient relax before a minor procedure or general surgery.

Antiseizure Medications

Barbiturates are also used to control seizures. Barbiturates that are hydantoins (e.g., phenytoin) delay sodium crossing the neural membranes. This decreases the potential for too much electrical activity and calms the cell. Succinimides are a class of antiseizure drugs that delay calcium moving over the neurons. Like hydantoins, they relax nerve cells.

Another type of antiseizure drug stimulates the neurotransmitter called gamma-aminobutyric acid (GABA) to suppress abnormal neural activity (see Fig. 11.2). Benzodiazepines can also intensify the effect of GABA transmitters in the brain.

Some drugs used to decrease seizures also help manage the symptoms of alcohol withdrawal.

A CLOSER LOOK: Seizures

Abnormal electrical activity in the brain can cause seizures. A patient may have a diagnostic test called electroencephalography (EEG) to detect seizure activity. Seizures may be mild (petit mal) or severe (grand mal). The most severe seizure is one that does not stop after a few minutes. It is called status epilepticus and requires immediate medical intervention—usually with IV benzodiazepines.

⬤ MEDICATIONS FOR BEHAVIORAL/EMOTIONAL/MOOD DISORDERS

Behavioral and emotional disorders are increasingly more common in the United States. Mood disorders are characterized by extreme emotions—very elevated (mania) and very low (depression). Some patients bounce between mania and depression, a condition called bipolar disorder. Several categories of drugs can be used to help patients with these disorders.

CNS Stimulants

Attention deficit disorder (ADD) and attention deficit with hyperactivity disorder (ADHD) are common in both children and adults. These disorders stem from the ineffectiveness of the impulse control center in the frontal cortex of the brain.

It may seem counterintuitive to give a distracted, unfocused, overactive patient a stimulant, but CNS stimulants cause the impulse control center to control impulses—thus calming the patient and increasing the ability to focus. People who do not have ADD/ADHD but are abusing a drug in this category find that it acts as a CNS stimulant.

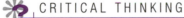 CRITICAL THINKING

> **If someone without ADHD uses a stimulant, they become hyperactive. Why does it have the reverse effect on the patient with ADHD?**

Sometimes an amphetamine, a type of CNS stimulant, is prescribed for obesity. Usually it is given 30 to 60 minutes before meals to speed up the metabolism, but only for short periods of time. It is best for weight loss that diet and exercise regimens be used concurrently with amphetamine use for weight loss.

CRITICAL THINKING

> **Why should obese patients not be routinely given amphetamines for weight loss?**

Antidepressants

Clinical depression is characterized by excesses of sleeping and eating, an inability to concentrate, avoidance of the companionship of other people, decreased interest in sex and activities one usually enjoys, and feelings of despair. Depression is usually a combination of genetic and environmental causes and can be devastating to the patient.

Antidepressants preserve neurotransmitters at the synapse. When neurotransmitters are depleted, the patient does not think as clearly as usual, and the mood becomes depressed.

Three categories of antidepressant agents are monoamine oxidase (MAO) inhibitors, tricyclics, and selective serotonin reuptake inhibitors (SSRIs).

MAO inhibitors

MAO inhibitors inhibit monoamine oxidase, an enzyme that terminates the action of neurotransmitters at the synapse. Inhibiting or stopping MAO improves the retention of neurotransmitters at the site. Unfortunately, this drug classification requires dietary exclusion of foods containing tyramine (Box 11.1). Because tyramine is common in many foods, these drugs are rarely prescribed.

 CRITICAL THINKING

> **If a patient on an MAO inhibitor went to a Super Bowl party, which foods would he or she be unable to eat?**

BOX 11.1   Foods High in Tyramine

Avocados	Papayas
Bananas	Paté, beef
Beer	Pepperoni
Bologna	Raisins
Chocolate	Salami
Dairy products, aged	Sausage
Fava beans	Soy sauce
Figs	Wine
Herring	Yeast
Hot dogs	

Tricyclic antidepressants

Tricyclic antidepressants (TCAs) are medications with a three-ring (tricyclic) chemical structure that keeps norepinephrine and serotonin at the nerve terminals, thereby helping electrical impulses cross the synapse (see Fig. 11.2). These drugs have been used for decades but have many more side effects than the currently more popular SSRIs.

Selective serotonin reuptake inhibitors

SSRIs prevent serotonin from being used up at the synapse. Low serotonin levels have been implicated in depression, and keeping serotonin at the synapse improves mood. Because they have so few side effects compared to MAO inhibitors and TCAs, they are frequently the first classification of drug prescribed for depression. However, each drug within the classification can affect the patient differently. If one drug does not work well for the patient, the prescriber may change the dosage or change to another medication.

CRITICAL THINKING

Why are antidepressants used to decrease pain?

Mood-Stabilizing Medications

Mood stabilizers (antimanic agents) stabilize the extreme mood shifts seen in patients with bipolar disorder. Therapy can decrease the number and intensity of manic episodes.

A common drug used to treat bipolar disorder is lithium. Lithium is a salt, so it is important that patients on lithium not get dehydrated and that they also avoid table salt. There is a small therapeutic range for lithium; lithium toxicity can be fatal, so blood lithium assays must be performed regularly. Signs of toxicity include drowsiness, blurred vision, confusion, sensitivity to light, tremors, muscle weakness, cardiovascular collapse, seizures, and coma.

CRITICAL THINKING

Why must a patient who is on lithium be careful not to become dehydrated?

Medications for Treating Psychoses

Psychoses are disorders in which the patient has abnormal thoughts, disorganized communication, and lack of interaction with the environment. Delusions (fixed, false beliefs), hallucinations (sensory experience not based on reality), paranoia (fear someone is trying to hurt you), and bizarre thoughts and behaviors are frequent symptoms of psychoses.

Antipsychotic mediations, called neuroleptics, treat the positive symptoms (doing things that are not normal) and negative symptoms (not having behaviors that normal patients do). Some antipsychotic medications are used for nausea and vomiting, dementia, agitation, and spasms as well as for psychoses. Be sure you know why the neuroleptic was prescribed.

MEDICATIONS FOR DEGENERATIVE DISORDERS

Dementia is a progressive, irreversible decline in mental function. Alzheimer's disease and vascular changes can cause dementia. At this time few drugs are available to treat dementia, and they produce only a minor reduction in symptoms of confusion and decreased memory.

CRITICAL THINKING

If a patient is diagnosed with dementia, what precautions may need to be taken in the home?

Parkinson's disease is a degenerative disorder of the CNS. When neurons that produce the neurotransmitter dopamine die, it leads to disorganization of muscle movements. Tremors, slow movement, rigid muscles, and balance problems are characteristic of this disease. Antiparkinsonian drugs focus on keeping dopamine and acetylcholine at the nerve synapse, thereby promoting the transmission of nerve signals. They are classified as dopaminergic (replacing or increasing dopamine) or cholinergic agents.

MEDICATIONS FOR LOCAL AND GENERAL ANESTHESIA

Anesthesia means loss of sensation. Local anesthesia creates a lack of feeling without loss of consciousness; general anesthetics cause patients to lose both feeling and consciousness.

Local Anesthesia

Local anesthesia can be applied to a surface to numb an area before a procedure. The local anesthetic blocks the entry of sodium ions into nerve fibers. Adequate amounts must be applied or injected to keep the area numb throughout the procedure. Local anesthetics are classified as esters or amides, depending on the structure of their molecules.

Amides, such as lidocaine and novocaine, tend to last longer, so they are more popular. Adverse effects and allergies are rare. The patient must be observed during the procedure to be sure the anesthetic is still in effect and for any negative reactions. Be sure to document your observations.

General Anesthesia

General anesthetics can be administered by intravenous (IV) infusion or inhalation. For longer procedures, an IV agent may be used initially, followed by inhalation therapy.

CRITICAL THINKING

Why would an IV anesthetic be given before an inhaled gas is administered by mask?

Inhaled general anesthetics are volatile agents that can depress respiratory and cardiovascular function, so patients must be carefully observed during procedures. An example is nitrous oxide, which is used for dental and brief surgical procedures. These agents can be combined with other medications to decrease dosages of both.

ALCOHOL

Alcohol, which is a CNS depressant, is rarely prescribed as a medication. However, it interacts with other medications and can have powerful effects on the body, including confusion, peripheral vasodilation, increased heart rate, electrolyte imbalances, decreased motor coordination, unsteady gait, and slurred speech. Prolonged use can permanently damage the CNS and liver.

Signs and symptoms of chronic alcoholism include irritability, tremors, GI disorders, frequent falling accidents, blackouts, memory loss, confusion, neural and muscular weakness, and conjunctivitis. Treatment includes disulfiram (Antabuse), behavior modification, vitamin B injections, and dietary changes (e.g., supplements to replace vitamins lost through poor nutrition).

Patients abusing alcohol should be assessed for respiratory problems, vomiting, convulsions, cerebral swelling, electrolyte imbalances, and tremors when withdrawing from alcohol.

SUMMARY

Medications that affect the central and peripheral nervous systems can be used to treat many brain and nervous system disorders, ranging from mild headaches to severe symptoms of Parkinson's disease. Always carefully assess any patient on medications that affect the neurological system—any drug that crosses the blood–brain barrier has the risk of creating severe side effects and permanent damage.

Activities

To make sure that you have learned the key points covered in this chapter, complete the following activities.

True or False
Write *true* if the statement is true. Beside the false statements, write *false* and correct the statement to make it true.

1. Parasympathomimetics have few therapeutic uses because of side effects. _____

2. Sympathomimetics are used to treat hypertension. _____

3. Beta blockers work on blood vessels. _____

4. Synapses are the most common site of drug action. _____

5. For more severe insomnia, benzodiazepines are prescribed. _____

6. Alpha blockers are prescribed for seizure disorders. _____

7. Some antiseizure drugs are used to manage alcohol withdrawal. _____

8. Benzodiazepines are used for anxiety. _____

9. Phenytoin delays calcium moving across nerves. _____

10. NSAIDs prevent migraine headaches. _____

Multiple Choice
Choose the best answer for each question.

1. The classification of drugs used to treat ADHD is
   a. Benzodiazepines
   b. CNS depressants
   c. CNS stimulants
   d. Narcotic analgesics

2. The classification of drugs usually used for routine dental procedures is
   a. Benzodiazepines
   b. Anesthetics
   c. Barbiturates
   d. Beta blockers

3. The classification of drugs used to prevent status epilepticus is:
   a. SSRIs
   b. NSAIDs
   c. Benzodiazepines
   d. Neuroleptics

4. The classification of drugs usually used for treating depression is:
   a. SSRIs
   b. EEGs
   c. Benzodiazepines
   d. Neuroleptics

5. Which of the following is *not* usually used for surgical procedures?
   a. Analgesics
   b. Anesthetics
   c. Antidepressants
   d. Antiinfectives

6. Which is a side effect of cholinergics?
   a. Flushing
   b. Confusion
   c. Blurred vision
   d. Slow heart rate

7. Which is *not* a side effect of SSRIs?
   a. Anxiety
   b. Tremor
   c. Sexual dysfunction
   d. Constipation

8. Which is *not* a side effect of anticonvulsant drugs?
   a. Dizziness
   b. Inflammation of the gums
   c. Sedation
   d. Increased blood pressure

9. Which of the following is used to decrease delusions and hallucinations?
   a. Antipyretics
   b. Antipsychotics
   c. Antidepressants
   d. Antiinfectives

10. Which is *not* a side effect of tricyclic antidepressants?
   a. Constipation
   b. Confusion
   c. Decreased appetite
   d. Decreased blood pressure

Application Exercises

Respond to the following scenarios on a separate sheet of paper.

1. Mirium Muhammed is very anxious about a surgery that is to be performed in 1 hour. **What techniques might you use to calm her?**
2. Hamsi Amro has ADHD. His family cannot understand why he is being given a CNS stimulant. **How would you explain this therapy to them?**
3. Perlita Mercedes is having surgery on her hand. The physician applied a topical anesthetic. **How can you tell if it is working?**
4. Ruth Schuknecht has tension headaches. Her sister takes Imitrex for migraines. She asks for Imitrex. **Explain to her why the nurse practitioner did not prescribe Imitrex for her.**
5. Dorothy Ko is pregnant and would prefer not to take any drugs during her labor. **Discuss alternatives for narcotics in labor.**

Virtual Field Trips

Go to the following websites to find the information. If a website is not available, try to find the information through another source.

1. Visit http://www.pdf.org and download information about the latest research on Parkinson's disease.
2. Go to http://alz.org and find how to reach your local chapter for support systems for Alzheimer's disease.

Essentials Review

For further study and practice with drug classifications learned in this chapter, complete the following table to the best of your ability.
Use resources such as a PDR, the Internet, or printed drug guides for help.

CLASSIFICATION	PURPOSE	SIDE EFFECTS	CONTRAINDICATIONS/PRECAUTIONS/INTERACTIONS	EXAMPLES	PATIENT EDUCATION
Cholinergics					
Salicylates					
Narcotics					
MAO Inhibitors					
Antipsychotics					

Cardiovascular System Medications

This chapter discusses medications that affect the cardiovascular system. The heart is a vital organ, and cardiovascular disorders can cause serious problems, such as chest pain or even death. Blood vessels throughout the body carry much-needed oxygen, hormones, and immune and clotting cells. Fortunately, cardiovascular disease has been well researched, and many medications exist to help patients.

OBJECTIVES

At the end of this chapter, the student will be able to:

- Define all key terms.
- Describe how cardiovascular drugs work in the body.
- List the side effects of cardiovascular drugs.
- Explain the effects of antianginals, antihypertensives, thrombolytics, anticoagulants, antiplatelets, antifibrinolytics, ADP receptor blockers, glucoprotein inhibitors, hematopoietics, ACE inhibitors, autonomic nervous system agents, diuretics, vasopressors, cardiac glycosides, sodium channel blockers, beta blockers, potassium channel blockers, calcium channel blockers, and antilipemic agents.

KEY TERMS

ACE inhibitors
Angina pectoris
Anoxia
Atherosclerosis
Contractility
CVA
Cyanosis
DVT
Dysrhythmias

Embolus
Fight-or-flight response
HDL
Heart failure
Hemostasis
HTN
Hyperlipemia
Infarction

Ischemia
LDL
Lumen
MI
Pernicious anemia
Shock
Thrombus
VLDL

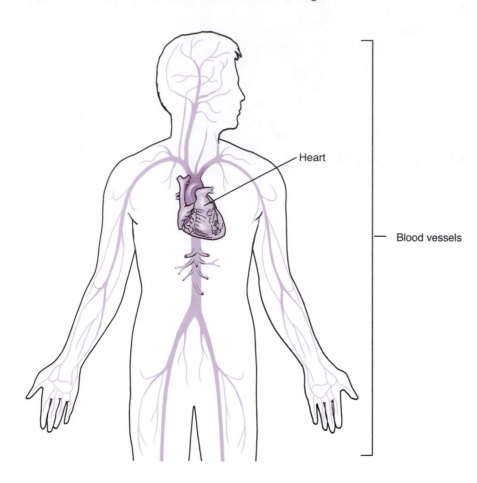

FIGURE 12.1. Cardiovascular system. The cardiovascular system includes the heart and blood vessels (arteries, veins, capillaries) that circulate blood throughout the body.

CARDIOVASCULAR MEDICATIONS

The cardiovascular system contains the vital parts of circulation—the heart and blood vessels (Fig. 12.1). Medications that affect this system are prescribed for a variety of illnesses. This section covers medications used to prevent myocardial infarction, stroke, and clotting; promote blood cell development; lower blood pressure; treat heart failure; regulate heart rhythm; treat shock, and treat lipid disorders. (See the Master the Essentials table for descriptions of the most common cardiovascular system drugs.)

MEDICATIONS FOR MYOCARDIAL INFARCTION, STROKE, AND CLOTTING

Chest pain can be a symptom of a total lack of oxygen (anoxia) or seriously reduced level of oxygen (hypoxia) in the heart muscle (myocardium). The lack or reduction of oxygen causes the tissues to not receive enough oxygen, which can lead to tissue injury (ischemia) or death (infarction). The telltale signs of a myocardial infarction (MI) are chest pain, sweating, pale skin, and blueness (cyanosis), particularly around the mouth. Keep in mind that chest pain can also be caused by noncardiovascular conditions, including broken ribs, gastrointestinal (GI) disorders, anxiety, or injured skeletal muscles.

Antianginal Medications
Antianginal drugs decrease chest pain (angina pectoris) by dilating arteries and veins. An example is nitroglycerin, which can be given by different routes, mainly under the tongue (sublingual) or on the skin (transdermal).

Master the Essentials: Cardiovascular Medications

This table shows the various classes of cardiovascular medications and key side effects, contraindications and precautions, and interactions for each class.

CLASS	SIDE EFFECTS	CONTRAINDICATIONS/ PRECAUTIONS	INTERACTIONS
Antianginals	Blurred vision, dry mouth, flushing, headache, hypersensitivity reaction, postural low blood pressure	Severe anemia, GI disease, glaucoma, intracranial pressure, low blood pressure	Alcohol, Viagra
Anticoagulants	Increased bleeding; blood irregularities; GI, liver, and kidney disease	Uncontrolled bleeding; heparin (an anticoagulant) does not cross the placenta but is used during pregnancy with caution	Acetaminophen, alcohol, anabolic steroids, antiinfectives, barbiturates, chloral hydrate, corticosteroids, estrogen, NSAIDs, tricyclic antidepressants, thyroid drugs
Antiplatelet agents	Diarrhea, dizziness, flushing, headache, nausea, rash, vomiting, weakness	Other medications that increase bleeding	ACE inhibitors, anticoagulants, anticonvulsants, NSAIDs, beta blockers, diuretics, methotrexate, oral hypoglycemics
Thrombolytics	Allergic reactions, bleeding, respiratory depression	Active bleeding, CVA within 2 months, recent intracranial or intraspinal surgery, intracranial neoplasm, uncontrolled hypertension	Antiplatelet agents, anticoagulants
Antifibrinolytics	Allergic reaction, anaphylaxis, dyspnea, confusion, bradycardia, rash	Known hypersensitivity, active intravascular clotting	Oral contraceptives
Hematopoietics (iron, vitamin B_{12})	Gastric irritation, liquid iron preparations can stain the teeth, allergic reactions	Known hypersensitivity; primary hemochromatosis, hemosiderosis, and hemolytic anemia (iron)	Antacids, tetracycline, H_2 blockers (iron); alcohol, neomycin, colchicines (vitamin B_{12})
ACE inhibitors	Blood irregularities, decreased blood pressure, light sensitivity, increased potassium, rash, decreased taste	Children, collagen disease, kidney impairment, lactation, pregnancy, vessel swelling	Antacids, digoxin, diuretics, lithium, NSAIDs, vasodilators

(table continued on page 222)

Master the Essentials: Cardiovascular Medications (continued)

CLASS	SIDE EFFECTS	CONTRAINDICATIONS/ PRECAUTIONS	INTERACTIONS
Beta-adrenergic blockers	Bronchodilation, uterine relaxation, vasodilation	Bronchospasm, HF, heart block, slow heart rate, some valvular diseases. Use with caution in the presence of diabetes mellitus, lactation, liver disease, pregnancy.	Bronchodilators, cimetidine, diabetic medications, digoxin
Diuretics	Hypotension, hyponatremia, hypokalemia, anorexia, nausea	Known hypersensitivity, anuria, breastfeeding, pregnancy	Oral hypoglycemics, lithium, corticosteroids, cardiac glycosides, NSAIDs
Calcium channel blockers	Decreased blood pressure, constipation, decreased heart rate, swelling	Children, lactation, liver or kidney disease, and pregnancy	ACE inhibitors, barbiturates, diuretics, lithium, rifampin, salicylates, sulfonamides
Phosphodiesterase inhibitors	Arrhythmias, nausea, vomiting, headache, fever, chest pain, hypotension	Known hypersensitivity, severe aortic or pulmonic valvular disease	Disopyramide, potassium-wasting diuretics
Cardiac glycosides	Arrhythmias, dizziness, electrolyte imbalances, GI upset, headache, irritability, lethargy, muscle weakness, tremors, seizures	Hypothyroidism, lactation, MI, pregnancy, impaired renal function. Monitor for high or low potassium, irregular rhythm, severe slow heart rate. If noted, discontinue drug.	Adrenergics, antacids, antiarrhythmics, diuretics, neomycin, phenobarbital, rifampin, sulfa drugs
Angiotensin receptor blockers	Dizziness, upper respiratory tract infection, palpitations	Known hypersensitivity, volume depletion, children	Cimetidine, fluconazole, digoxin, phenobarbital
Sodium channel blockers	New or worsened arrhythmia, dizziness, nausea, headache, fatigue, palpitations, dyspnea	Breastfeeding, heart block, pregnancy, known hypersensitivity, severe renal or liver disease	Other antiarrhythmics, anticholinergics, digoxin, warfarin, cimetidine
Potassium channel blockers	Hypotension, nausea, anorexia, malaise, fatigue, tremor, pulmonary toxicity	Known hypersensitivity, severe sinus node dysfunction, second or third degree heart block, severe aortic stenosis, severe pulmonary hypertension	Sympathomimetics, antihypertensives, warfarin, digoxin, procainamide

CLASS	SIDE EFFECTS	CONTRAINDICATIONS/ PRECAUTIONS	INTERACTIONS
Vasopressors	Angina, apnea, difficulty breathing, dizziness, headache, necrosis, pallor, palpitations, tremor, weakness, arrhythmias	Ventricular arrhythmias, hypoxia, acidosis	MAO inhibitors, phenytoin, tricyclic antidepressants, oxytocic drugs
HMG-CoA reductase inhibitors	Asthenia, headache, abdominal pain, nausea, vomiting, constipation, diarrhea, myalgia, rash	Known hypersensitivity, liver disease, elevated liver enzymes, pregnancy, lactation	Itraconazole, erythromycin, protease inhibitors, nefazodone, cyclosporine, antacids, cimetidine
Bile acid sequestrants	Constipation, abdominal pain, nausea, vomiting, headache, dizziness	Complete biliary obstruction, known hypersensitivity, pregnancy, lactation	Anticoagulants, corticosteroids, cardiac glycosides, iron
Fibric acid derivatives	Hypersensitivity, adverse GI effects similar to bile acid sequestrants, arrhythmias	Gallbladder disease, hepatic or renal dysfunction, pregnancy, peptic ulcer disease, breastfeeding	Anticoagulants, sulfonylureas

Teach the patient to put one nitroglycerin tablet under the tongue, wait 5 minutes, then put another under the tongue if the chest pain is not relieved. The patient should wait 5 minutes more and take a third tablet if the chest pain continues. If the pain continues, emergency medical services should be called; the patient must be evaluated to see if he or she is having an MI. The transdermal patch of nitroglycerin gives a maintenance dose to prevent MI, whereas the sublingual tablets are used during an acute episode of chest pain.

Angina can be treated by more than just medicine (see Fast Tip 12.1).

If chest pain is caused by skeletal muscle illness, not heart muscle problems, pain relievers such as nonsteroidal antiinflammatory drugs (NSAIDs) may be effective. Be sure to teach patients that they should have heart problems ruled out (excluded as a diagnosis) before medicating chest pain with NSAIDs.

Anticoagulants, Antiplatelet, Thrombolytic, and Antifibrinolytic Medications

A stroke or cerebrovascular accident (CVA) occurs when the brain is deprived of oxygen and blood flow for several minutes. CVAs are a major cause of death and disability. MIs are caused by ischemia of heart muscle; CVAs are caused by ischemia of the brain. For this reason, medications that prevent ischemia can be prescribed to prevent stroke as well as MI.

Fast Tip 12.1 Nonpharmacological Treatment for Angina

All of these strategies can help treat angina: decreasing dietary fats, lowering blood pressure, coping better with stress, exercising, decreasing alcohol consumption, smoking cessation, and decreasing dietary sodium. If these changes do not improve heart function, nitrates may be prescribed.

◯ *Fast Tip 12.2* Patient Teaching About Anticoagulants

Patients on anticoagulants need to be cautioned that, if they are injured, clotting will likely be delayed. They should be taught to:

• Use an electric razor to avoid injury.
• Reduce dietary intake of green leafy vegetables, green tea, hummus, and other foods that are high in vitamin K, an anticoagulant.
• Watch for signs of abnormal bleeding, such as frequent bruising, bleeding gums, and black, tarry stool.
• Keep appointments to have blood drawn to monitor the effect of anticoagulants.

Anticoagulants and antiplatelet drugs prevent the formation of clots. Thrombolytics dissolve clots that have already formed. Aggressive treatment of thrombolytic stroke with anticoagulants and thrombolytics (as well as antihypertensives, discussed later) can increase survival. Thrombolytics can also be used to prevent CVAs and MIs. Antifibrinolytics prevent the destruction of fibrin and thus promote clot formation—the opposite effect.

Anticoagulants and antiplatelet medications

Anticoagulants prevent blood from clotting. Antiplatelet drugs prevent platelets from creating clots. The clotting process is a complex one, with several stages. Anticoagulants interrupt the clotting mechanism and ensure that blood flows smoothly through vessels. However, if a patient on anticoagulants has a break in the skin or mucosal integrity, bleeding can be copious because the clotting mechanism is disturbed (see Fast Tip 12.2).

Aspirin is used as an antiplatelet modifier. Because it is an over-the-counter (OTC) medication, patients may not understand how potent it can be in interfering with clotting. Always ask a patient whether OTC medications, including aspirin, are being taken.

Two other antiplatelet medications are adenosine diphosphate (ADP) receptor blockers and glycoprotein IIb/IIIa inhibitors. ADP receptor blockers interfere with the plasma membrane of platelets. An example of this thrombus-prevention drug is clopidogrel (Plavix). These medications provide long-term prevention against clot formation.

Glycoprotein IIb/IIIa inhibitors prevent the enzyme that aggregates platelets from working. They are sometimes given before cardiac procedures to stop clots from forming during surgery or a procedure.

Patients on antiplatelet medications should also be taught the signs of bleeding and what precautions to take.

Thrombolytic medications

If other medications fail to prevent clots from blocking blood vessels, thrombolytics can dissolve them. A clot in a vessel is known as a thrombus. A clot that breaks loose and travels is an embolus.

A clot can form in the heart, lung, or brain or in the peripheral circulation. If a thrombus forms in a peripheral vein, as is the case with a deep vein thrombosis (DVT), the embolus can travel and cause an MI, a pulmonary embolus, or a stroke.

Thrombolytics can also be used to clear intravenous (IV) catheters and cannulas blocked with blood, but they must be used with extreme caution. If the blood has been in the cannula too long, injecting the drug can break off the clot instead of dissolving it.

Antifibrinolytic medications

Uncontrolled bleeding is just as dangerous as clotting. Clots must be dissolved quickly to prevent ischemia and infarction; however, a patient can die of uncontrolled bleeding, so frequent testing is necessary to ensure that the dose is a therapeutic one. The most common tests are the prothrombin time (PT), activated partial thromboplastin time (aPTT), and internationalized normalized ratio (INR). These tests are also used with anticoagulant, antiplatelet, and antithrombolytic therapy.

A CLOSER LOOK: Deep Vein Thrombosis

After surgery, a patient may develop DVT because of inactivity. Physicians may prescribe not only anticoagulants to prevent clots but also tight stockings that cover most of the leg. These stockings compress the veins and aid the smooth return of blood to the heart, even if the veins in the leg are weakened. They are called "antiembolic stockings." Antiembolic stockings are usually prescribed in addition to, not instead of, medications.

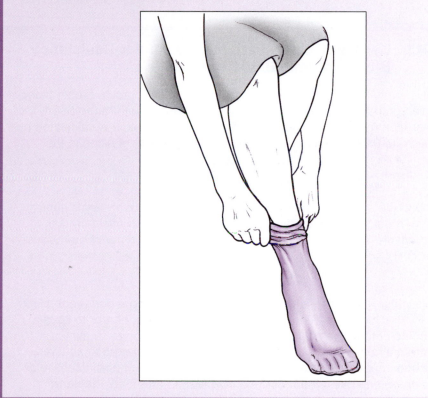

Antifibrinolytics do the opposite of thrombolytics. They help form clots when the patient is losing too much blood, thereby providing hemostasis (stopping the bleeding). You may remember that "anti" means against and "lytic" means to break down. These drugs go up against the breakdown of fibrin—thus allowing fibrin to form a clot. They are used to treat hemorrhage.

Blood loss can also be treated with other hemostatic drugs, such as vitamin K and desmopressin acetate (DDAVP). They help regulate the clotting process. Vitamin K is an antidote for anticoagulant overdose, because it promotes clotting.

MEDICATIONS THAT PROMOTE BLOOD CELL DEVELOPMENT

Some medications stimulate the growth of blood cells. Hematopoietics are used to treat anemias such as sickle cell anemia and pernicious anemia (vitamin B_{12} deficiency). They are also used to treat patients with a low iron level in the blood, which decreases the ability of the red blood cells to carry oxygen.

Examples of hematopoietics are ferrous sulfate (iron) and cyanocobalamin (vitamin B_{12}). Many patients cannot absorb vitamin B_{12} in the GI tract, so injectable vitamin B_{12} is usually given to facilitate blood cell development. This, in turn, promotes oxygen delivery to the cells and boosts the patient's energy.

● MEDICATIONS THAT DECREASE BLOOD PRESSURE

Cardiac output, peripheral resistance, and blood volume interact to create blood pressure. Cardiac output is the product of the heart rate and the stroke volume (amount of blood that is pumped with each heartbeat). Peripheral resistance is determined by the size and flexibility of the arteries. Therefore, the force of the heart's contraction, the amount of blood that is pumped, and the resistance, or "give," of the blood vessels all influence blood pressure. The kidneys also play a key role by regulating circulating fluid volume.

A CLOSER LOOK: Cardiac Output, Peripheral Vascular Resistance, Blood Volume, Blood Pressure

Cardiac output, peripheral resistance, and blood volume all interact to create blood pressure. Cardiac output (CO) relates to the volume of blood that fills the heart, the force of the heart contraction, and the ability of the heart to relax. It is calculated by multiplying heart rate (HR) and stroke volume (SV), the amount of blood in the left ventricle.

$$CO = HR \times SV$$

Remember that the sympathetic and parasympathetic nervous systems control the heart rate, so medications that affect the heart rate may also affect cardiac output. Blood pressure is the product of cardiac output (CO) and peripheral vascular resistance (PVR).

$$BP = CO \times PVR$$

Peripheral vascular resistance is how much force there is in the peripheral blood vessels. If the PVR is higher than normal, the heart has to work harder to keep appropriate cardiac output, the volume of blood the heart pumps each minute.

Stroke volume may be referred to as preload, and PVR is referred to as afterload. If a medication decreases the preload of the heart, the *contractility* (ability of the heart to contract) improves. If a medication decreases afterload, the heart works more efficiently.

Poor heart action, atherosclerosis (fatty plaques in the arteries), kidney failure, narrowed peripheral blood vessels caused by diabetes mellitus, and chronic stress can cause hypertension.

Hypertension (HTN), or high blood pressure, is a major cause of death and disability. Chronic high blood pressure can reduce the kidney's ability to get rid of excess fluid, which then puts a strain on circulatory organs.

Antihypertensives, which reduce blood pressure, include angiotensin-converting enzyme (ACE) inhibitors, autonomic nervous system agents, diuretics, and calcium channel blockers. Many of these drugs are also used to treat heart failure, which is discussed in the next section.

ACE inhibitors block the renin-angiotensin pathway from the kidneys to decrease blood pressure. Autonomic nervous system agents, such as adrenergic blockers (see Chapter 11), relax the "fight or flight" stress response. They can act on alpha- and beta-adrenergic receptors. Diuretics clear excess fluid from the body. Calcium channel blockers block calcium from contracting the muscle in the blood vessels.

To understand how these drugs work, be sure you recall how blood pressure is regulated.

ACE Inhibitors

In addition to reducing blood pressure, ACE inhibitors help reduce the possibility of heart failure by blocking the action of the renin-angiotensin system. These drugs stop the enzyme that converts

A CLOSER LOOK: Blood Pressure Regulation

Blood pressure regulation is a complex process. The primary regulation is carried out by the medulla oblongata (the vasomotor center in the brain), chemoreceptors, and baroreceptors. Chemoreceptors recognize oxygen and carbon dioxide levels and pH in the blood. Baroreceptors sense pressure in the large blood vessels. Both types of receptors pass on their information to the medulla, which then tells the body how to respond.

The endocrine system also plays a role through the renin-angiotensin system, shown below. This system increases blood pressure through its effects on the blood vessels and the kidneys.

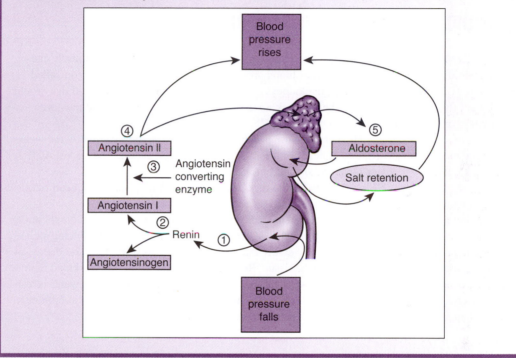

angiotensin I to angiotensin II. This causes a reduction in the release of the hormone aldosterone, which leads to less sodium and water retention.

Beta-Adrenergic Blockers

Beta-adrenergic blockers are autonomic nervous system agents that decrease the fight or flight response that causes blood vessels to constrict and the heart to pound faster. They are used to manage hypertension and angina pectoris, slow the heart rate, prevent MIs, reduce congestion associated with heart failure, and treat glaucoma. Reducing the body's perception that it is in a threatening situation can improve cardiovascular function.

Diuretics

Diuretics regulate blood pressure by encouraging the kidneys to excrete fluid. Less fluid in the body creates less blood volume and thus less pressure in the blood vessels — decreased peripheral vascular resistance. Diuretics are also used in the treatment of heart failure.

When diuretics work effectively, the patient may lose valuable minerals, so potassium and other supplements are frequently prescribed. Diuretics, although relieving heart failure and decreasing blood pressure, can also significantly disrupt the lives of patients by necessitating frequent trips to the bathroom. A patient may need assistance in planning activities around the dosing.

There are ways to decrease blood pressure without medications. Weight reduction, ceasing tobacco use, decreasing salt (sodium) intake, limiting alcohol, reducing stress, and exercising are all ways to regulate blood pressure.

CRITICAL THINKING

What is the role of stress in hypertension?

Calcium Channel Blockers

Calcium channel blockers affect muscle contraction. They decrease the level of contraction in the muscles in the arteries, triggering a series of responses: dilation of the arteries, decreased peripheral vascular resistance (PVR), reduced workload for the heart, and reduced blood pressure. Calcium channel blockers are used to treat angina and certain tachyarrhythmias, as well as hypertension. Drugs in this class that are indicated for the treatment of hypertension include amlodipine, diltiazem, nifedipine, and verapamil hydrochloride.

MEDICATIONS FOR HEART FAILURE

Chronic high blood pressure can place a great deal of stress on the heart muscle. The muscle can weaken and fail to push a normal amount of blood around the body, leading to a condition called heart failure (HF). When that happens, the kidneys don't receive enough blood, and fluid that would normally get flushed out of the body builds back up in the blood. This additional fluid puts even greater strain on the heart and leads to worsening HF.

There is no cure for chronic HF, but some drugs can decrease the symptoms caused by the weakened heart muscle. Drugs used to treat heart failure include vasodilators, cardiac glycosides, ACE inhibitors, angiotensin receptor blockers, and beta blockers.

Signs and symptoms of HF are anxiety, restlessness, cyanotic and clammy skin, fast heart rate, lower-leg swelling, rapid breathing, persistent cough, and a forward-leaning posture.

In addition to taking medications, patients can decrease their symptoms and risk of complications by quitting smoking, exercising, reducing weight, decreasing salt consumption, and reducing stress. The nicotine in tobacco contracts the blood vessels and increases blood pressure. Exercise decreases stress and causes increased blood flow to the tissue. Reducing body fat reduces the workload required to move an overweight body. With salt goes water; so if the patient retains a lot of salt, water is also retained. Increased fluid retention increases blood pressure. Decreasing stress reduces the fight or flight mechanism, thus decreasing blood pressure.

Vasodilators

Vasodilators decrease oxygen demand on the heart by decreasing resistance in the vessels (vascular resistance), which makes it easier for the heart to pump more effectively. In essence, blood vessels open up, blood pressure drops, and there is less pressure on the heart. Phosphodiesterase inhibitors, a type of vasodilator, cause vasodilation and increase the force of contraction by blocking the enzyme phosphodiesterase.

Cardiac Glycosides

Cardiac glycosides, which are made up of three sugars, or glycosides, strengthen the heart's contractility. In a fight or flight situation, constricting peripheral blood vessels would reduce blood loss if injury occurred. However, this is not a desired effect in the presence of cardiovascular disease. Cardiac glycosides increase the strength of heart contractions, whereas other drugs relax the resistance in the peripheral vessels (reduced afterload). Therefore, combining these drugs makes the cardiovascular system more efficient. Cardiac glycosides come from plants, such as purple and white foxglove.

DRUGS FOR ABNORMAL HEART RHYTHMS

Dysrhythmias (heart rhythm irregularities) can be caused by increased blood pressure, cardiac valve disease, coronary artery disease, decreased potassium consumption, heart failure, diabetes mellitus, stroke, MI, and certain medications (see Fast Tip 12.3).

⬤ *Fast Tip 12.3* Do Not Miss Dysrhythmias
_____

Be sure you accurately check a patient's pulse for a full minute so you do not miss a dysrhythmia that would prevent the patient from benefiting from medication therapy.

Drugs used to treat dysrhythmias are classified by how they act to improve the heart rhythm.

• Sodium channel blockers (class I)
• Beta-adrenergic blockers (class II)
• Potassium channel blockers (class III)
• Calcium channel blockers (class IV)

Sodium Channel Blockers

Sodium channel blockers slow the rate of electrical conduction by inhibiting sodium. Sodium is necessary to facilitate nerve impulses and muscular contraction. Blocking sodium transfer therefore inhibits irregular rhythms. Sodium also is the main contributor to osmotic pressure and hydration.

Beta-Adrenergic Blockers

Beta-adrenergic blockers slow electrical conduction in the heart and return the heart rhythm to normal. They can also be used to decrease oxygen demands for the heart by decreasing the fight or flight response.

Potassium Channel Blockers

Potassium channel blockers change the heart rhythm by affecting potassium—a necessary element for contraction of cardiac muscle. If too much potassium is lost through the use of diuretics or a poor diet, the patient may need to take potassium supplements or eat foods high in potassium, such as oranges, sweet potatoes, and bananas.

Calcium Channel Blockers

Calcium channel blockers, which block calcium ions, dilate heart vessels and thus decrease the workload of the heart.

⬤ MEDICATIONS FOR SHOCK

Shock is a collapse of the cardiovascular system. It can be caused by failure of the heart to pump (cardiogenic), loss of blood volume (hypovolemic), vasodilation due to central nervous system (CNS) dysfunction (neurogenic), or microbe invasion (septic). Treatment of shock primarily targets the underlying causes. Signs and symptoms of shock are listed in Figure 12.2.

Drug therapy for shock includes vasopressors to increase blood pressure and cardiotensive drugs to increase cardiac output.

Anaphylactic shock is another type of shock caused by an overactive response to a threat to the body such as an allergen. Signs and symptoms include breathing difficulty, bronchoconstriction, decreased cardiac output, edema, increased heart rate, hives, itching, and vasodilation. It is treated with epinephrine.

⬤ DRUGS FOR LIPID DISORDERS

Many Americans eat a lot of fat. Excess fat can be deposited in the walls of the blood vessels, causing hyperlipemia. Plugged vessels can lead to atherosclerosis, high blood pressure, and HF.

Not all lipids or fats are the same. High-density lipids (HDL) act as cannonballs and clean out blood vessels. Low-density lipids (LDL) are more like snowflakes, depositing fat in the vessels. Very low-density lipids (VLDL) are the worst. They are so small they actually wedge themselves inside the blood vessel walls and are difficult to clear.

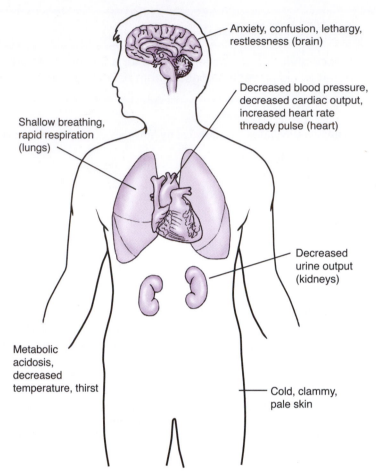

Anxiety, confusion, lethargy, restlessness (brain)

Decreased blood pressure, decreased cardiac output, increased heart rate thready pulse (heart)

Shallow breathing, rapid respiration (lungs)

Decreased urine output (kidneys)

Metabolic acidosis, decreased temperature, thirst

Cold, clammy, pale skin

FIGURE 12.2. Signs and symptoms of shock. Shock can affect every system in the body.

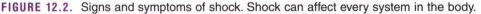

> ⊙ *Fast Tip 12.4* Nonpharmacologic Treatment for Lipidemia
>
> Nonpharmacologic ways to decrease lipids include smoking cessation, decreasing dietary fats and cholesterol, avoiding stress, exercising, maintaining a healthy weight, and periodic blood cholesterol screening.

HMG-CoA reductase inhibitors, commonly referred to as statins, decrease blood levels of lipids. They encourage the liver to make less cholesterol and increase the number of LDL receptors in the liver. Increased LDL receptors grab the circulating LDL from the blood. Other drug classes that act to decrease serum lipid levels are bile acid sequestrants and fibric acid derivatives. Bile acid sequestrants lower LDL blood levels by forming complexes with bile acids, thus causing the liver to make more bile acids from cholesterol. Fibric acid derivatives are used mainly to lower triglyceride levels.

You can help your patients by teaching them about nonpharmacologic approaches for managing lipidemia (see Fast Tip 12.4).

SUMMARY

The cardiovascular system is vital for life. If blood flow through the blood vessels or the electrical activity of the heart is impaired, the patient can die. Many drugs are available to manage cardiovascular disease. They can decrease chest pain; prevent MIs, stroke, and clotting; facilitate blood cell development; decrease blood pressure; reduce heart failure; regulate heart rhythm; treat shock; and reduce fats in the blood.

Activities

To make sure that you have learned the key points covered in this chapter, complete the following activities.

True or False

Write *true* if the statement is true. Beside the false statements, write *false* and correct the statement to make it true.

1. Anticoagulants prevent clot formation. _____

2. Antifibrinolytics destroy clots. _____

3. Blocking the renin-angiotensin pathway increases blood pressure. _____

4. Diuretics remove excess fluid. _____

5. VLDLs are the best kind of lipids. _____

6. Exercise can decrease blood lipid levels. _____

7. Ischemia is tissue death. _____

8. Potassium is found in bananas. _____

9. Antilipemic agents interact with some fruits. _____

10. Baroreceptors sense pressure in the heart. _____

Multiple Choice

Choose the best answer for each question.

1. Which destroy clots?
   a. Anticoagulants
   b. Antiplatelets
   c. Antifibrinolytics
   d. Thrombolytics

2. Aspirin is *not* an:
   a. Antipyretic
   b. Anticoagulant
   c. Analgesic
   d. Anesthetic

3. Which are used to treat heart failure?
   a. Anticoagulants
   b. Diuretics
   c. Antiinfectives
   d. Thrombolytics

4. Which are *not* a treatment for stroke?
   a. Anticoagulants
   b. Antiinfectives
   c. Antihypertensives
   d. Thrombolytics

5. Which of the following means lack of blood flow to tissues?
   a. Diuresis
   b. Embolus
   c. Infarction
   d. Ischemia
   e. Immunoglobin

6. Which medications decrease cholesterol?
   a. Statins
   b. Diuretics
   c. Thrombolytics
   d. Antifibrinolytics

7. Which of the following interferes with ions?
   a. Calcium channel blockers
   b. Statins
   c. Thrombolytics
   d. Digoxin

8. All are good patient teaching ideas *except*:
   a. Cease smoking
   b. Decrease salt intake
   c. Change positions slowly
   d. Stop taking the medication when better

9. Calcium channel blockers do all these *except*:
   a. Dilate coronary arteries
   b. Increase heart rate
   c. Decrease blood pressure
   d. Prevent action of calcium

10. Which of the following means injury to heart muscle?
   a. CVA
   b. MI
   c. CHF
   d. DVT
   e. HTN

Application Exercises

Respond to the following scenarios on a separate sheet.

1. Steve Spinner has just had his first heart attack. Although he agrees to take the medications the physician prescribes, he asks you what behaviors he could adopt to further reduce the risk of another heart attack. **What do you teach him?**
2. Lorraine Pond has just been given a prescription for a diuretic. **At what time of day should she take it?**
3. Randall Waller has just been hospitalized after surgery. He wants to know why he has to wear such tight stockings and also take medications. **What do you tell him about his antiembolic stockings and the medication therapy?**
4. A.J. Cardounel has hypertension. **What are some of the factors that may be causing it? Which can he change?**
5. Belinda Rose has been prescribed an anticoagulant. **What precautions should she take?**

Virtual Field Trips

Go to the following websites to find the information. If a website is not available, try to find the information through another source.

1. Go to your favorite drug information site and record the classification of the following:

   a. Lasix

   b. Apresoline

   c. Lanoxin

   d. Nitrobid

   e. Zocar

   f. Streptase

   g. Plavix

   h. Inderal

   i. Quinidine

   j. Heparin sodium

2. Go to http://www.procrit.com and print a list of side effects of cancer medications on blood cells.
3. Visit http://www.lipidsonline.org and print a slide show about hyperlipidemia.
4. Find a website of your choice and create an educational tool to decrease behaviors that could lead to heart attacks.
5. Visit http://www.americanheart.org and find a support group for heart patients in your area.

Essentials Review

For further study and practice with drug classifications learned in this chapter, complete the following table to the best of your ability. Use resources such as a PDR, the Internet, or printed drug guides for help.

CLASSIFICATION	PURPOSE	SIDE EFFECTS	CONTRAINDICATIONS/PRECAUTIONS/INTERACTIONS	PATIENT EDUCATION	EXAMPLES
Anticoagulants					
Antiplatelet agents					
ACE inhibitors					
Diuretics					
Calcium channel blockers					
Vasopressors					

Immunologic System Medications

The immunologic system protects the body from disease. Specialized cells attack invading microbes and clean out the remains of cells damaged in the attacks. Usually medications are used to boost the body's immune system, but sometimes drugs are given to suppress an immune response. For example, allergic reactions and rejection of transplanted organs need to be suppressed by medications. Keeping the immune system healthy keeps the body healthy.

OBJECTIVES

At the end of this chapter, the student will be able to:

- Define key terms.
- List the side effects of antiinfective drugs used to treat bacterial, viral, and fungal infections.
- Discuss the effects of chemotherapy and how to help the patient cope with side effects.
- Explain the effects of antihistamines, sympathomimetics, antiinflammatories, immunosuppressants, alkylating agents, antimetabolites, antitumor antibiotics, hormones, hormone antagonists, plant extracts, and biological response modifiers.

KEY TERMS

Aerobe	Booster	Malignant
Anaerobe	C & S	Metastasis
Attenuated	Chemotherapy	Superinfection
Bactericidal	CSF	Titer
Bacteriostatic	Lymphatic	TNF
Benign		

● MEDICATIONS THAT AFFECT THE IMMUNE SYSTEM

A healthy immune system is necessary to protect us from microbes such as bacteria, fungi, and viruses. An unhealthy immune system can attack the body, leading to such diseases as rheumatoid arthritis (see Chapter 17) and cancer. (See the Master the Essentials table for descriptions of the most common immunologic system drugs.)

Be sure you understand how the immune system functions before you read about the medications that affect it.

A CLOSER LOOK: The Immune Response

When the body is invaded by microbes or another antigen (foreign substance), it marshals an attack against these invaders. Inflammation is the natural response to limit the spread of microbes or injury.

The first response is a local one at the site of the invasion (e.g., a cut). Chemicals released during inflammation include bradykinin (vasodilator that causes pain), complement (protein that destroy antigens), histamine (released by mast cells—causes smooth muscle contraction, blood vessel dilation, and itching), leukotrienes (released by mast cells—same effects as histamine), and prostaglandins (released by mast cells to increase capillary permeability, attract leukocytes to the inflammation site, and increase pain).

The immune system also launches an attack throughout the body by secreting antibodies (immunoglobins) that are specific to the invading antigen.

After the attack of the microbe is over, some B cells (memory cells) remember the battle and help to launch future attacks against those particular invaders. Vaccines are administered to encourage the production of these memory cells.

T cells, also called CD cells, are lymphocytes—cells that do not produce antibodies but instead create cytokines. Some cytokines create inflammation, and others attack the invader directly.

● ANTIINFLAMMATORY MEDICATIONS

Antiinflammatory medications shut off the body's inflammatory response. They may be used in patients with such conditions as anaphylaxis, ankylosing spondylitis, rheumatoid arthritis, ulcerative colitis, Crohn's disease, dermatitis, diabetes mellitus (type 1), glomerulonephritis, Hashimoto's thyroiditis, multiple sclerosis, peptic ulcers, allergic rhinitis, and systemic lupus erythematosus.

Allergies are an overresponse of the body's defenses to substances that may not be a threat to the body. Examples of sensitizing substances are pollen, animal dander, mold, mildew, certain foods, dust, and cigarette smoke. Patients may also have allergic reactions to food or medications.

Signs and symptoms of a mild allergy such as allergic rhinitis, with which you are probably familiar, are sneezing, nasal congestion, and watery eyes. Patients with serious reactions, such as anaphylactic shock (the most serious form of a reaction), may experience urticaria (hives), swelling, itching, or difficulty breathing. These patients can die if not treated promptly.

Medications used to treat allergic reactions include antihistamines, glucocorticoids, nasal decongestants, nonsteroidal antiinflammatory drugs (NSAIDs), and immunosuppressants.

Antihistamines

Antihistamines, as the name suggests, block the histamine response, thereby decreasing swelling, itching, and congestion. These drugs are also referred to as H_1-receptor antagonists. Their effects include relaxation of the respiratory, vascular, and gastrointestinal smooth muscle.

Master the Essentials: Immunologic System Medications

This table shows the various classes of immunologic medications and key side effects, contraindications and precautions, and interactions for each class.

CLASS	SIDE EFFECTS	CONTRAINDICATIONS/PRECAUTIONS	INTERACTIONS
Antihistamines	CNS depression (sedation, dizziness, muscle weakness), epigastric distress, dry mouth	Known hypersensitivity, breastfeeding, MAO inhibitors, glaucoma, hypertension	CNS depressants, anticholinergics, aminoglycosides, salicylates, epinephrine
Glucocorticoids (systemic)	Behavioral changes, hyperglycemia, increased susceptibility to infection, osteoporosis, hypertension	Known hypersensitivity, systemic fungal infection	Phenytoin, salicylates, NSAIDs, vaccines, estrogen, antihypertensives
Nasal decongestants	Arrhythmias, hypertension, headache, nausea; sneezing, dryness (topical)	Known hypersensitivity, MAO inhibitors, hypertension	Beta blockers, MAO inhibitors, tricyclic antidepressants
NSAIDs	Nausea, vomiting, hypersensitivity reactions, vertigo, insomnia, rash	Known hypersensitivity, renal disease, GI bleeding, allergic reaction to sulfonamides	ACE inhibitors, fluconazole, phenobarbital, cyclosporine, corticosteroid, anticoagulants
Immunosuppressants	Leukopenia, thrombocytopenia, nephrotoxicity, hyperkalemia, hypertension, diarrhea, nausea	Known hypersensitivity, pregnancy, breastfeeding	Allopurinol, aminoglycosides, other immunosuppressants, calcium channel blockers, cardiac glycosides
Penicillins	Blood changes, CNS effects, diarrhea, hypersensitivity, kidney and liver disorders, nausea, vomiting	Known hypersensitivity, decreased renal function, electrolyte imbalances	Antagonizes antacids and foods. Probenecid potentiates penicillin. May decrease the action of oral contraceptives.
Cephalosporins	Bleeding, diarrhea, hypersensitivity, liver dysfunction, kidney disease, nausea, phlebitis, respiratory distress, seizures, vomiting	Known hypersensitivity, children, kidney impairment, lactation, pregnancy. Not for long-term use.	Alcohol and diuretics
Tetracyclines	Allergic hypersensitivity, CNS malfunction, diarrhea, decreased bone growth in a fetus or child, discolored teeth, light sensitivity, thrombophlebitis, nausea, superinfection, vomiting	Children, direct sunlight, esophageal illness, kidney and liver disease, lactation, pregnancy	Antacids, antidiarrheal agents, calcium, dairy products, iron, magnesium, oral contraceptives, zinc
Macrolides	Anorexia, cramps, diarrhea, nausea, superinfection, urticaria, vomiting	Alcoholism and liver damage	Cyclosporine, digoxin, Halcion, Tegretol, theophylline, warfarin

(table continued on page 238)

Master the Essentials: Immunologic System Medications (continued)

CLASS	SIDE EFFECTS	CONTRAINDICATIONS/PRECAUTIONS	INTERACTIONS
Aminoglycosides	Blurred vision, CNS symptoms, ear damage, kidney disease, paralysis (including respiratory paralysis), rash, urticaria	Decreased kidney function, dehydration, infancy, high-frequency hearing loss, lactation, pregnancy, tinnitus, vertigo	Antiemetics, general anesthesia, ototoxic drugs
Quinolones	CNS effects, crystallemia, diarrhea, toxicity in sunlight, nausea, superinfection, vomiting	Cardiovascular disorders, children, kidney disease, lactation, pregnancy	Antacids, calcium, Coumadin, iron, magnesium, probenicid, theophylline, zinc
Sulfonamides	Fever, crystalluria, nausea, vomiting, diarrhea, rash, photosensitivity	Known hypersensitivity, impaired kidney or liver function, lactation, pregnancy	Anticoagulants, antidiabetics, local anesthesia, cyclosporine
Antituberculosis medications	Diarrhea, dizziness, hypersensitivity, liver damage, nausea, numbness, red-orange secretions, vomiting	Alcoholism, children, lactation, liver or kidney disease, pregnancy	Alcohol, anticoagulants, corticosteroids, digoxin, estrogen, phenytoin
Antifungals (systemic)	Anemia, chills, decreased blood pressure, dizziness, fever, headache, low blood potassium, kidney damage, malaise, muscle and joint pain and weakness, rapid heart rate, sensitivity to light	Children, liver damage, penicillin hypersensitivity, pregnancy, porphyria	Alcohol, anticoagulants, oral contraceptives, phenobarbital
Antivirals	Confusion, diarrhea, headache, kidney disease, nausea, rash, urticaria, vomiting	Children, dehydration, lactation, kidney disease, neurological disease, pregnancy	Probenecid, nephrotoxic agents, cytotoxic agents, anticholinergics
Antiretrovirals	Fat redistribution, hypoglycemia, gastrointestinal upset, kidney stones	Known hypersensitivity, breastfeeding, pregnancy, kidney or liver impairment	Alcohol, oral contraceptives
Alkylating agents	Allergic reactions, nausea, vomiting, diarrhea, bone marrow suppression, pulmonary fibrosis, hepatotoxicity	Known hypersensitivity, pregnancy, breastfeeding	Anticoagulants, phenobarbital, digoxin
Antimetabolites	Alopecia, bone marrow depression, diarrhea, nausea, neurotoxicity, rash, reproductive ability loss, pulmonary fibrosis, vomiting	Pregnancy, breastfeeding, hepatic impairment	Probenecid, NSAIDs, alcohol, salicylates

CLASS	SIDE EFFECTS	CONTRAINDICATIONS/PRECAUTIONS	INTERACTIONS
Antitumor antibiotics	Alopecia, anorexia, bone marrow suppression, cardiotoxicity, nausea, pneumonitis, rash and scaly skin, ulceration of the skin and mouth, vomiting	Known hypersensitivity, pregnancy, renal impairment, heart disease, breastfeeding	Cyclophosphamide, myelosuppressive drugs, hepatotoxic medications, digoxin, phenytoin, oxygen
Plant extracts	Alopecia, constipation, diarrhea, nausea, necrosis, neurotoxicity, rash, sensitivity to light, ulcers in the mouth or GI system, vomiting, white blood cell deficiency	Pregnancy, breastfeeding, bacterial infection, severe granulocytopenia, liver impairment	Mitomycin, phenytoin, erythromycin, digoxin
Hormones	Hot flashes, decreased sex drive, nausea, vomiting	Pregnancy, thromboembolic disorders, breastfeeding, undiagnosed vaginal bleeding	Warfarin, bromocriptine
Biological response modifiers	Anemia, bleeding, difficulty breathing, fever, muscle aches and pain, infection, mouth infection, nausea, vomiting, diarrhea, malnutrition, loss of appetite, hair loss, damage to ear and peripheral nervous system, kidney and heart disease, tingling, loss of reflexes, confusion, personality changes, bone marrow suppression, GI upset	Known hypersensitivity, pregnancy. Because of intense side effects, antiemetics may be needed to prevent vomiting.	Protease inhibitors, antihypertensives, corticosteroids
Monoclonal antibodies	Infusion reactions, arrhythmias, angina, renal failure, bleeding, nausea, thrombocytopenia, rash, abdominal pain, malaise	Known hypersensitivity, pregnancy, breastfeeding	Anticoagulants
Immunomodulators	Headache, fever, nausea, vomiting, fatigue, myalgia, depression	Known hypersensitivity, depression, kidney or liver disease, autoimmune disorders	Theophylline; neurotoxic, hematotoxic, or cardiotoxic drugs
Radioactive isotopes	Radiation sickness, nausea, vomiting, rash	Pregnancy, breastfeeding	None reported

Glucocorticoids

Glucocorticoids are administered intranasally to combat allergic rhinitis or systemically for acute or severe inflammation. Because of the serious side effects and danger of long-term suppression of the immune system, glucocorticoids must be used only as prescribed and discontinued gradually.

Nasal Decongestants

Nasal decongestants can alleviate nasal congestion either orally or intranasally by drying secretions. They cause vasoconstriction on the adrenergic receptors in the nose by affecting the sympathetic tone of the blood vessels. The mucous membranes shrink, thereby promoting drainage. These drugs are typically used for only 3 to 5 days; otherwise, "rebound" nasal congestion occurs and the patient continues to suffer.

NSAIDs

NSAIDs are the most common treatment for inflammation. NSAIDs also have antipyretic and analgesic properties. They work by inhibiting prostaglandin synthesis. NSAIDs can be purchased over-the-counter (OTC). As with all OTC drugs, they must be taken as directed. Also, many drugs in this class have similar mechanisms, but patient responses vary. Someone may respond poorly to one NSAID but report great relief from another.

Immunosuppressants

The only medications used for long-term therapy of inflammatory diseases are immunosuppressants. Because long-term suppression of the immune system renders the body vulnerable to infection and certain cancers, they are used primarily to prevent or treat rejection of organ transplants. However, immunosuppressants can also be used to treat rheumatoid arthritis and psoriasis.

⬤ ANTIINFECTIVE MEDICATIONS

Bacteria are microbes that come in a variety of shapes and do not require a host (e.g., person or animal) to reproduce. They are named based on their shapes, and all are potentially vulnerable to antibiotics, or antiinfectives. If the specific bacterium cannot be identified, the prescriber orders a broad-spectrum antibiotic, one that is effective against many types of bacteria. Sometimes a specific bacterium is resistant to antibiotics and therefore difficult to treat. An example of a bacterium-caused disease is otitis media (middle ear infection).

Antiinfective drugs are classified by their mechanisms of action or chemical structure. They target the processes of the invading organism. Some go after protein synthesis. Some inhibit DNA or RNA synthesis. Still others destroy the cell wall.

Bacteria can change, or mutate. Because there is such a wide range of bacteria, it is vital to prescribe the correct antibiotic. A culture and sensitivity (C & S) test can help determine which antibiotic would be most effective against the microbe (Fig. 13.1).

Unfortunately, antibiotics may also kill healthy or normal flora while killing bacteria. These normal flora kill fungi and other microbes. This destruction of the body's own bacteria can create another infection on top of the original one, called a super infection.

Viruses and parasites can also cause infections.

Antibiotics

Antibiotics include penicillins, cephalosporins, tetracyclines, macrolides, and aminoglycosides. Although not truly antibiotics, sulfonamide medications are typically listed in this category too.

Penicillin medications

Penicillins are used to treat many common infections. They kill gram-positive and gram-negative bacteria by destroying cell walls. They are the oldest and least expensive antibiotics available. However, many people are allergic to the penicillins, so other antibiotics are used.

A CLOSER LOOK: All About Bacteria

Bacteria are characterized by their shape, how they stain, and whether they need oxygen to survive.

Shape. Bacteria shaped like rods are called bacilli. Example of a rod-shaped bacterium is gonorrhea. Those shaped like spheres are called cocci. Strep throat is caused by streptococci. Spiral-shaped bacteria are called spirilla. Syphillis and Lyme disease are illnesses caused by spirilla.

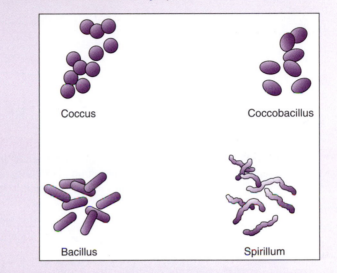

Coccus   Coccobacillus

Bacillus   Spirillum

Staining. When stained with violet dye in the laboratory, some bacteria hold onto the purple color in their thick cell walls. They are known as gram-positive bacteria. Those with thinner walls do not retain the stain, and so are called gram-negative bacteria. Different medications are used for these two types.

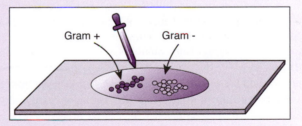

Gram +   Gram -

Oxygen. Some bacteria like to live in oxygen-rich environments (e.g., the lungs) and others do not. Oxygen-loving microbes are known as *aerobes.* Those that prefer to live without oxygen are *anaerobes.* They inhabit other parts of the body (e.g., gastrointestinal tract), where oxygen is not as prevalent as it is in the lungs.

Cephalosporin medications

Cephalosporins are similar to penicillins. They are more expensive but are useful for people who cannot tolerate penicillins. Cephalosporins are organized into three generations, based on their activity. First-generation cephalosporins are used mainly for patients allergic to penicillin. They act against gram-positive bacteria. Second-generation cephalosporins are commonly used to treat nosocomial pneumonia and pelvic or intraabdominal infections. Third-generation cephalosporins act against gram-negative bacteria.

Tetracycline medications

Tetracyclines were commonly used during the 1950s and 1960s, but many bacteria have become resistant to them. These drugs prevent bacteria from making protein (protein synthesis). They are useful against both gram-negative and gram-positive microbes.

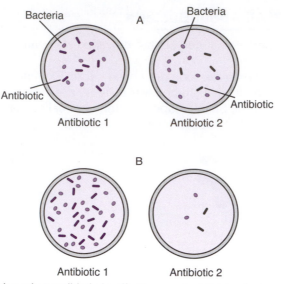

FIGURE 13.1. To determine what antibiotic is effective against the bacteria, a culture and sensitivity test is done. (A) Various antibiotics are applied to the same bacteria spread in petri dishes. (B) The antibiotic that kills the bacteria in the petri dish is selected to treat the patient.

Macrolide medications

Erythromycin and other macrolides are prescribed for infections that are resistant to penicillins. They inhibit bacterial protein synthesis and may either kill bacteria (bactericidal) or inhibit growth (bacteriostatic).

Aminoglycoside medications

Aminoglycosides are more toxic than other antibiotics. They are ideal against aerobic gram-negative bacteria, mycobacteria, and some protozoans. Patients taking aminoglycosides should have blood levels of the antibiotic monitored periodically to assess for efficacy and toxicity.

Quinolone medications

Quinolones such as ciprofloxacin are bacteriostatic. They prevent bacteria from reproducing. They can be given intravenously, ophthalmically, or orally. They are commonly used orally to treat urinary tract infections.

Sulfonamide medications

Sulfonamides are mainly used to treat acute urinary tract infections. They do not kill the invading microbes but prevent their growth and reproduction. Many patients are allergic to sulfonamides. Older sulfonamides had serious side effects, but modern versions are not as toxic.

Antitoxins

Antitoxins are toxic bacteria used to fight other microbes. Examples of antitoxins include diphtheria, tetanus, and botulism.

One bacterium, *Mycobacterium tuberculosis*, causes a highly contagious infection, tuberculosis (TB). Tubercles remain in a patient's body for a lifetime and can be reactivated if not treated. For this reason, many patients with immunologic disorders such as acquired immunodeficiency syndrome (AIDS) can die of TB. Pharmacologic treatment of TB requires exact adherence to a regimen of several drugs over 16 to 24 months. These medications can also be given to close companions of infected patients to prevent infection in them.

Antifungal Medications

Fungi, yeast-like plants, require different antiinfective medication for destruction. Fungi can live on the skin or inside the body. Unlike bacteria, fungi can be single-celled or multicellular organisms that have a complex structure. The human body can usually fight off fungal infections unless the immune system is compromised by the human immunodeficiency virus (HIV) or other microbes.

Topical antifungal medications can treat fungal infections on the skin. If the fungi are growing in the body, systemic antifungal drugs can protect the internal organs.

Proliferation of fungi can create opportunistic infections that prey on the body's reduced normal flora. Fungi can cause tinea pedis (commonly known as athlete's foot) or candidiasis (yeast infection).

Medications That Fight Viruses

Viruses are so small you need a microscope to see them. They infect bacteria, plants, and animals. Viruses use humans as breeding hosts. AIDS, rabies, and herpes are all caused by viruses. Medications that fight viruses include antiviral and antiretroviral drugs. The choice is based on the type of virus infecting the patient.

Antiviral medications

Antiviral therapy is difficult because viruses replicate (reproduce) and mutate rapidly. Each antiviral drug works specifically on certain viruses, just as the body attacks each virus according to the T cells' or CD cells' specific instructions. Antiviral drugs can treat influenza (the flu) or herpes simplex. Most other viruses have not yet been conquered.

Antiretroviral medications

Antiretrovirals are needed against retroviruses such as HIV. This virus specifically attacks the invading T4, or CD4, cells, rendering the host powerless to fight its reproduction. Many patients develop AIDS as a result of HIV infection. Because HIV is a virus that mutates easily, it is imperative that patients with AIDS take several medications according to a specific regimen to fight the retrovirus, prevent its reproduction, and protect their own immune system.

Vaccines

Vaccines are a means of giving someone immunity from a disease. In addition, some humans are naturally immune to certain human illnesses, a condition called "inborn immunity." All other immunity is acquired, either naturally or artificially.

Both naturally and artificially acquired immunity may be active or passive. Active natural immunity is created when a microbe invades and the body learns to fight it. This immunity is permanent. Passive natural immunity comes from a mother passively giving it to the fetus through the placenta. It is temporary.

Artificially acquired immunity requires injection of antigens or antibodies. This is where vaccines come in. Active artificial immunity comes from giving the patient a vaccination of live, attenuated (weakened) or dead viruses, or toxoids, and allowing the patient to form antibodies. This protection may be semipermanent (for years) or permanent (forever). Passive artificial immunity comes when we give antibodies from a donor directly to a patient to teach the patient's immune system how to fight. This protection is temporary.

Vaccines act by provoking memory B cells to prepare for a future attack from a similar microbe. Boosters (later doses) can be given to boost the immune system into continuing its protection. To see if the body has produced enough antibodies in response to a vaccination, a blood titer, or level, may be determined.

Vaccines can have side effects, including fever and redness and pain at the injection site. Severe reactions, called anaphylaxes, are possible, so patients must always be observed for at least 15 minutes after a vaccination or an allergy shot. Assess the patient for rash or difficulty breathing. Document your observations even if the patient tolerated the procedure well.

Parasites

Parasites are organisms that live on or in another organism (host) and can cause diseases, such as malaria. Malaria, worms, and other parasitic diseases are rarely seen in the United States and Canada. Antiparasitic drugs include antimalarials, antiprotozoans, antihelmintics (against worms), pediculicides (against lice), and scabicides (against scabies). Nits are lice eggs, which must be destroyed to prevent skin breakdown and infection. Medication and combing (and perhaps cutting) hair can kill lice eggs before they hatch (see Chapter 14).

CHECK UP

Use your research skills (Internet or otherwise) to fill in the following vaccination chart.

AGENT	TRADE OR GENERIC NAME	ROUTE	SITES	SIDE EFFECTS
BCG				
DTP				
Haemophilus influenzae B (Hib)				
Hepatitis A				
Hepatitis B				
HPV				
Influenza				
MMR				
Pneumococcus				
Polio				
RhoGAM				
Rubella				
Tetanus toxoid				
Varicella				

DRUGS TO FIGHT CANCER

Cancer is a disease caused by a disorderly and uncontrolled division of cells. Many chemicals, such as nicotine and alcohol, can trigger a cell to begin dividing abnormally. Normally the body can spot an abnormal cell and get rid of it. In some individuals, however, the body can't make that identification. As a result, it can't get rid of the abnormal cell and cancer results.

Cancer cells typically divide much faster than normal and can spread to surrounding or distant body areas, a process called *metastasis*. For instance, cancers of the breast frequently metastasize to the brain, bones, or liver.

A CLOSER LOOK: Types of Tumor

Tumors are classified as benign or malignant.

Tumors that are often annoying to the patient but not fatal can be called *benign.* Benign tumors grow slowly and do not metastasize. They may be removed if they impede the function of surrounding tissues; they do not usually grow back when removed.

Malignant tumors are called cancer. They must be treated, or the patient will die. They spread as nonfunctional tissues that compete with healthy tissue for the blood and nutrient supply. Malignant cancers are treated with surgery, radiation, and/or chemotherapy. Of course, a patient always has the right to choose not to be treated.

Sarcomas, carcinomas, and other malignant cancers must be completely eliminated, or they can return. For this reason, a powerful treatment, chemotherapy, is often prescribed. Chemotherapy, usually a combination of several antineoplastic (anticancer) and cytotoxic (destructive to cells) drugs, is frequently given in several doses for maximum effectiveness. These drugs act as toxins, or poisons, to the malignant cells, but can kill or damage healthy cells as well, causing patients to be weakened, sickened, or otherwise negatively affected by chemotherapy.

Among the choices for treating cancer are alkylating agents, antimetabolites, antitumor antibiotics, plant extracts, hormones, biological response modifiers, monoclonal antibodies, immunomodulators, and radioactive isotopes. These agents are usually given parenterally: intramuscularly (IM), subcutaneously (SC), intravenously (IV), or intrathecally.

Chemotherapy frequently causes vomiting when taken orally, so antiemetics are usually given. Frequently, antiemetics are not effective, so most chemotherapy is given IV over a period of time. Whether allied health professionals are allowed to administer IV chemotherapy varies according to state, facility, and level of training. Because chemotherapy is usually a long process, patient education about IV therapy, care of venous lines, and how to recognize signs and symptoms of infection is vital.

CANCER-FIGHTING AGENTS

There are a number of types of cancer-fighting agents, including alkylating agents, antimetabolites, antitumor antibiotics, plant extracts (alkaloids), hormones, biological therapies, and radioactive isotopes.

Alkylating Agents

Alkylating agents attach to DNA and alter the shape of the DNA, preventing it from reproducing normally. Because blood and bone marrow cells are especially sensitive to them, alkylating agents are ideal for treating leukemia. Types of alkylating agents are nitrogen mustards, nitrosoureas, triazenes, alkyl sulfonates, and ethylenimines/methylmelamines.

Antimetabolite Medications

Antimetabolites disrupt critical cell pathways. When cancer cells try to construct DNA or proteins, they inadvertently use antimetabolites, which kill the cells. Folic acid antagonists, purine analogs, and pyrimidine analogs are all antimetabolite drugs.

Antitumor Antibiotics

Bacteria are used to create antibiotics that can kill cancer cells. Many of these agents cause cell death by altering the DNA molecules. Although these drugs have properties of antibiotics, they are used for their cytotoxic effects.

Plant Extracts/Alkaloids

Plant extracts, or alkaloids, called mitotic inhibitors, prevent cell division. Plants used for this purpose include periwinkle, the mandrake plant, the Pacific yew, and a shrub called *Campothecus accuminata*. These drugs are called mitotic inhibitors because they prevent formation of the mitotic spindle, and the cells cannot complete mitosis. This causes cell death.

Hormones

Hormones can help the brain and other organs in the body communicate and are very powerful. Some hormones can significantly impair the growth of some tumors. Tumors that depend on hormones for growth can be eradicated by large amounts of an opposing hormone. For example, tumors that enjoy growth under the effects of estrogen can be killed by testosterone, and vice versa.

Biological Therapy

Biologicals—marvels of medicine—do not actually kill cancer cells but, rather, boost the body's own immune system. However, biological therapy also alters the nature of the response and often produces severe side effects. Three drug classes fall under this heading: biological response modifiers, monoclonal antibodies, and immunomodulators.

One type of biological therapy is the biological response modifier, which boosts the immune system. The exact mechanisms by which these drugs exhibit antitumor effects is not clear. Biological response modifiers include the interleukins.

Monoclonal antibodies are substances that specifically target tumor cells. Whereas toxic substances are nonselective and kill any rapidly growing cells, monoclonal antibodies specifically go after cancer cells.

A third form of biological therapy employs immunomodulatory cytokines, which are messenger proteins that deliver messages within the cells. In some cancer patients, these cytokines are not functional. The interferons are immunomodulator drugs.

Radioactive Isotopes

Radiation can also be used to kill cancer cells. In addition to external irradiation, radioactive isotopes can be swallowed as capsules or solutions, or they can be implanted. Always be extremely careful when handling these dangerous substances. Follow your facility's policy about isolating the patient and the patient's body fluids after administering radioactive isotopes.

Special Handling of Chemotherapeutic Medications

Antineoplastic agents are toxic to cells, but can also be dangerous or even fatal to those who administer them and thus require special handling. Exposure to chemotherapy poses risks to reproductive health as well as causing other problems. For that reason, gloves should be worn while administering, handling, or transporting antineoplastic agents, so that agents don't become absorbed through the skin. Ensure that packages of hazardous drugs are well labeled and secured properly. Although protocols vary by location, follow all safety measures and do not perform any task out of your scope of practice. Regulations always include wearing protective clothing, strictly following safety measures, and rigidly observing protocols for drug preparation and delivery (Box 13.1).

Do not forget to educate the patient, family members, and other health care workers about safety issues related to handling toxic substances. Note that women who are pregnant or breastfeeding—or even trying to conceive—should not receive chemotherapy. Always ask fertile women if they might be pregnant before giving chemotherapy.

Complications of Chemotherapy

Infiltration—accidental leakage of medication into surrounding tissue—is always a risk with IV therapy. These substances are particularly toxic if they infiltrate tissues. Always assess the IV site for swelling or coolness. The potential for infiltration increases when you increase the rate of the IV too quickly or put pressure on the vein. If infiltration occurs, the IV catheter must be removed and a new IV started at a different location.

If the patient complains of burning pain or aching in the vein, the chemotherapy might have irritated and damaged the vein wall, causing phlebitis and thrombosis. You may need to obtain an order to dilute the strength of the medication, lower the infusion rate, or change the site.

BOX 13.1 Special Handling of Chemotherapeutic Drugs

- Always give as ordered and have another colleague double-check the order.
- Frequently assess IV site.
- Help patient with oral hygiene as needed.
- Assess for malnutrition related to nausea, vomiting, and diarrhea.
- Administer an antiemetic, as necessary.
- Encourage soft, mild foods.
- Offer cool liquids.
- Measure input and output.
- Inquire about pregnancy before administering to women.
- Assess for complications.
- Use standard precautions to decrease infection in patient and protect yourself.
- Assess vital signs, as ordered.
- Educate the patient about the effects of the therapy.
- Dispose of chemotherapeutic products according to facility standards.

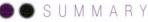 S U M M A R Y

The immune system plays a key role in keeping you alive and healthy by blocking or fighting off foreign substances. Sometimes the body's immune system can fail or react inappropriately, requiring the use of medications. Cancer is the uncontrolled growth of destructive cells and the failure of the immune system to stop the growth. Toxic substances are used against cancer growth, helping to destroy the malignant cells. Agents used to treat cancer must be carefully administered because of hazards to the health professional. Take precautions such as wearing gloves while handling antineoplastic medications.

Activities

To make sure that you have learned the key points covered in this chapter, complete the following activities.

True or False

Write *true* if the statement is true. Beside the false statements, write *false* and correct the statement to make it true.

1. Anaphylaxis is caused by a decreased immune system. _____

2. Side effects of anticancer drugs include nausea, diarrhea, vomiting, and hair loss. _____

3. Systemic glucocorticoids are used to suppress transplant rejection. _____

4. Antifungals can only be applied topically. _____

5. Metastasis is the spread of cancer beyond its organ of origin. _____

Multiple Choice

Choose the best answer for each question.

1. Which prevent organ transplant rejection?
   a. Antibiotics
   b. Antifungals
   c. Antiretrovirals
   d. Immunosuppressants

2. Which is *not* a sign or symptom of anaphylaxis?
   a. Itching
   b. Decreased heart rate
   c. Difficulty breathing
   d. Swelling

3. Which vaccination uses a toxoid?
   a. Varicella
   b. MMR
   c. DTP
   d. Pneumoccocus
   e. Hib

4. Which vaccination prevents chickenpox?
   a. Varicella
   b. MMR
   c. DTP
   d. Pneumococcus
   e. Hib

5. Transferring immunity from mother to fetus is called
   a. Naturally acquired passive immunity
   b. Artificially acquired passive immunity
   c. Naturally acquired active immunity
   d. Artificially acquired active immunity

Application Exercises

Respond to the following scenarios on a separate sheet.

1. Denise Woodson has just received a prescription for antibiotics. She is also on birth control pills. **What patient education do you need to give?**
2. Betty Monroe has been treated with an antibiotic for 10 days and calls to say that she now has a fungal infection. **Explain to her why this happened.**
3. Jennifer Dickerson brings her baby in for a vaccination. She asks how vaccinations work. **How do you respond?**
4. Brenda Massey has the flu and demands an antibiotic. The prescriber does not give her one. **Explain to her why antibiotics do not work on viruses.**
5. Louie Garcia has come in for his first round of IV chemotherapy. **What patient education should you give him?**

Virtual Field Trips

Go to the following websites to find the information. If a website is not available, try to find the information through another source.

1. Go to your favorite drug information site and record the classification of the following:

   a. 5-FU

   b. Erythromycin

   c. Taxol

   d. Methotrexate

   e. Mycostatin

   f. Chlor-Trimeton

   g. Cortaid

   h. Interferon

   i. Nix

   j. AZT

2. Visit http://www.aidsmeds.com or http://www.aids.org and research drugs currently used for patients with acquired immunodeficiency syndrome.
3. Surf to http://www.cancer.org and download a patient teaching aid about cancer.
4. Go to http://www.procrit.com and print a list of side effects of cancer medications.

For further study and practice with drug classifications learned in this chapter, complete the following table to the best of your ability. Use resources such as a PDR, the Internet, or printed drug guides for help.

CLASSIFICATION	PURPOSE	SIDE EFFECTS	CONTRAINDICATIONS/PRECAUTIONS/INTERACTIONS	EXAMPLES	PATIENT EDUCATION
Antiinfectives					
Antibacterials					
Penicillins					
Cephalosporins					
Tetracyclines					
Macrolides					
Aminoglycosides					
Quinolones					
Sulfa drugs					
Antituberculosis drugs					
Antiinfectives					
Antivirals					
Antiretrovirals					
Anticancer drugs					
Alkylating agents					
Antimetabolites					
Antitumor antibiotics					
Plant extracts/ alkaloids					
Hormones					
Biological response modifiers					
Radioactive isotopes					

Integumentary System Medications

The integumentary system includes the skin (the largest organ of the body), hair, and nails. Integumentary medications are placed directly on the affected area unless a systemic problem requires a systemic medication. For example, if a patient has a small pimple, it may be treated directly with a topical antibiotic. However, if the patient has urticaria, or hives, because of an allergic reaction to something in the body, a systemic medication may be needed.

OBJECTIVES

At the end of this chapter, the student will be able to:

- Define all key terms.
- List the effects of medications on the integumentary system.
- Describe the types of medication that are administered to and through the skin: antiinfectives, oral contraceptives, immunosuppressants, antihistamines, and antipruritics.
- Contrast the effects of systemic versus topically applied medications.

KEY TERMS

Acne
Alopecia
Comedos
Condyloma
Débride
Eczema
HPV
Keratinization
Melanocyte

Nevus (nevi)
Nits
Nodule
Papule
Psoriasis
Rosacea
Seborrhea
Verruca(e)

● INTEGUMENTARY SYSTEM

The skin covers the entire body with only a few openings, such as the eyes and ears. Injury can damage the skin and open a pathway for infection.

Examples of dangers to the skin include abrasions, blisters, calluses, cracks, cuts, irritated areas, inflamed areas, lesions, scrapes, sores, rashes, and sunburn. Skin can become infected or infested with bacteria, fungi, parasites, or viruses.

Some patients are especially susceptible to integumentary weaknesses. Some are genetically predisposed (more likely) to especially delicate skin and skin tumors. Additionally, those who have fair skin and repeated exposure to the sun are more vulnerable to skin damage. Other environmental hazards may also cause skin discoloration, hair loss (alopecia), oily skin lesions (seborrhea), scaly patches (psoriasis), warts (verrucae—which are caused by viruses), moles (nevi), and tumors.

Skin disorders are classified as infectious, inflammatory, or cancerous. The medications used are based on the diagnosis in that classification. (See the Master the Essentials table for descriptions of the most common integumentary system drugs.)

● MEDICATIONS USED TO TREAT INFECTIONS

As you know, bacteria, parasites, viruses, and fungi can invade the body. Antibiotics are used topically or systemically to fight bacteria, and fungi are fought with antifungals, either topically or systemically.

Bacteria

Acne is an inflammatory disorder that affects the sebaceous glands. Bacteria can cause acne, which is found in many adolescents as well as adults. Puberty causes seborrhea, a condition caused by an overproduction of skin oils. Abnormal keratinization, or hardening of the epithelial tissue, also occurs. A bacterium, *Propionibacterium acnes*, grows inside the sebaceous glands and makes an irritating, acidic substance. The skin produces inflamed bumps in response to this irritation.

Open comedos, or blackheads, are oil glands plugged with melanin granules. Closed comedos, or whiteheads, are white rather than black because they are produced just below the skin and lack melanin. Deeper lumps called nodules involve inflammation deep below the skin. Severe inflammation and pus can cause pain and deformity.

Rosacea is a type of skin irritation without pus. Small bumps, or papules, create a reddened color to the skin. Even though they do not contain pus, they may produce pain because of the thickening and swelling. The patient with rosacea appears flushed, especially on the nose and cheek. Sunlight, stress, and hot temperature can aggravate rosacea. Alcohol, spicy foods, and hot beverages can also exacerbate it.

Medications used to treat acne and rosacea can be applied topically to the areas of irritation, frequently the face and neck. The active ingredient in these drugs may be vitamin A, an acid, or an antibiotic.

Over-the-counter (OTC) acne medications usually contain benzoyl peroxide as a cream, gel, or lotion. Benzoyl peroxide is bacteriostatic and inhibits bacterial growth.

Retinoids contain vitamin A, which increases the body's resistance to infection by reducing the oil production that clogs the pores. They reduce both the function of the sebaceous glands and keratinization. Because of serious associated side effects, the use of oral retinoids, such as isotretinoin (Accutane), is reserved for patients with severe acne who do not respond to other topical agents.

For severe acne, salicylic acid, sulfur, or resorcinol may be used to remove the infected skin through shedding. Systemic antibiotics are sometimes necessary in extreme cases.

Oral contraceptives have been effective in decreasing the symptoms of acne as well and are sometimes prescribed for this purpose. The hormones in some oral contraceptives can help stop acne from forming by reducing the amount of androgens that the body produces.

Master the Essentials: Dermatologic Medications

This table shows the various dermatologic medications and key side effects, contraindications and precautions, and interactions.

CLASS	SIDE EFFECTS	CONTRAINDICATIONS/ PRECAUTIONS	INTERACTIONS
Benzoyl peroxide	Peeling, erythema, edema	Hypersensitivity	Tretinoin
Retinoids	Photosensitivity, local reactions (topical); depression, suicidal ideation, pseudotumor cerebri, pancreatitis, visual changes, hepatotoxicity, hypertriglyceridemia (oral)	Hypersensitivity, pregnancy	Other topical products, photosensitizers
Scabicides and pediculocides	Eczema, rash, redness, itching, burning	Hypersensitivity	Oils, pentobarbital, phenobarbital, diazepam
Salicylic acid	Local irritation	Hypersensitivity; prolonged use; irritated skin; moles, birthmarks, or warts with hair growth; mucous membranes	Use with sulfur may cause additive effects.
Topical antifungals	Burning, stinging, pruritus, erythema	Hypersensitivity	None reported
Topical corticosteroids	Burning, itching, irritation	Hypersensitivity; use on the face, groin, or axillae; pregnancy	None reported
Topical immunomodulators	Burning, pruritus	Hypersensitivity, pregnancy, breastfeeding	Formal studies have not been performed.
Antipsoriatic agents	Irritation to surrounding skin; discoloration of skin, hair, or fabrics	Hypersensitivity, use on the face, renal disease, pregnancy, breastfeeding, hypercalcemia (calcipotriene)	Topical corticosteroids
Topical fluorouracil	Erythema, burning, vesicle formation, insomnia, photosensitivity, malaise	Hypersensitivity, pregnancy	None reported

Parasites

Itch mites, called *Sarcoptes scabiei,* cause scabies by burrowing into the skin. Lice, which cause pediculosis, live in hair and feed on blood. Scabicides and pediculicides are used to treat mite and lice infestations, respectively. These drugs are applied directly to the area of infestation.

Lice lay eggs called nits. After applying a pediculicide, the hair where the nits live should be combed with a special fine-toothed comb and the site inspected for at least 1 week after treatment to be sure all the nits are dead. Because bedding and clothing may hold eggs, they must be thoroughly cleaned.

Viruses

Viruses can be difficult to eradicate. The human papillomavirus (HPV) that causes warts is especially troublesome. When warts are found on the genitals, they are called condylomas; otherwise they are called verrucae. HPV can lie dormant in the system and flare up if not completely treated. The goal of wart treatment is to destroy the affected skin superficially. Cryosurgery with liquid nitrogen or topical products containing salicylic acid may be necessary.

Herpes simplex virus type 1 (HSV-1) typically causes cold sores, or fever blisters, on the mouth and lips. Herpes simplex type 2 (HSV-1) is a sexually transmitted virus and usually affects the genital mucosa. Both HSV-1 and HSV-2 are treated with oral antivirals. Herpes zoster, or shingles, is a reactivation of the varicella-zoster virus that causes chickenpox. This is also treated with oral antiviral medications, which are covered in Chapter 13.

Fungal Infections

Fungal infections that affect the dermatologic system include tinea infections and candidiasis. In tineal infections, dermatophytes invade keratin and can infect the hair, nails, and skin. Topical antifungals, such as clotrimazole (Lotrimin) or terbinafine (Lamisil), may be used when the infection is present on the trunk, extremities, groin, or feet. If the infection is on the scalp, oral agents may be needed.

Candidal infections, also known as yeast infections, are caused by *Candida albicans.* This infection is associated with a pruritic red rash that may be painful. When it occurs in the mouth, this infection is commonly known as thrush; white plaques are usually present on the oral mucosa. Topical antifungals such as nystatin may be ordered.

● MEDICATIONS USED TO TREAT INFLAMMATORY CONDITIONS

Inflammatory conditions of the skin include burns, atopic dermatitis, and psoriasis.

Burns

Burns can damage the skin by removing water from the skin, causing it to blister, or by removing the skin entirely. They are classified as first, second, or third degree (Fig. 14.1).

Sunburn is a common first degree burn. The skin becomes red and painful to touch. People with few melanocytes (darkening cells) and thus fair skin are especially prone to sunburn.

Nonpharmacological treatment for sunburn includes applying cool water for 20 minutes and applying an herb called aloe vera. Applying butter or lard to a sunburn causes more damage and should not be done.

If a blister forms over the burn and the burn is yellow in appearance, it is classified as a second degree burn. It is important to cover second degree burns and administer an antibiotic, as prescribed. If the blister breaks, the dressing over the burn can act as a barrier against infectious organisms.

A third degree burn is a severe burn that affects all layers of skin as well as subcutaneous tissue and possibly even muscle and bone. The patient with a third degree burn has serious loss of skin integrity and is at great risk for infection and water loss. Immediate treatment of severe burns includes maintaining the patient's airway, giving oxygen, and administering intravenous (IV) fluids, as needed. Sometimes a dressing that débrides (or removes) tissue is prescribed to get rid of the dead tissue. Remember that this dressing also removes healthy tissue and must be applied only to the wound as ordered. An antimicrobial nonstick dressing may be ordered. Other dressings may be ordered to absorb exudates or stimulate healthy new granulation tissue to form. Systemic medications ordered may include analgesics, antiinflammatory agents, and antibiotics.

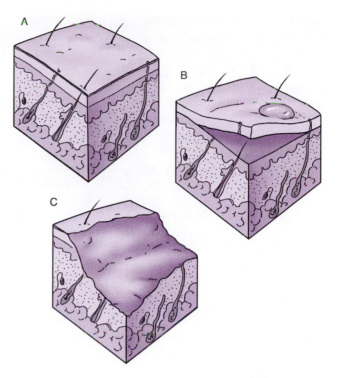

FIGURE 14.1. Burn degrees. (A) Burning of the top layer of skin is called a first degree burn; it commonly causes red skin and swelling. (B) A burn that causes a blister is a second degree burn; the blisters may open and ooze a clear fluid. This burn is often very painful. (C) A burn that removes the skin and tissue beyond it is a third degree burn; the area looks brown, even charred. The patient may or may not complain of pain.

Atopic Dermatitis

Atopic dermatitis is also called eczema. It is an allergic disorder usually associated with other atopic diseases, such as asthma or allergic rhinitis. It causes cutaneous inflammation that is evidenced by extremely dry patches of skin that itch. Initial methods of treatment include avoiding allergens, removing irritants, and maintaining hydration. Agents that may be needed include topical corticosteroids or topical immunomodulators, such as tacrolimus or pimecrolimus. Oral antihistamines such as diphenhydramine (Benadryl) may relieve itching but can cause mood changes, bone defects, or hematologic problems if used for prolonged periods.

Psoriasis

Psoriasis is a chronic inflammatory skin disease in which an altered immune system causes the life cycle of skin cells to be shortened (Fig. 14.2). This results in a buildup of skin cells on the surface, and the dead cells take on a flaky white appearance atop a reddened (erythematous) plaque. Treatment of psoriasis may include topical corticosteroids, low-dose antihistamines, salicylic acid, or phototherapy. Specific antipsoriatic agents include anthralin and calcipotriene, which are topical preparations. Oral or injectable methotrexate is used for severe disease unresponsive to other therapy.

Nonpharmacological therapies include using natural substances found in lagoons of volcanic eruptions. Many countries have spas that claim to have healing pools of water that cure both psoriasis and dermatitis.

⬤ MEDICATIONS USED TO TREAT CANCER

Cancer can occur anywhere in the body. The skin is our outer defense system and thus susceptible to injury, which can lead to damaged tissue that can eventually cause cancer. If a *nevus* (mole) or discolored area changes color, grows, or becomes less rounded on its borders, a physician should be notified. A biopsy may be ordered. The good news is that, with frequent observation by a trained professional, skin cancers can usually be diagnosed in an early stage.

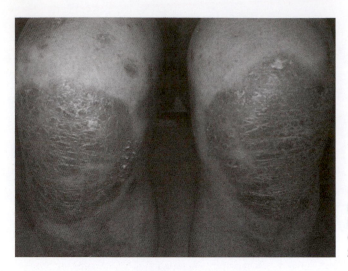
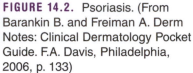

FIGURE 14.2. Psoriasis. (From Barankin B. and Freiman A. Derm Notes: Clinical Dermatology Pocket Guide. F.A. Davis, Philadelphia, 2006, p. 133)

The three major types of skin cancer are basal cell carcinoma, squamous cell carcinoma, and malignant melanoma. Basal cell carcinoma (Fig. 14.3) is the most common form of skin cancer and rarely spreads (metastasizes). Treatment may require surgical excision, but topical preparations such as fluorouracil or imiquod (a topical immunomodulator) may be used. Liquid nitrogen cryotherapy is also an option.

Squamous cell carcinoma (Fig. 14.4) arises from malignant keratinocytes. This form of skin cancer can metastasize. Surgical removal is the treatment of choice, and radiation therapy may be needed.

The incidence of malignant melanoma is quickly rising (Fig. 14.5). This is an unpredictable cancer that spreads through the lymphatic system and blood. Treatment includes surgery, radiation, and chemotherapy.

FIGURE 14.3. Basal cell carcinoma. (From Barankin B. and Freiman A. Derm Notes: Clinical Dermatology Pocket Guide. F.A. Davis, Philadelphia, 2006, p. 70)

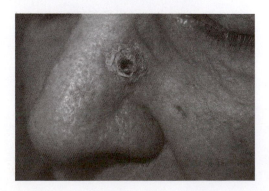

FIGURE 14.4. Squamous cell carcinoma. (From Barankin B. and Freiman A. Derm Notes: Clinical Dermatology Pocket Guide. F.A. Davis, Philadelphia, 2006, p. 150)

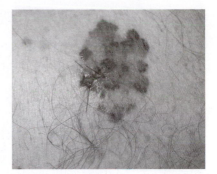

FIGURE 14.5. Melanoma. (From Barankin B. and Freiman A. Derm Notes: Clinical Dermatology Pocket Guide. F.A. Davis, Philadelphia, 2006, p. 116)

●●● SUMMARY

The skin is the major defense organ of the body. Skin disorders can cause pain, itching, body image disturbances, and embarrassment. A disorder such as malignant melanoma is life-threatening. A thorough skin assessment can help find problems early. An understanding of treatments and available medications is essential.

Activities

To make sure that you have learned the key points covered in this chapter, complete the following activities.

True or False
Write *true* if the statement is true. Beside the false statements, write *false* and correct the statement to make it true.

1. Scabicides kill lice._____

2. Pediculicides only kill nits._____

3. Vitamin K is used to treat acne._____

4. Rosacea is a form of measles._____

5. OTC drugs can cure acne._____

Multiple Choice
Choose the best answer for each question.

1. A sunburn is an example of a:
   a. First degree burn
   b. Second degree burn
   c. Third degree burn
   d. Fourth degree burn

2. A nit is:
   a. A louse egg
   b. A nodule
   c. A form of acne
   d. Earwax

3. A blackhead is called a:
   a. Comedo
   b. Psoriasis lesion
   c. Verruca
   d. Nevus

4. Retinoids contain vitamin:
   a. E
   b. C
   c. D
   d. A

5. Shingles is caused by:
   a. Herpes simplex type 1
   b. Herpes simplex type 2
   c. Herpes zoster
   d. Herpes roster

Application Exercises
Respond to the following scenarios on a separate sheet.

1. Gisela Winne has been given an order of birth control pills for her acne. She is outraged that she should be put on birth control pills for a skin problem. **What would you say?**

2. Flavia Owen has a wound that needs to be débrided. **How would you explain what this means?**

3. Bill Jinkins has acne. He asks why he has to wash his face before he applies acne cream. **What would you answer?**

4. Breanoh Lafayette has very fair skin. She asks why she has to use such a strong sunscreen when her darker-skinned friends do not. **What would you say?**

Virtual Field Trips

Go to the following websites to find the information. If a website is not available, try to find the information through another source.

1. Visit your favorite website and write the classification of each of the following.

   a. Kwell

   b. Retin-A

   c. Nix

   d. Accutane

   e. Floxin

2. Go to your local health department or similar website and create a patient teaching aid on lice infestation removal.

3. Visit the American Academy of Dermatology (http://www.aad.org/default.htm) and learn the ABCDs of melanoma.

4. Visit MedlinePlus (http://medlineplus.gov/) and review the important warning regarding isotretinoin (Accutane).

For further study and practice with drug classifications learned in this chapter, complete the following table to the best of your ability. Use resources such as a PDR, the Internet, or printed drug guides for help.

CLASSIFICATION	PURPOSE	SIDE EFFECTS	CONTRAINDICATIONS/PRECAUTIONS/INTERACTIONS	EXAMPLES	PATIENT EDUCATION
Topical antibiotics					
Topical antifungals					
Topical corticosteroids					
Antipsoriatic agents					

Pulmonary System Medications

*F*rom the first breath our body takes, the body depends on the respiratory or pulmonary system to bring oxygen to the cells and dispose of carbon dioxide. If this system works improperly, immediate medication may be needed. Thus, many pulmonary medications are delivered by inhalation to maximize delivery to the lungs.

OBJECTIVES

At the end of this chapter, the student will be able to:

- Define all key terms.
- Detail the action of pulmonary medications.
- List the side effects of pulmonary medications.
- Describe how administering pulmonary medications through different routes affects their action.

KEY TERMS

Alveoli	Expiration
Antihistamine	Glucocorticoid
Antiinfluenza agent	Hypoxia
Antispasmotic	Inspiration
Antitussive	Mast cell stabilizer
Beta-adrenergic agent	Mucolytic
CO_2	O_2
COPD	PPD
Decongestant	Respiration
Dyspnea	Smoking cessation
Expectorant	Status asthmaticus

● PULMONARY MEDICATIONS

The pulmonary system is responsible for respiration—bringing oxygen (O_2) into the blood stream and removing waste in the form of carbon dioxide (CO_2) from it. (See the Master the Essentials table for descriptions of the most common pulmonary system drugs.)

A CLOSER LOOK: Respiration

The pulmonary and musculoskeletal systems work together during the process of respiration. The muscles need an O_2 supply (and CO_2 removal) to survive. A large muscle called the diaphragm facilitates breathing. When the diaphragm contracts, the lungs are compressed, expelling CO_2 up through the bronchus and trachea into the air. The now mostly empty lungs then inhale O_2 from the air. The outward movement of air is called expiration. The inward movement of air is called inspiration, and it requires energy.

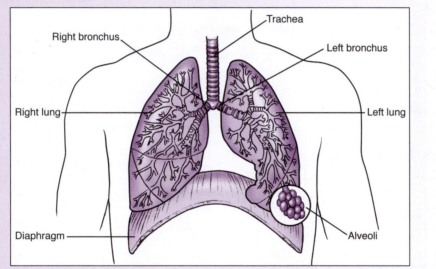

The brain regulates the rate and depth of breathing, depending on the needs of the body. That is why when you exercise and need more oxygen, you breathe faster.

The exchange of CO_2 and O_2 occurs at the level of the alveoli (tiny air sacs in the lungs). Anytime alveolar function is impaired, CO_2 builds up and oxygenation declines. Changes in alveolar function occur with smoking and diseases such as asthma.

Oxygen is vital to every cell in the body. Four to six minutes without breathing causes a person to die. That is why when someone has serious trouble breathing (dyspnea) it is a medical emergency (see Fast Tip 15.1).

Diseases such as asthma, chronic obstructive pulmonary disease (COPD), and tuberculosis can cause dyspnea or impair the lung's ability to do its job. Medications can help these patients improve their pulmonary function (Table 15.1).

The medications used depend on what part of the pulmonary system is affected. Some medications liquefy secretions, and others completely dry up secretions. Some medications act locally, and some act systemically (Box 15.1).

Mast Cell Stabilizers

Mast cell stabilizers inhibit mast cells from releasing inflammatory mediators such as histamine. These drugs decrease swelling, inflammation, itching, and capillary permeability. They are used to prevent

Master the Essentials: Respiratory Medications

This table shows the various classes of respiratory medications and key side effects, contraindications and precautions, and interactions for each class.

CLASS	SIDE EFFECTS	CONTRAINDICATIONS/PRECAUTIONS	INTERACTIONS
Mast cell stabilizers	Throat irritation, bad taste, wheezing, cough	Hypersensitivity	None reported
Antiinfluenza agents	Anorexia, bronchitis, diarrhea, dizziness, dry mouth, headache, insomnia, nervousness, vertigo	Hypersensitivity, kidney or liver impairment, pregnancy, breast-feeding, underlying respiratory disease	Acetaminophen, aspirin, cimetidine
Antitussives	Constipation, dizziness, respiratory depression, sedation, urinary retention	Asthma, COPD, addiction-prone patients, hypersensitivity	MAO inhibitors, other CNS depressants
Expectorants	Vomiting, diarrhea, abdominal pain	Hypersensitivity	None reported
Anticholinergics	Agitation, confusion, dizziness, drowsiness, headache, increased heart rate, thickened secretions, bronchitis	Hypersensitivity, cardiac instability, glaucoma, prostatic hypertrophy	Use with other anticholinergics is not recommended.
Xanthines	Dysrhythmias, CNS stimulation, GI distress, increased blood glucose and heart rate, urinary frequency	Diabetes mellitus, glaucoma, peptic ulcer, pregnancy, hypersensitivity	Barbiturates, hydantoins, ketoconazole, loop diuretics, beta blockers, calcium channel blockers, oral contraceptives
Beta-adrenergic agonists	CNS stimulation; increased appetite, blood glucose, and blood pressure	CV disorders, diabetes mellitus, hyperthyroidism, kidney problems, seizure disorders	MAO inhibitors, tricyclic antidepressants, cardiac glycosides, beta blockers
Decongestants	Hypersensitivity reaction, anxiety, decreased cardiac output, decreased urine output, electrolyte imbalances, headache, nervousness, racing heart rate, seizures, tremor	CV disorders, diabetes mellitus, hyperthyroidism, lactation, pregnancy, hypersensitivity	Other sympathomimetics, MAO inhibitors, beta blockers, methyldopa
Glucocorticoids	Cough, dry mouth, hoarseness, oral fungal infection, throat irritation, headache, dizziness	Viral, bacterial, or fungal infections; heart failure, cirrhosis, diabetes mellitus, hypertension, hypothyroidism, renal failure	Barbiturates, phenytoin, oral contraceptives

(table continued on page 264)

Master the Essentials: Respiratory Medications (continued)

CLASS	SIDE EFFECTS	CONTRAINDICATIONS/PRECAUTIONS	INTERACTIONS
Mucolytics	Drowsiness, mouth inflammation, runny nose, bronchospasm, nausea, vomiting	CV disease, diabetes mellitus, ineffective cough, lactation, pregnancy, thyroid abnormalities	Activated charcoal
Oxygen	Alveolar changes, blindness in premature infants, confusion, hypoventilation	Avoid using high doses in patients with COPD.	None reported
Nicotine	Cardiac irritability, local irritation, headache	Hypersensitivity, pregnancy, breastfeeding	Alcohol, benzodiazepines, beta blockers, insulin

the occurrence of asthma attacks. They do not cure the disease, but they do decrease the body's reaction to asthma triggers, such as air pollutants, respiratory infections, chemicals, food allergies, pollen, dust, mold, animal dander, and stress.

Cromolyn sodium and nedocromil sodium are examples of mast cell stabilizers. These medications should not be used for acute asthma attacks. They are administered via a nebulizer or metered-dose inhaler. They also come in an intranasal form for seasonal allergies.

Antiinfluenza Agents

Medications can ease the signs and symptoms of influenza. These drugs are usually taken for 2 to 5 days. Although it is better to prevent the patient from getting influenza through vaccination, these agents can reduce the duration of the illness. Examples of drugs used to treat influenza include zanamivir (Relenza) and oseltamivir phosphate (Tamiflu).

Antitussives and Expectorants

As the name indicates, antitussives stop coughs. If a cough is dry and thus not productive, an antitussive may be indicated. Some narcotic analgesics, such as codeine, are effective antitussives in low dosages.

When secretions are present, expectorants are used to boost the ability to cough out secretions. Expectorants can also soothe respiratory tract mucous membranes.

Bronchodilator Medications

Bronchodilators relieve acute bronchospasm and include anticholinergics, xanthines, methylxanthines, and beta-adrenergic agonists. They relax the smooth muscle of the bronchi, allowing the patient to breathe more easily. When taken by inhalation, these drugs work immediately on the pulmonary system. When taken orally, the body takes longer to feel the effect but the action is of longer duration—producing side effects for longer periods of time as well.

Fast Tip 15.1 Fast Relief for Dyspnea

Pulmonary medications are usually given by inhalation for quick action. A nebulizer or inhaler is used for this purpose.

TABLE 15.1 Common Pulmonary Diseases

PULMONARY DISEASE	OVERVIEW	SYMPTOMS	MEDICATIONS
Asthma	Asthma is a disease caused by increased reaction of the tracheobronchial tree to stimuli, which results in episodic narrowing and inflammation of the airways. Although the cause is not always known, the airways are chronically inflamed.	Breathlessness, air hunger, coughing, and dyspnea are common symptoms. If asthma continues for a long period of time, *status asthmaticus,* or asthma that does not stop, becomes a medical emergency.	*Antiasthmatic* medications target both the bronchoconstriction and the inflammation.
COPD	The main diseases included under COPD are chronic bronchitis and emphysema. Chronic bronchitis is an inflammation of the bronchial tree. In response to irritation, mucus floods the bronchi and impairs breathing. Emphysema occurs after years of chronic inflammation when the bronchioles lose elasticity and the alveoli dilate beyond effectiveness. COPD is usually caused by tobacco smoking—both direct and second-hand. Irritants and pollutants in the air can also cause COPD. It cannot be cured.	Dyspnea and coughing, particularly a cough that is productive (brings up mucus)	A patient with COPD can expect to need a variety of drugs to treat infections because the patient has damaged the first line of defense—the lungs. The patient will also need drugs to decrease the bronchospasm that is created by the chemical irritation and to control the chronic cough that comes from irritating the pharynx. *Mucolytics* and *expectorants* are usually indicated, along with oxygen therapy.
Tuberculosis	Tuberculosis (TB) is an infection caused by *Mycobacterium tuberculosis*, a gram-positive bacterium.	A persistent cough, night sweats, and weight loss.	The TB bacterium is gram-positive but frequently resists treatment with traditional antibiotics. For that reason, it is often treated with a combination of drugs. Treatment must continue for as long as 6–9 months.

BOX 15.1 **Classification of Pulmonary Medications**

Anticholinergics—dilate bronchi
Antiinfluenza agents—reduce influenza symptoms
Antitussives—stop coughing
Beta-adrenergic agonists and xanthines—open up the bronchi
Decongestants—remove fluid buildup in the respiratory passages
Expectorants—produce a more productive cough
Glucocorticoids—decrease inflammation
Mast cell stabilizers—prevent asthma attacks
Mucolytics—loosen mucus
Oxygen—provides additional needed oxygen to the lungs
Smoking cessation drugs—help people stop smoking

Anticholinergics

Parasympatholytics or anticholinergics dilate bronchi by decreasing the cholinergics that cause bronchospasm. Because they stimulate the sympathetic nervous system, you can expect a "fight or flight" response, including increased heart rate and blood pressure. This effect also dries up lung secretions, thereby decreasing congestion and improving pulmonary function. An example of an anticholinergic bronchodilator is ipratropium bromide.

Xanthines

Xanthines, also called methylxanthines, include theophylline and aminophylline. These drugs relax smooth muscle and relieve bronchospasm. Because patients metabolize them at different rates, the dosage must be carefully adjusted based on patient reaction. They have a narrow safety margin, so careful monitoring is essential. Oral forms should be taken on an empty stomach with a full glass of water for faster absorption. However, taking it on a full stomach decreases gastric upset.

Beta-adrenergic agonists

Beta-adrenergic agonists are bronchodilators that are commonly used for treating asthma. They stimulate beta-2 receptor sites in the sympathetic nervous system, which results in bronchial dilation. Short-acting agents include albuterol and isoproterenol; they are mainly used "as-needed." A long-acting agent, such as salmeterol, is used to keep asthma controlled.

Decongestants

Decongestants cause blood vessels in the mucous membranes in the nose to tighten, reducing nasal passage drainage. They are available as nasal sprays and oral medications. Use of the topical form provides immediate relief of nasal mucosal swelling and congestion.

Glucocorticoids

Glucocorticoids suppress inflammation. They are usually taken daily as prophylaxis against asthma but are not used for acute episodes.

If taken longer than 10 days, oral glucocorticoids may have severe adverse effects due to suppressing the immune system. These drugs should be taken at the lowest dose that is effective for as short a time as possible.

Mucolytics

Mucolytics liquefy lung secretions so they are easier to cough out. They do this by changing the composition of the mucus. Combined with expectorants, mucolytic agents help remove irritating substances from lungs. Acetylcysteine is an example of a mucolytic.

Oxygen

Oxygen is used as therapy for low oxygenation, or hypoxia. Chronic use includes management of COPD; acute use is needed to treat dyspnea and carbon monoxide poisoning. Oxygen can be delivered by nasal cannula, mask, endotracheal tube, hood, or tent.

It is important not to give more O_2 than ordered. For instance, patients with COPD tend to retain CO_2. This leads to higher than normal levels of CO_2 and lower than normal levels of O_2 in the blood. Normally the body reacts to higher levels of CO_2 by prompting the lungs to breathe deeper and faster to blow off the excess CO_2. In patients with COPD, however, the body has adapted to the long-term higher levels of CO_2, causing these patients to breathe from a lowered O_2 level. So giving a patient with COPD more O_2 than is prescribed can actually shut off this adaptive mechanism and cause the patient's breathing to stop or slow markedly.

Smoking Cessation

Because tobacco smoking is addictive and causes so many illnesses (e.g., emphysema, lung cancer, and bronchitis), drugs have been developed to facilitate smoking cessation. Combined with hypnosis and behavioral therapy, they can be extremely effective. Because it is very difficult to quit completely and suddenly ("cold turkey"), smoking cessation aids deliver small, consistant doses of nicotine to help the individual gradually withdraw from nicotine use.

It is important that you teach patients not to smoke while using nicotine patches to avoid a nicotine overdose. Also, patients should not wear nicotine patches when inside magnetic resonance imaging equipment. Other routes for nicotine include inhalation, gum, and nasal spray.

SUMMARY

The pulmonary system must function properly for the patient to be healthy. Many medications exist to help heal a malfunctioning system. They focus on opening the bronchi, drying secretions, decreasing the histamine response, treating influenza, getting oxygen into the lungs, stopping coughs, loosening mucus, and forcing secretions out. Smoking cessation drugs help patients stop a habit that could lead to significant complications and even death.

Activities

To make sure that you have learned the key points covered in this chapter, complete the following activities.

True or False

Write *true* if the statement is true. Beside the false statements, write *false* and correct the statement to make it true.

1. Glucocorticoids are used during acute asthma attacks. _____

2. Expectorants are used to suppress cough. _____

3. Emphysema can be cured with O_2. _____

4. Bronchodilation is a symptom of asthma. _____

5. Bronchioles are where O_2 and CO_2 are exchanged. _____

Multiple Choice

Choose the best answer for each question.

1. When teaching a patient about oxygen therapy, which of the following is correct?
   a. Oxygen is combustible.
   b. Oxygen should be administered at less than 4 L/min.
   c. Nebulizers must be attached for oxygen therapy.
   d. Oxygen is not portable.

2. Asthma occurs in the:
   a. Brain
   b. Bronchi
   c. Alveoli
   d. Pharynx

3. Which loosen secretions for productive cough?
   a. Beta-adrenergic agents
   b. Glucocorticoids
   c. Mast cell stabilizers
   d. Mucolytics

4. Which test looks for the presence of *Mycobacterium tuberculosis*?
   a. Rheumatoid factors
   b. Viral load
   c. Bone scan
   d. PPD

5. All of the following are acceptable routes for oxygen *except*:
   a. Nasal cannula
   b. Tent
   c. Nasogastric tube
   d. Mask

Application Exercises

Respond to the following scenarios on a separate sheet.

1. While you are teaching a CPR class, a student, Carmen Thornton, asks you why exhaled CO_2 into the victim does not harm the victim. **What do you answer?**

2. Willie Jefferson has asthma. When he takes his asthma medication, he says he feels "like his heart is going to jump out of his chest." **How do you explain this side effect to him?**

3. Sandi Durkee has emphysema. The doctor has prescribed O_2 therapy. **What must you do to set up this treatment for her?**

4. Julian Hollifield has COPD. He wants to know why he cannot use more than the prescribed flow of O_2 per minute. **What would you say to him?**

5. Thiekoro Cisse shares his inhaler with other members of the band in which he plays. **How would you counsel him?**

Virtual Field Trips

Go to the following websites to find the information. If a website is not available, try to find the information through another source.

1. Go to http://www.lungusa.org (the site of the American Lung Association) and get tips for smoking cessation.

2. Surf to the website of your choice and find the classifications of:

   a. Serevent

   b. Sudafed

   c. Theo-Dur

   d. Prednisone

   e. Cromolyn

   f. Caffeine

   g. Pnemovax

   h. Oxygen

   i. Allegra

   j. Claritin

   k. Robitussin

For further study and practice with drug classifications learned in this chapter, complete the following table to the best of your ability. Use resources such as a PDR, the Internet, or printed drug guides for help.

CLASSIFICATION	PURPOSE	SIDE EFFECTS	CONTRAINDICATIONS/PRECAUTIONS/INTERACTIONS	PATIENT EDUCATION	EXAMPLES
Anticholinergics					
Antiinfluenza agents					
Antitussives					
Beta-adrenergic agonists					
Decongestants					
Glucocorticoids					
Mast cell stabilizers					
Mucolytics					
Oxygen					
Nicotine					

16

Gastrointestinal System Medications

*T*he gastrointestinal system is actually a very long tube through which food is passed, nutrients are absorbed, and waste is removed. The main organs of digestion are the stomach, small intestine, and large intestine. Accessory organs such as the liver and pancreas assist these organs by secreting enzymes to break down food into vital nutrients. Gastrointestinal medications have diverse purposes, including coating the stomach, relieving nausea and vomiting, inducing vomiting, reducing acid in the stomach, protecting teeth, killing microbes, promoting good nutrition, reducing diarrhea and constipation, suppressing the appetite, and reducing gas.

OBJECTIVES

At the end of this chapter, the student will be able to:

- Define all key terms.
- Describe how these medications affect the gastrointestinal (GI) system: anorectal preparations, anorexiants, antacids, antibiotics, antiemetics, antiflatulence agents, antihelmintics, antispasmodics, lipase inhibitors, emetics, H_2-receptor agonists, laxatives, mouth cleansers, nutritional supplements, prokinetic agents, prostaglandins, and proton pump inhibitors.
- Identify drugs used to treat GI disorders, including GERD and peptic ulcer disease.
- Describe side effects, contraindications, and potential drug interactions of GI medications.

KEY TERMS

Alimentary canal
Crohn's disease
Constipation
Emesis
Epistaxis
Diarrhea
Fissure
Flatulence
GERD
H_1
H_2

HCl
H. pylori
Halitosis
Heartburn
Hemorrhoid
Morbidly obese
Nausea
Peristalsis
Stomatitis
Ulcer
Ulcerative colitis

● GASTROINTESTINAL SYSTEM

The gastrointestinal (GI), or digestive, system consists of a long tube that goes from the mouth to the anus, with accessory organs attached (Fig. 16.1). This alimentary canal is responsible for bringing nutrients into the body, selecting what to absorb, and choosing what to reject. In other words, the three major functions of this body system are digestion, absorption, and excretion. The goal is to allow nutrients from food to be used as cellular energy.

Food is taken in by the mouth and broken down into a form usable to the body, first by mechanical digestion (chewing) and then by chemical digestion (enzymes). Specific enzymes perform specific functions with respect to digesting the three complex organic molecules found in foods: fats, proteins,

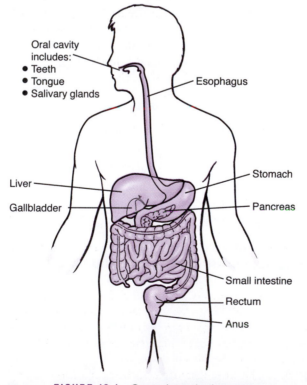

FIGURE 16.1. Gastrointestinal system.

TABLE 16.1 **Functions of the Major Digestive Organs**	
Stomach	• Stores food. • Mixes food with hydrochloric acid. • Passes this mixture, called chyme, into the small intestine.
Small intestine	• Carbohydrates, fats, and proteins are broken down here. • Pancreatic enzymes and bile from the liver aid in digestion. • End products of digestion are absorbed into the bloodstream through mucous membranes.
Large intestine	• Absorbs extra water and electrolytes. • Eliminates waste products (feces).

and carbohydrates. These enzymes work at various sites along the GI tract. Food particles are moved from the mouth, through the oropharynx, through the esophagus, into the stomach, and then through the small intestines and large intestines via peristalsis (wave-like movements). If this process is impeded, toxic substances can build up. Infection can develop when the normal flora living in the alimentary canal is disturbed.

Review Table 16.1 to better understand the role of the major digestive organs.

The stomach's environment is high in hydrochloric acid (HCl). Reflux (backflow) of HCl into the esophagus can lead to ulcers, or mucosal breakdown. When the mucosa is penetrated, it creates an excellent environment for infection to spread, especially when one considers that food moving through the digestive tract comes from outside sources and may carry harmful microorganisms. Although the HCl and normal flora of the digestive tract kill some organisms, the GI system can still be a major site of infection.

Digestion is the process of converting food into chemical substances that can be used by the body. However, depending on our food choices, we can damage the GI system. Bad or "junk" food can damage the system by overworking the pancreas, liver, and gallbladder. Extreme undereating can lead to anorexia nervosa, and extreme overeating can cause obesity. Other ways to damage the GI system include using medications that change the acidity of the stomach and eating food or other substances that contain harmful microbes, such as worms, viruses, or bacteria.

● GASTROINTESTINAL MEDICATIONS

Gastrointestinal medications are used to treat specific disorders of the GI system or to control certain signs and symptoms, such as abdominal pain, change in bowel habits, heartburn, gas, indigestion, weight loss, nausea, vomiting, difficulty swallowing, loss of appetite, and blood or mucus in the feces. (See the Master the Essentials table for descriptions of the most common GI system drugs.)

Gastrointestinal drugs work to increase or decrease the function of the system by changing the muscle tone, replacing deficient enzymes, or increasing or decreasing the emptying time or rate of passage through the system. Some drugs serve to move food through the system at a desirable rate and to have enzymes ready to aid in the process of digestion.

Timing of GI medication administration is important too. Some medications are taken to coat the stomach lining or reduce gastric acidity and need to be taken on an empty stomach. Other medications need to be taken with food to be absorbed properly. Some foods such as grapefruit can affect the absorption of medications if taken simultaneously. It is important to understand the impact of the food we eat and the other medications we take on the GI system.

The following section details the most common complaints and disorders of the GI system and which drugs are used to manage them.

Master the Essentials: Gastrointestinal Medications

This table shows the various classes of gastrointestinal medications and key side effects, contraindications and precautions, and interactions for each class.

CLASS	SIDE EFFECTS	CONTRAINDICATIONS/PRECAUTIONS	INTERACTIONS
Antacids	Constipation, diarrhea (especially with magnesium compounds), electrolye imbalances, flatulence, kidney stones, osteoporosis	Heart failure, dehydration, kidney or liver disease	Antibiotics, salicylates
Anorexiants	Palpitations, arrhythmias, dry mouth, hair loss, blurred vision, decreased blood pressure, dizziness, drowsiness	Arteriosclerosis, heart disease, hypertension, glaucoma, pregnancy	MAO inhibitors, SSRIs, TCAs
Antidiarrheals	Nausea, vomiting, drowsiness; constipation (kaolin and pectin)	Hypersensitivity, bloody diarrhea	Alcohol, opiates, barbiturates, sedatives, metoclopramide; digoxin, allopurinol (kaolin and pectin)
Antiemetics	Drowsiness, agitation, confusion, constipation, dry mouth, nausea, anorexia	Sensitivity, severe emesis, seizure disorder, pregnancy, prolonged QTc interval (5-HT$_3$ receptor antagonists)	Anticholinergics, lithium, CNS depressants
Antiflatulents	None reported	None reported	None reported
Antifungals (nystatin)	Nausea, vomiting, diarrhea	Hypersensitivity, pregnancy	None reported
Antihelmintics	Abdominal pain, diarrhea	Hypersensitivity, pregnancy	Carbamazepine, hydantoins
Antispasmodics	Palpitations, vision disturbances, headache, nervousness	Hypersensitivity, glaucoma, bowel obstruction, urinary retention	Digoxin, phenothiazines, tricyclic antidepressants
Bowel evacuants	Nausea, abdominal fullness, bloating, cramping	GI obstruction, ileus, gastric retention, bowel perforation, pregnancy	Administration of oral drugs within 1 hour may be flushed from the GI tract.
Emetics	Diarrhea, drowsiness	Semiconscious or unconscious patient; if corrosives ingested	Do not administer syrup of ipecac and activated charcoal concomitantly.
Gallstone solubilizing agents	Headache, abdominal pain, diarrhea, dyspepsia, nausea	Hypersensitivity, intermittent acute cholecystitis, gallstone pancreatitis	Antacids, bile acid sequestrants, oral contraceptives

CLASS	SIDE EFFECTS	CONTRAINDICATIONS/PRECAUTIONS	INTERACTIONS
Gallstone solubilizing agents	Headache, abdominal pain, diarrhea, dyspepsia, nausea	Hypersensitivity, intermittent acute cholecystitis, gallstone pancreatitis	Antacids, bile acid sequestrants, oral contraceptives
GI stimulants	Extrapyramidal symptoms, dizziness, drowsiness, fatigue, headache, insomnia, restlessness	GI hemorrhage, pheochromocytoma, sensitivity	Alcohol, cimetidine, cyclosporine, digoxin, levodopa, MAO inhibitors, anticholinergics
H. pylori agents	Diarrhea, tinnitus, infection, mild GI problems	Kidney or liver insufficiency	Salicylates, digoxin, anticoagulants
H_2-receptor antagonists	Constipation, diarrhea, nausea, headache, malaise, rash	Hypersensitivity, liver impairment	Antacids, benzodiazepines, opioids, phenytoin, beta blockers, calcium channel blockers, cyclosporine
Laxatives/stool softeners	Diarrhea, nausea, vomiting, cramping, bloating, flatulence	Hypersensitivity, nausea, vomiting, fecal impaction, intestinal obstruction	Antacids, H_2 antagonists, proton pump inhibitors
Lipase inhibitors	Flatulence, fecal urgency, oily stool, incontinence, abdominal pain	Hypersensitivity, malabsorption syndrome, cholestasis	Pravastatin, warfarin
Prostaglandins	Diarrhea, abdominal pain	Pregnancy, history of allergy to prostaglandins, heart disease	Antacids
Proton pump inhibitors	Headache, abdominal pain, nausea, constipation, diarrhea	Hypersensitivity, liver disease	Clarithromycin, sucralfate, benzodiazepines, azole antifungals, digoxin, hydantoins
Sucralfate	Constipation, diarrhea, nausea, vomiting, flatulence, rash	Renal failure	Antacids, anticoagulants, digoxin, H_2 antagonists, hydantoins

Medications to Treat Constipation

Many of the drugs we discussed in the previous chapters can slow body systems. For example, medications that change smooth muscle tone affect the movement of food through the body. Whenever peristalsis slows down, constipation or infrequent, hard stools, can result. Medications that remove fluid from the body can lead to hard stool. If the colon reabsorbs too much fluid, the feces become hard and the alimentary canal does not clear. Laxatives are drugs that promote bowel movements. A cathartic is an even stronger medication that facilitates fast emptying of the colon. Laxatives can also be used for diagnosing GI disorders. They should not be used for weight loss. Laxatives can be classified as bulk-forming agents, osmotics, stimulants, or stool softeners.

Nonpharmacological treatments for constipation include exercise, laughing, increasing dietary fiber, drinking more fluids, decreasing consumption of dairy products, and drinking warmed prune juice.

Bulk-forming laxatives increase bulk and water content. They are made to resemble dietary fiber. They should be made of a medium consistency and taken with fluids. Prunes and bran have the same effects. Bulk-forming laxatives are the best laxatives to be taken during pregnancy; they absorb water, thereby facilitating movement through the bowels. By making a larger bulk to move through the colon, these laxatives help purge the body of feces. They take 12 hours to 3 days to purge the bowel. Psyllium (Metamucil) is an example of a bulk-forming laxative.

Lubricant laxatives such as mineral oil increase the water-to-fecal mass. They can cause leakage from the rectum and are usually taken in the form of suppositories. Lubricant laxatives have an oily nature. They ease the passage of stool and are usually given rectally. They take 6–8 hours to work.

Osmotic laxatives increase the amount of water in the large intestines and usually work within 2–12 hours. They are contraindicated in patients with hypertension, edema, or congestive heart failure. Milk of magnesia is a mild osmotic saline laxative. Osmotic laxatives irritate the bowels to increase peristalsis. Salt ions can suck water toward themselves, thus lubricating the GI tract. They take 2–12 hours to work, depending on the dose.

Stimulant laxatives stimulate peristalsis in 6–8 hours. Side effects include cramping, diarrhea, flatulence, and nausea. Senna, aloe, and cascara sagrada discolor urine. Castor oil should not be used during pregnancy or lactation. Stimulant laxatives act directly on the intestinal mucosa and irritate the bowel.

Stool softeners decrease the consistency of stool by decreasing surface tension. Docusate (Colace) is a detergent stool softener. Stool softeners attract water and fat to the stools, thus softening them and improving the passage of stool through the colon.

Bowel evacuators are cleansing solutions that are used before diagnostic tests to remove stool. They are made as mixes similar to body fluids, so material held in the bowel is rejected. Usually the patient is asked to drink 1 gallon of fluid mixed with a bowel evacuator within 2–3 hours. Bowel evacuators have side effects of bloating, nausea, and fullness. An example of a bowel evacuant is polyethylene glycol solution (MiraLax).

CRITICAL THINKING

Patients can become dependent on laxatives. What are some nonpharmacological treatments for constipation?

Medications to Treat Diarrhea

The opposite of constipation is diarrhea (an increase in the frequency and fluidity of bowel movements). Almost all individuals have diarrhea at one time or another, but if it occurs over several days the body can lose too much fluid and electrolytes.

Diarrhea is a symptom, not a disease. Certain chemicals, inflammation, infections, and other medications can cause diarrhea. Antiinfective therapy frequently causes diarrhea. Anxiety and circulatory disorders can cause diarrhea as well.

Stools of excessive volume and fluidity are more than just a bother. The cramping that frequently accompanies diarrhea can be very painful. Diarrhea can signal that the person has eaten spoiled or contaminated food and has an intestinal infection. In small children and the elderly, diarrhea can cause life-threatening loss of valuable electrolytes.

Opioid-related antidiarrheals are highly effective. They inhibit GI motility, decrease peristalsis, and slow the functions of the system. An example is loperamide (Imodium). Side effects include dizziness, dry mouth, agitation, numbness, drowsiness, and tachycardia.

Adsorbents, such as bismuth (Pepto-Bismol) or kaolin and pectin (Kaopectate), are taken after every bowel movement to adsorb toxins or bacteria and to coat the walls of the GI tract. Treatment of diarrhea may also include antibiotics, antiinflammatories, or antiparasitics.

Medications to Treat Nausea and Vomiting

Nausea, although an uncomfortable feeling that vomiting is imminent, is not dangerous. Sometimes nausea is caused by unusual smells, pregnancy hormones, or emptiness of the stomach. Vomiting (emesis) occurs when the patient ejects the contents of the stomach.

Antiemetics decrease nausea and vomiting and are also used to treat motion sickness. Examples of antiemetics include phenothiazines such as prochlorperazine; antihistamines such as diphenhydramine and meclizine; trimethobenzamide; cannabinoids; phosphorated carbohydrate solution; and 5-hydroxytryptamine-3 (5-HT$_3$, serotonin) receptor antagonists such as ondansetron.

Phenothiazines block dopamine receptors in the area of the brain that stimulates vomiting. The action of antihistamines in decreasing nausea and vomiting is unclear. Trimethobenzamide is an anticholinergic that can be given orally, rectally, or by intramuscular injection. It is thought to act on the chemoreceptor trigger zone. Cannabinoids, derivatives of marijuana, are used sparingly because of the high potential for abuse. They are controlled drugs. Phosphorated carbohydrate solution (Emetrol) contains dextrose, fructose (a type of sugar), and phosphoric acid. It decreases the hyperactivity of the smooth muscle of the gastric mucosa. This drug should not be used by patients with diabetes mellitus because of the fructose content. 5-HT$_3$ receptor antagonists are commonly used to prevent and treat the nausea and vomiting associated with chemotherapy.

Medications to Treat Gastroesophageal Reflux Disease

If the cardiac sphincter is loose, stomach acid can move upward into the esophagus, causing irritation to the mucosa. This can result in gastroesophageal reflux disease (GERD). The burning sensation that the patient feels when acid damages the esophagus is heartburn. Heartburn does not actually involve the heart, but pain is localized near the heart and patients often report that it feels like their heart is burning.

Antacids, as the name implies, counteract acids. They are given to decrease the amount of hydrochloric acid (HCl) in the stomach and create a more alkaline environment. This neutralizes the acid and protects the vulnerable mucosa. Therefore, they relieve the pain and destruction associated with GERD. Except for sodium bicarbonate (baking soda), they are not readily absorbed and do not alter the systemic pH. Some antacids may need to be taken regularly to condition the stomach to decreased acid. Timing of these medications is critical; they must be given before food. Sometimes antacids are given in suspensions, which must be shaken, or chewable tablets. Chewable tablets are usually taken with a glass of water or milk. Action occurs within 30 minutes to 3 hours. Antacids are usually taken 1 hour before H$_2$-receptor blockers. Chronic use of antacids can induce gastric secretory cells to increase acid secretion. Patients should be cautioned not to overuse sodium bicarbonate because of its systemic effect, and that changing gastric acid pH may affect absorption of other medications.

Antacids are also used to lower elevated acid levels due to spicy foods and to decrease the nausea related to pregnancy hormones. Many mild antacids, such as Tums and Rolaids, are available over the counter.

Gastric stimulants or prokinetic agents stimulate gastric activity in the patient with decreased peptic activity. They decrease esophageal sphincter pressure and increase gastric emptying, which improves peristalsis. An example of a GI stimulant is metoclopramide (Reglan).

Medications to Treat Ulcers

The stomach secretes HCl to break down food into amounts small enough to allow easy absorption. However, the stomach can create too much acid, which erodes the mucosal layer and can lead to a peptic ulcer. Acid from the stomach can spill into the duodenum and erode the mucosa there as well.

Patients at high risk for ulcers are patients with blood type O, cigarette smokers, those infected with *Helicobacter pylori*, and those who do not cope well with stress. Alcohol, caffeinated foods and beverages, and certain drugs [corticosteroids, aspirin, nonsteroidal antiinflammatory drugs (NSAIDs)] can also increase the risk of a peptic ulcer.

In the past, patients with peptic ulcers were encouraged to drink lots of milk because it was thought that ulcers were related to the acidity of the stomach and milk is alkaline. Now it's known that *H. pylori* grows very well in milk, and milk was perhaps one of the worst treatments to recommend. This is why it is important for allied health professionals to keep current on treatments supported with research.

Medications used to treat ulcers include mucosal protectants such as sucralfate (Carafate), which is aluminum hydroxide and sulfated sucrose. They cover and protect the ulcer and thus promote healing, but they must be taken on an empty stomach. Side effects include constipation and vitamin deficiency.

Misoprostal (Cytotec) is a prostaglandin that inhibits gastric acid secretion. It is used to reduce the risk of NSAID-induced ulcers. This drug must not be used during pregnancy.

Antispasmodics (which are actually anticholinergics) decrease secretions and gastric mobility. They reduce gastric spasm and slow gastric motility. They are also used to treat GERD, ulcerative colitis, diverticulitis, biliary spasm, and irritable bowel syndrome. Examples include atropine sulfate and glycopyrrolate.

H_2-receptor antagonists include the drugs cimetidine and ranitidine. These drugs block histamine from binding to parietal cells, preventing the parietal cells from secreting gastric acid. H_2-receptor antagonists can be given without regard to meals but should not be given within 1 hour of an antacid.

Antibiotics fight *H. pylori*, which is a bacterium that can damage the GI tract. It is associated with 75% of gastric ulcers and with 90% of duodenal ulcers. When the *H. pylori* is killed, the ulcer has a chance to heal. Antibiotics used to treat *H. pylori* include amoxicillin, clarithromycin, metronidazole, and tetracycline. These agents are never used alone but in different combinations together. It is important that patients complete the entire 7- to 14-day regimen to totally remove *H. pylori*, even if the patient feels better. Bismuth compounds can also be prescribed, because they are bacteriostatic and stop *H. pylori* from sticking to the mucosa.

Proton pump inhibitors reduce the acidity of the stomach by binding to stomach enzymes. Because they act on enzymes that cause increased acidity, these medications tend to protect the stomach for a time. They inhibit hydrogen and potassium ions and are used as short-term treatment for GERD and benign peptic ulcers. They are frequently combined with antibiotics to act against *H. pylori*. Side effects include abdominal pain, headache, constipation, diarrhea, and nausea. Examples of proton pump inhibitors are omeprazole and pantoprazole.

Antacids and GI stimulants are also often used in the treatment of ulcers.

CRITICAL THINKING

What risks for peptic ulcers involve lifestyle, not genetics? What lifestyle changes should a patient with a peptic ulcer make?

Medications to Treat Gallstones

Cholelithiasis, or the abnormal condition of having stones in the gallbladder, is caused by cholesterol or calcium forming a calculus (stone). Cholesterol cannot be seen on radiographs, but calcium stones can. Symptoms of gallstones are bloating, gas, and nausea. Ursodiol is a gallstone-solubilizing agent. It is a naturally occurring bile acid that decreases the production of cholesterol and inhibits absorption of cholesterol by the intestines. Therapy can take up to 2 years; but if partial dissolution of the gallstones is not seen by 12 months, this treatment is likely to be unsuccessful.

Medications to Treat Obesity

Increasing obesity rates in North America are prompting many physicians to prescribe medications to decrease appetite. Many factors cause obesity: metabolic abnormalities, overeating, insulin resistance, and a sedentary lifestyle. A person is considered morbidly obese when he or she is 20% above ideal body weight. Obesity causes increased workload for the pancreas, which helps digest carbohydrates, and the liver, which helps digest fats. It also causes an increased workload in the circulatory system. Lifestyle changes are the best way to reduce obesity, but anorexiants are sometimes necessary. Examples of anorexiants are sibutramine (Meridia) and phentermine.

Appetite suppressants, which give a feeling of fullness and sometimes create nausea, can be used with caution to decrease food intake and thus decrease obesity potential. They mimic the sympathetic system, so most are controlled substances. They are only for short-term use.

Lipase inhibitors such as orlistat (Xenical) can also be used in the management of obesity. These drugs bind to the enzyme lipase, so the intestines cannot break down dietary fat. Instead, fats are eliminated in the feces. This reduces the amount of fat absorbed into the body, thereby reducing serum lipids.

✳ CRITICAL THINKING

What are some lifestyle changes that can lead to reduced weight?

Medications to Treat Hemorrhoids

If the anus, a sphincter at the end of the rectum, becomes irritated, it may need an anorectal preparation to decrease swelling of varicose veins (hemorrhoids) or to soothe cracks (fissures). An example of a hemorrhoid cream is Preparation H. Some of these preparations contain lanolin or mineral oil, which acts as an emollient to lubricate the anus.

Medications to Treat Flatulence

Flatulence is gas released by the GI tract. Sometimes flatulence is caused from foods rather than disease. Patients who complain of flatulence should be cautioned to decrease consumption of cabbage, onions, and beans and to use straws for drinking. Flatulence is more common with air swallowing, diverticulitis, peptic ulcer, irritable bowel syndrome, and dyspepsia. *Antiflatulents* may also be used with gastroscopy and bowel radiography. The main drug in this class in simethicone.

Medications to Treat Fungal Infections of the GI Tract

Oral candidiasis (thrush) is a fungal infection of the mucous membranes of the mouth. Nystatin is the main drug used for its treatment. It is available as a suspension or a troche (lozenge). Regardless of the form used, it should be kept in the mouth as long as possible to coat the affected area. Troches should not be chewed or swallowed whole.

Intestinal candiadiasis is also treated with nystatin, but in tablet form. In this instance, the drug should be swallowed whole.

Medications to Treat Intestinal Parasites

Antihelmintics kill intestinal parasites, such as roundworm and pinworm. Laxatives may be given at the same time to expel the dead parasites. Side effects are abdominal cramps, headaches, anorexia, nausea, and vomiting.

✳ CRITICAL THINKING

Why is it important to cook chicken, beef, pork, and fish thoroughly?

Medications to Induce Vomiting and Treat Drug Overdose

Vomiting may or may not be beneficial, depending on the circumstance. If caused by food poisoning, vomiting is therapeutic because it helps rid the body of toxins. Antiemetics stop vomiting, and emetics promote it. Emetics, such as syrup of ipecac, induce vomiting in 80%–90% of patients within 20–30 minutes. Syrup of ipecac has been widely used to induce vomiting in poisoning incidents outside the hospital. It has fallen in disfavor lately, but activated charcoal—which attracts the toxin to it before stomach contents are pumped out—is still used to promote safe expulsion of toxins. Emetics should not be used if the ingested substance is corrosive or the patient has decreased alertness, a history of convulsions, or is in shock. Emetics should never be administered to infants or with milk, which inactivates them.

Nutritional Supplements

Poor nutrition can result in poor health. Malnutrition can be caused by lack of availability of food, excessive dieting, poor dietary choices, or illnesses that reduce appetite. Medications that reduce nausea and vomiting can improve nutritional status. Furthermore, nutritional supplements such as a multivitamin can compensate for a lack of vitamins in food.

Nutritional supplements may not sound like drugs, but they are frequently prescribed to improve nutrition in patients who are malnourished. Liquid nutritional supplements can help improve health. Examples include Boost and Ensure. Store brands are available, but be sure to ask the prescriber whether substitutions are allowed. Some prescribers want specific nutrients found only in certain supplements. The patient can usually choose the flavor of the supplement, however.

Mouthwashes and Other Oral Treatments

Mouthwashes or gargles are used to decrease halitosis (bad breath) or stomatitis (inflammation of the mouth). Fluoride preparations can prevent tooth decay by hardening the tooth enamel. They are prescribed in tablets, drops, or gargles. For a patient without saliva, saliva substitutes are prescribed. Oral topical anesthetics can be used for teething pain and mouth ulcers. Hydrogen peroxide is an over-the-counter agent that acts as a weak antibacterial agent in the mouth. Dentifrices or toothpastes are used to clean teeth, decrease plaque, and prevent gum disease. Some have whitening elements as well.

SUMMARY

For the body to function correctly, what is put in the GI system is important. Too large a quantity of food can lead to obesity, and too small a quantity can lead to malnutrition. Medications can have a powerful effect on our bodies. Although they might help cure disease, they can also disrupt the delicate GI system.

Activities

To make sure that you have learned the key points covered in this chapter, complete the following activities.

True or False
Write *true* if the statement is true. Beside the false statements, write *false* and correct the statement to make it true.

1. Pica is intestinal gas. _____

2. Morbidity means to die. _____

3. The alimentary canal is another name for the GI tract. _____

4. GERD is a sexually transmitted disease. _____

5. Gastric ulcers are usually caused by eating the wrong foods. _____

Multiple Choice
Choose the best answer for each question.

1. Movement through the intestines is called:
   a. Halitosis
   b. Pica
   c. Peristalsis
   d. Fissure

2. Which causes gastric ulcers?
   a. GERD
   b. Halitosis
   c. *Helicobacter pylori*
   d. Flatulence

3. Which of the following is *not* a type of laxative?
   a. Bulk-forming
   b. Osmotic
   c. Stool softeners
   d. Lubricants
   e. Proton pump inhibitors

4. Which is used to treat motion sickness?
   a. Laxatives
   b. Antiemetics
   c. Emetics
   d. Proton pump inhibitors
   e. Prostaglandins

5. Which can cause pregnancy loss?
   a. Emetics
   b. Laxatives
   c. Antiemetics
   d. Prostaglandins
   e. Mouthwashes

Application Exercises

Respond to the following scenarios on a separate sheet.

1. Butler Butterworth is having a gastric bypass surgery, with the surgeon removing most of Mr. Butterworth's stomach. **How will that affect the absorption of drugs he takes?**
2. Ratcliffe Savides wants to lose weight. He wants to be put on Xenical but continue his lifestyle. **What do you need to teach him?**
3. Marilyn Rhodes takes Dulcolax every night to have bowel movements. **Is this a good practice? Why or why not?**
4. Joyce Coffey says that her mother always drank milk to treat her stomach ulcer. She does not understand why she is taking antibiotics and told not to use milk to treat the ulcer. **What would you say?**

Virtual Field Trips

1. Go to http://www.ific.org and download an article about obesity.
2. Surf to http://www.obesityhelp.com and calculate your body mass index.
3. Visit Dr. Phil McGraw on http://DrPhil.com and download some weight loss tips.

For further study and practice with drug classifications learned in this chapter, complete the following table to the best of your ability. Use resources such as a PDR, the Internet, or printed drug guides for help.

CLASSIFICATION	PURPOSE	SIDE EFFECTS	CONTRAINDICATIONS/PRECAUTIONS/INTERACTIONS	EXAMPLES	PATIENT EDUCATION
Antacids					
Antidiarrheals					
Antifungals (nystatin)					
Antispasmodics					
Emetics					
GI stimulants					
H. pylori agents					
H$_2$-receptor antagonists					
Prostaglandins					
Proton pump inhibitors					

Musculoskeletal System Medications

*T*he skeleton, including the muscles, provides the scaffolding for the body. Without muscles the body cannot move or interact with the environment. Therefore, these systems must remain healthy for the body to function.

OBJECTIVES

At the end of this chapter, the student will be able to:

- Define all key terms.
- Describe how musculoskeletal drugs work.
- List side effects of musculoskeletal drugs: anticholinergics, antispasmodics, antiarthritics, antiinflammatory agents, glucocorticoids, antigout agents, ERT/HRT, and muscle relaxants.
- Discuss the origins of muscle disorders.
- Describe how calcium storage affects the body.

KEY TERMS

Antispasmodic
Bisphosphonates
Calcitonin
DMARDs
Dystonia
Endogenous
ERT
Gout

HRT
Hypocalcemia
Osteoarthritis
Osteomalacia
Osteoporosis
Rheumatoid arthritis
Rickets
Spastic

● MUSCULOSKELETAL MEDICATIONS

The musculoskeletal system consists of muscles and bones (Fig. 17.1) and depends on the nervous and endocrine systems for signals to cue it to function. Coordinated and strong movement requires healthy nerve signals, adequate hormonal stimulation, and healthy muscle tissue. In addition, the skeleton not only gives the body structure, it stores minerals that, in turn, help muscles move. The endocrine system must be healthy to control the deposit of these minerals. (See the Master the Essentials table for descriptions of the most common musculoskeletal system drugs.)

Musculoskeletal disorders can be categorized into those of muscle and those of bone. Medications are used to treat musculoskeletal disorders in both of these areas.

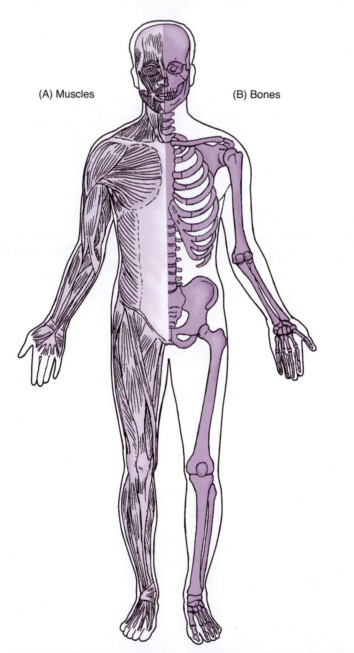

(A) Muscles   (B) Bones

FIGURE 17.1. The musculoskeletal system is made up of (A) muscles and (B) bones that form the skeleton. It gives the body its structure and is the force behind movement.

Master the Essentials: Musculoskeletal Medications

This table shows the various classes of musculoskeletal medications and key side effects, contraindications and precautions, and interactions for each class.

CLASS	SIDE EFFECTS	CONTRAINDICATIONS/ PRECAUTIONS	INTERACTIONS
Antigout drugs	Acute gouty attacks, headache, GI symptoms	Hypersensitivity, uric acid kidney stones, blood dyscrasias, active peptic ulcer	Antibiotics, antineoplastics, warfarin, salicylates, oral antidiabetics
Antiinflammatory drugs	Albumin in urine, blood in urine, bronchospasm, constipation, dizziness, epigastric pain, increased bleeding time, hypersensitivity reactions, gastroesophageal reflux disorder (GERD), GI ulcers and bleeding, headache, tinnitus and hearing loss, vision disturbances	Anemia, asthma, children with viral infections, clotting disorders, disorders of the CV and GI systems, GERD, lactation, liver and kidney failure, pregnancy, sulfonamide hypersensitivity, thyroid disorders	Alcohol, anticoagulants, corticosteroids and other steroids, oral hypoglycemics
Bisphosphonates	Headache, abdominal pain, bone pain	Hypersensitivity, hypocalcemia, esophageal stricture or achalasia	Calcium supplements, antacids, ranitidine, aspirin
Calcitonin	Rhinitis, nasal irritation (nasal spray); hypertension, dizziness, injection site reactions, nausea, vomiting	Clinical allergy to drug, pregnancy, breastfeeding	None reported
Calcium supplements	Constipation, headache, nausea, vomiting; confusion, delirium, stupor, coma (severe hypercalcemia)	Hypercalcemia, ventricular fibrillation	Iron salts, quinolones, tetracyclines
Cholinesterase inhibitors	Bradycardia, hypotension, convulsions, rash, increased saliva, weakness, muscle cramps	Hypersensitivity, peritonitis, mechanical intestinal or urinary obstruction	Succinylcholine, aminoglycosides, anesthetics, antiarrhythmics, corticosteroids, magnesium
COX-2 inhibitors	Headache, insomnia, rash, abdominal pain, diarrhea, dyspepsia, upper respiratory infection	Hypersensitivity to sulfonamides	Fluconazole, rifampin, theophylline, ACE inhibitors

(table continued on page 288)

Master the Essentials: Musculoskeletal Medications (continued)

CLASS	SIDE EFFECTS	CONTRAINDICATIONS/ PRECAUTIONS	INTERACTIONS
Muscle relaxants/ antispasmodics	Anxiety, ataxia, blurred vision, confusion, decreased blood pressure and respirations, diarrhea, dizziness, drowsiness, dry mouth, headache, slurred speech, tremor, urinary incontinence, weakness	Asthma, lactation, muscular dystrophy, myasthenia gravis, pregnancy	Alcohol, analgesics, antihistamines, psychotropics
Vitamin D	Headache, weakness, nausea, dry mouth, constipation	Hypercalcemia, vitamin D toxicity, decreased kidney function, hypervitaminosis D	Digoxin, verapamil, ketoconazole, mineral oil, thiazide diuretics, phenytoin

Medications Used to Treat Muscular Disorders

Muscle disorders can originate in the brain or in the muscle tissue itself. Some brain disorders that can affect muscles are brain or spinal cord injury, cerebral palsy, stroke, and multiple sclerosis. Muscle spasms can develop from these disorders or from the use of psychotropic drugs.

Antispasmodic medications

Certain conditions (e.g., injury to a muscle in the back, muscular dystrophy) cause patients' muscles to move in uncoordinated, or spastic, ways. Other patients have dystonia, an abnormal tension in one area of the body, such as the limbs, neck, face, eyes, neck, or spine.

CRITICAL THINKING

How might impaired mobility of the legs affect an individual?

Muscle relaxants relieve muscle stiffness, and antispasmodics relieve muscle spasms. Both work on the central nervous system (CNS) to inhibit the neurological activity that causes the spasms or rigidity. Sometimes antispasmodics are used with benzodiazepines or other CNS drugs to maximize effectiveness and help patients live productive, mobile lives.

Other antispasmodics focus on the muscle itself. Botulinum toxin type A is a toxic substance derived from the bacterium *Clostridium botulinum* that can cause food poisoning in high dosages. However, researchers have found that in lower doses it acts as an effective muscle relaxant. Botulinum toxin blocks acetylcholine release, thus paralyzing the muscle. With the muscle relaxed, the patient can do strengthening exercises to promote muscle strength. This treatment reaches maximum effectiveness within 6 weeks and needs to be repeated every 3–6 months. Because botulinum toxin causes pain, it is usually administered with a local anesthetic.

Other medications used to treat muscle disorders

Myasthenia gravis is a progressive disease of skeletal muscle fatigue and weakness caused by loss of acetylcholine receptors. This autoimmune disease can be debilitating. Cholinesterase inhibitors, such as neostigmine, block cholinesterase and thus facilitate acetylcholine accumulation.

Fibromyalgia is a disorder of chronic pain in muscles and soft tissue surrounding joints. This rheumatologic illness is difficult to manage. Treatment includes decreasing the contributory factors (e.g., lack of exercise, poor coping response to stress), physical therapy, antidepressants, antiinflammatory medications, trigger-point injections, and narcotic analgesics.

Medications Used to Treat Skeletal Disorders

The skeleton is a repository for minerals such as calcium. Calcium is needed for nerves, bones, and muscles to function properly. If not enough calcium is stored in bones, the bones can break. If too much calcium is stored, not enough is available for the bloodstream.

The endocrine system, through the action of the parathyroid and thyroid glands, ensures the proper amount of circulating and stored calcium. The parathyroid glands secrete parathyroid hormone, which pulls calcium from bones into the bloodstream. The thyroid gland secretes calcitonin, which puts calcium into the bones (Fig. 17.2). The two glands work together to keep calcium levels in balance. If either gland fails, musculoskeletal disorders can result.

Medications for abnormal calcium levels

Calcium supplements are prescribed for hypocalcemia, or low blood calcium. Vitamin D may be added to facilitate calcium usage.

When calcium is not stored in bones, the bones can become soft (leading to osteomalacia or rickets) or filled with holes (leading to osteoporosis). Because the bones are not firm, they break easily. Thus, a bone can break with little stress or pressure. Sometimes patients fall and then break a bone—and sometimes they break a bone and then fall.

Risk factors for hypocalcemia include smoking, lack of exercise, high alcohol consumption, anorexia nervosa, estrogen or testosterone deficiency, poor nutrition, and obesity.

Sometimes calcium and vitamin D are used to prevent bone breaks, as is the case with osteoporosis. Bone density tests can be done to assess the risk for osteoporosis.

Some drugs inhibit bone resorption of calcium. Estrogen replacement therapy (ERT), also called hormone replacement therapy (HRT), can reduce the degree of osteoporosis but has side effects, including breast and uterine cancer and blood clots. Hence, these drugs are used with caution. If

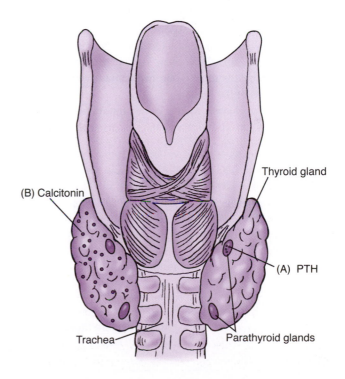

FIGURE 17.2. Action of parathyroid hormone (PTH) and calcitonin. PTH and calcitonin help keep calcium in the body in balance. (A) The parathyroid glands secrete PTH, which pulls calcium from the bones into the bloodstream. (B) The thyroid gland secretes calcitonin, which puts calcium into the bones.

a patient prefers not to take ERT, she may choose to take a bisphosphonate, a similar medication that doesn't cause the side effects that can occur with ERT. These drugs are similar to bisphosphate salts, which are found naturally (endogenously) in the body. An example of a bisphosphonate is alendronate sodium (Fosamax).

CRITICAL THINKING

Why might a woman choose to take HRT? Why might she choose not to take it?

Patients with hypocalcemia may also be given calcitonin, which is available as a nasal spray or an injectable form. Calcitonin can come from humans or fish such as salmon.

Although too little bone calcium can cause fractures, too much bone calcium is a problem as well. Paget's disease is a chronic disease that debilitates patients by creating enlarged bones. A patient with Paget's disease resorbs bone excessively, but the new bone is weak and fragile. The bones are deformed, leading to pain and fractures. Paget's disease can be diagnosed by a blood test. Treatment is calcitonin and bisphosphonates, which encourage strong bone formation. Patients with Paget's disease may also take supplemental calcium and vitamin D, as needed.

Medications for bone inflammation

Arthritis (Table 17.1) and gout can cause inflammation of the bones. Gout is caused by a buildup of uric acid in the blood or joints. Antiarthritic drugs are specific for treating this type of disorder.

Nonsteroidal antiinflammatory drugs (NSAIDs) reduce inflammation, which is helpful to the patient with gout, osteoarthritis, or rheumatoid arthritis. Aspirin, acetaminophen, and other analgesics are used both topically and orally for pain. Stronger pain relief can be obtained by combining analgesics and antidepressants.

Cyclooxygenase-2 (COX-2) inhibitors [celecoxib (Celebrex)] suppress inflammation but can increase the risk of heart problems in certain patients. They cannot be used by patients who are allergic to sulfa drugs.

If antiinflammatory drugs do not reduce the inflammation adequately, disease-modifying antirheumatic drugs (DMARDs) may be used in patients with rheumatoid arthritis. These medications suppress the autoimmune response and so also suppress immunity systemically. One example is gold salt. Given by injection or sometimes orally, it prevents joint damage and disability. Gold is used infrequently because other DMARDs, such as methotrexate and sulfasalazine, are more effective.

Gout is treated with antigout medications, which inhibit uric acid buildup in the bloodstream and synovial fluids of the joints.

Glucocorticosteroids reduce inflammation but do not cure the diseases. Because they reduce the body's ability to fight infection, they are used only for short-term therapy.

TABLE 17.1 Types of Arthritis

TYPE	CAUSE	AGE AFFECTED
Osteoarthritis	Degeneration (erosion) of bones where they meet, or articulate, at the joints	Strikes people middle-aged or older. Extremely sedentary and extremely active people are at increased risk.
Rheumatoid arthritis	Autoimmune reaction: the body's immune system attacks the joints, causing inflammation.	Can affect children, but most sufferers are women who are 30–50 years old when symptoms first start.

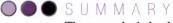 S U M M A R Y

The musculoskeletal system must function well to achieve proper motion and electrolyte storage in the body. Muscles may malfunction by being weak or too tight. Bones can be weakened by lack of calcium, or they can have too much calcium. Medications for the muscular system act in the brain or in muscle, depending on where the problem is. Diseases can weaken or inflame bones, or they can retain or get rid of too much calcium. There are many drugs available to help heal malfunctions in the musculoskeletal system.

Activities

To make sure that you have learned the key points covered in this chapter, complete the following activities.

True or False

Write *true* if the statement is true. Beside the false statements, write *false* and correct the statement to make it true.

1. Both vitamin D and calcium are needed for healthy nerves, muscles, and bones. _____

2. Paget's disease produces weak bones. _____

3. Calcium and vitamin D supplements are used to treat hypocalcemia. _____

4. Antispasmodic drugs treat spasticity only in the brain. _____

5. Gold injections work for all forms of arthritis. _____

Multiple Choice

Choose the best answer for each question.

1. Fibromyalgia is a:
   a. Rheumatologic disease
   b. Gout
   c. Joint degeneration
   d. Calcium disorder

2. Which is excessive buildup of bone tissue?
   a. Fibromyalgia
   b. Gout
   c. Paget's disease
   d. Myasthenia gravis

3. Which has an accumulation of uric acid?
   a. Fibromyalgia
   b. Gout
   c. Paget's disease
   d. Myasthenia gravis

4. Which suppresses inflammation?
   a. Glucocorticosteroid
   b. Antispasmodic
   c. Calcitonin
   d. Parathyroid hormone

5. Which one puts calcium into bones?
   a. Glucocorticosteroid
   b. Antispasmodic
   c. Calcitonin
   d. Parathyroid hormone

Application Exercises

Respond to the following scenarios on a separate sheet.

1. Jason Briggs is about to receive a Botox injection. He asks you, "Why are you injecting food poisoning into me?" **What would you say?**

2. Barbie Pritzlaff has had her thyroid and parathyroid glands removed because of cancer. **What consequences does that have on her bone and blood calcium levels?**

3. Joette Lehberger is entering menopause. **Why might she need supplemental calcium?**

4. Bhavna Patel has osteoarthritis. She came in for gold injections. **How would you explain how gold decreases inflammation?**

5. Vicki Chaukley is taking NSAIDs for osteoarthritis. She has developed a bleeding ulcer, and the physician tells her to stop taking them. **What other choices are open to her?**

Virtual Field Trips

Go to the following websites to find the information. If a website is not available, try to find the information through another source.

1. Visit http://www.arthritisconnection.com and http://www.arthritis.org and download information about Celebrex.

2. Surf to the website of your choice and find the classifications of:

   a. Ultram

   b. Fosamax

   c. Gold thioglucose

   d. Citracal

   e. Flexeril

For further study and practice with drug classifications learned in this chapter, complete the following table to the best of your ability. Use resources such as a PDR, the Internet, or printed drug guides for help.

CLASSIFICATION	PURPOSE	SIDE EFFECTS	CONTRAINDICATIONS/PRECAUTIONS/INTERACTIONS	PATIENT EDUCATION	EXAMPLES
Muscle relaxants					
Calcium and vitamin D					
COX-2 inhibitors					

CHAPTER 18

Endocrine System Medications

The body cannot carry on life processes without communication among its parts. The endocrine system communicates messages between systems and organs. It is involved in how the body uses energy, when the body sleeps, and how effectively the body reproduces.

OBJECTIVES

At the end of this chapter, the student will be able to:

- Define all key terms.
- List actions of endocrine hormones.
- Describe what happens to the body when a hormone is over- or under-produced.
- Discuss why hormones must be taken as directed.
- List the functions of the reproductive hormones.
- Describe the effects of medications to treat endocrine disorders, including thyroid hormone, antithyroid agents, insulin, oral antidiabetic drugs, and corticosteroids.

KEY TERMS

Acromegaly	ERT
ACTH	Estrogen
Addison's disease	Fight or flight response
ADH	FSH
Androgen	GH
Calcitonin	Gigantism
Cretinism	Graves' disease
Cushing's disease	HRT
Diabetes insipidus	Hyperglycemia
Diabetes mellitus	Hypoglycemia
Dwarfism	ICSH

IDDM
LH
Melatonin
Myxedema
Negative feedback system
NIDDM
Oxytocin
Parathormone
Progestin

Prolactin
Prostaglandin
Releasing factor
SIADH
Somatotropin
T_3
T_4
TSH
Vasopressin

● ENDOCRINE SYSTEM MEDICATIONS

The endocrine system sends messages throughout the body by secreting hormones. Several components make up this system (Fig. 18.1), which is controlled by the hypothalamus. The hypothalamus secretes chemicals called releasing factors that trigger the release of hormones from the pituitary gland. The pituitary gland is known as the master gland because it secretes most of the body's hormones (Table 18.1). A later chapter covers medications used to treat reproductive disorders. (See the Master the Essentials table for descriptions of the most common endocrine system drugs.)

The hypothalamus is the body's switchboard—it tells the pituitary gland what hormones to send out to the body. When a hormone level becomes too high, the body tells the hypothalamus, which in turn tells the pituitary to stop producing the hormone. This is called a negative feedback system.

The endocrine system includes the pineal gland—a small gland found in the brain that secretes melatonin. Melatonin helps a patient sleep; hence, when the pineal gland fails, sleep is impaired. Melatonin or sleeping pills (see Chapter 12) may be prescribed to correct this disorder.

Medications used to treat disorders of the endocrine system can be divided into those for thyroid and parathyroid disorders, those for pancreatic disorders, and those for adrenal disorders.

Medications for Thyroid and Parathyroid Disorders

The thyroid gland cues individual cells to work. It is an "on" switch for the body. When the thyroid fails to work properly, the patient has less energy and every cell of the body is affected.

The thyroid produces two hormones: triiodothyronine (T_3) and thyroxine (T_4). Decreased levels of these two hormones indicate hypothyroidism. Prolonged hypothyroidism can lead to a skin and tissue disorder called myxedema, which may prove difficult to treat. A decrease of thyroid hormone secretion in utero and early infancy causes cretinism (slowed brain growth) in children. Rapid treatment can prevent mental retardation and growth retardation.

To treat hypothyroidism, patients take hormones prepared from natural sources, such as dried bovine or porcine thyroid gland, or synthetically manufactured tablets. T_3 can be broken down from T_4 by the patient's body, so usually only T_4 is prescribed.

Too much thyroid hormone causes Graves' disease, characterized by bulging eyes, hyperactive metabolism, goiter (enlarged thyroid), and weight loss. The thyroid can be inhibited in secreting T_3 and T_4 by thyroidectomy. Radioactive sodium iodide-131 can be used to stop thyroid functioning. Antithyroid drugs, such as propylthiouracil or methimazole, can also be used.

The thyroid gland also regulates blood and bone calcium. It does so by secreting calcitonin. Calcitonin helps force calcium ions into bone. If the patient has insufficient calcitonin, the blood calcium level remains high and the bone calcium level remains low, leading to bone fractures. Replacement hormones help with both energy and calcium storage, but the prescriber may prescribe only calcium supplements.

Master the Essentials: Endocrine Medications

This table shows the various classes of endocrine medications and key side effects, contraindications and precautions, and interactions for each class.

CLASS	SIDE EFFECTS	CONTRAINDICATIONS/ PRECAUTIONS	INTERACTIONS
Anabolic steroids	Acne, hirsutism, depression, altered libido, edema, glucose tolerance, aggression, liver cancer, atherosclerosis	Breast cancer, prostate cancer, pregnancy, hypercalcemia, liver failure	Oral anticoagulants, oral hypoglycemic agents
Antithyroid drugs	Paresthesias, headache, rash, agranulocytosis	Hypersensitivity, pregnancy, breastfeeding	Anticoagulants
Corticosteroids	Adrenocortical insufficiency, anxiety, cessation of menses, constipation, decreased wound healing, decreased growth in children, diarrhea, dizziness, fluid and electrolyte imbalances, GI upset, headache, hyperglycemia, increased eye pressure, increased infection, muscle pain and weakness, osteoporosis, psychosis, petechiae	Pregnancy, lactation, children; history of clots, seizures, or immuno-suppression. Not used for long-term therapy. Cautious use with infection, hypothyroidism, cirrhosis, increased blood pressure, congestive heart failure, emotional instability, diabetes, glaucoma, or GI upset. Do not use in patients with a history of clots, seizures, or immuno-suppression.	Barbiturates, contraceptives, diuretics, NSAIDs, vaccines
Insulin	Headache, increased sweat, irritability, tingling, tremor, blurred or double vision, weakness, hypoglycemia, hypokalemia	Hypoglycemia, sensitivity, kidney impairment, liver impairment	Alcohol, MAO inhibitors, salicy-lates, anabolic steroids
Oral antidiabetic agents	Hypoglycemia; abdominal pain (alpha-glucosidase inhibitors); nausea, vomiting, metallic taste (metformin); aplastic anemia, rash, nausea (sulfonylureas); swelling, weight gain (thiazolidinediones)	Hypersensitivity, diabetic ketoacidosis, cirrhosis; inflammatory bowel disease (alpha-glucosidase inhibitors); kidney or liver dysfunction (metformin)	Alcohol, MAO inhibitors, corticos-teroids, salicylates, warfarin
Thyroid medications	Palpitations, fast heart rate, irregular heart beat, increased blood pressure, nervousness, tremor, headache, insomnia, weight loss, diarrhea, abdominal cramps, intolerance of heat, fever, menstrual irregularities	Adrenal insufficiency, diabetes, cardiovascular disease	Adrenergics, insulin, oral antico-agulants, oral hypoglycemics

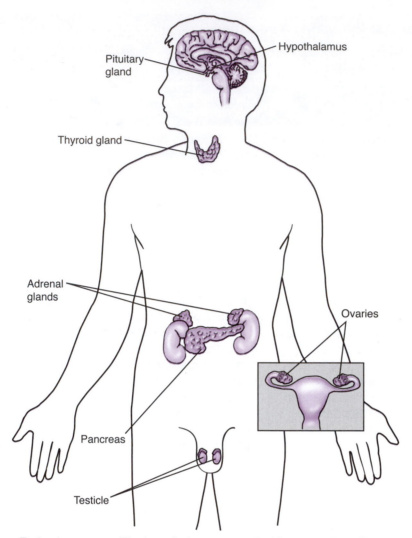

FIGURE 18.1. Endocrine system. The hypothalamus controls this system by telling the pituitary gland which hormones to secrete. Hormones have a wide range of effects on body organs, including the thyroid, pancreas, adrenals, and reproductive organs (testes and ovaries).

CRITICAL THINKING

How does removal of the thyroid gland affect calcium in the body?

The parathyroid glands, which are embedded in the thyroid gland, also help regulate calcium balance. They counter calcitonin with parathormone, which pulls calcium out of the bones into the bloodstream.

Medications for Pancreatic Disorders

The pancreas regulates blood glucose by secreting two hormones: insulin (which decreases blood glucose) and glucagon (which increases blood glucose). The liver helps the pancreas determine the blood glucose levels, so the liver and pancreas must be functional to control the blood glucose.

The pancreas functions by secreting the correct amount of each hormone. If that doesn't happen, the patient may develop one of two very serious problems. Too much glucose in the blood (hyperglycemia) can lead to problems with wound healing, high blood pressure, and nerve damage, among others. Too little glucose in the blood (hypoglycemia) can cause death.

TABLE 18.1   Hormones Secreted by the Pituitary Gland

HORMONE	TARGET ORGANS AND EFFECT	TOO MUCH CAUSES...	TOO LITTLE CAUSES...
Front or Anterior Pituitary			
Adrenocorticotropic hormone (ACTH)	Regulates release of epinephrine and glucocorticoids from the adrenal glands, which determines "fight or flight" responses of the autonomic nervous system	Cushing's disease	Addison's disease
Thyroid-stimulating hormone (TSH)	Regulates release of hormones in the thyroid, which affects energy	Graves' disease	Myxedema in adults, cretinism in children
Somatotropin, or growth hormone (GH)	Regulates growth of bone, muscles, and other tissues by affecting the liver and adipose tissue	Gigantism (abnormally tall stature; patient becomes a "giant") Acromegaly (growth of hands and feet after puberty when growth is supposed to stop) Treatment of acromegaly: medications that suppress growth hormones	Dwarfism (abnormally short stature) Treatment: growth hormones
Prolactin	Stimulates milk production in the mammary gland	Overproduction of breast milk in women Milk production in a non-nursing patient can be a sign of a pituitary tumor. Parlodel is used to suppress lactation in women who choose not to breastfeed, but a side effect is increased fertility.	Underproduction of milk in women; baby has difficulty nursing
Follicle-stimulating hormone (FSH)	Stimulates sperm production in men and egg production in women	Increased fertility	Men: sterility Women: irregular or absent menses

(table continued on page 300)

TABLE 18.1 **Hormones Secreted by the Pituitary Gland** (continued)

HORMONE	TARGET ORGANS AND EFFECT	TOO MUCH CAUSES...	TOO LITTLE CAUSES...
Luteinizing hormone (LH)	Stimulates release of the ripened egg in women (ovulation); also helps in the production of female hormones (estrogens and progestins)	Multiple gestations (e.g., twins, triplets)	Infertility (woman cannot ovulate, so cannot conceive)
Interstitial cell-stimulating hormone (ICSH)	Stimulates production of androgens (the male hormone testosterone)	Aggressiveness, excessive hair	Feminine attributes in men (e.g., high voice, small muscles)
Back or Posterior Pituitary			
Antidiuretic hormone (ADH)	Conserves fluids by changing the permeability of the kidneys	Syndrome of inappropriate antidiuretic hormone (SIADH); too much fluid is retained. Treatment: diuretics	Diabetes insipidus; too much fluid is excreted by the kidneys, which causes dehydration. Treatment: desmopressin (DDAVP)*
Oxytocin	Contracts the uterus and milk ducts in the breasts of women; contracts the prostate gland in men	The uterus or prostate can contract so much that it ruptures (rarely)	Labor may be slowed or milk expulsion constricted. Treatment: Pitocin (oxytocin in synthetic form) may be given IM or IV to the laboring or postpartum patient to increase the force of uterine contractions.

*DDAVP is also used to help chronic bed-wetters stop urinating at night and to stop bleeding in hemophiliacs.

Diabetes mellitus is a disease characterized by hyperglycemia. Diabetes is classified as type 1 or type 2. With type 1 diabetes, destruction of the beta cells of the pancreas causes a decrease or lack of insulin secretion. With type 2 diabetes, patients have insulin resistance; that is, their bodies do not respond well to insulin. Patients with type 1 diabetes require insulin for treatment, whereas patients with type 2 may be managed with diet alone or with oral diabetic (antihyperglycemic) agents (Table 18.2). Some antihyperglycemic drugs encourage the pancreas to release insulin, and others encourage the liver to tell the pancreas to release insulin. Which drug is prescribed varies depending on the patient's individual problem. Oral antidiabetic drugs are categorized as follows: sulfonylureas such as glimepiride, alpha-glucosidase inhibitors such as acarbose, metformin, thiazolidinediones such as pioglitazone, and meglitinides such as nateglinide.

CRITICAL THINKING

Why might too much glucose in the blood affect wound healing and nerve health?

TABLE 18.2 Types of Diabetes

DIABETES TYPE	CONTRIBUTING FACTORS	INSULIN PRODUCTION	TREATMENT
Type 1: insulin-dependent diabetes mellitus (IDDM)	Family history Pancreatic trauma	Pancreas makes little or no insulin.	Insulin is destroyed in the stomach, so patients are dependent on inhalable or subcutaneously injectable insulin. Diet modification and exercise
Type 2: non-insulin-dependent diabetes mellitus (NIDDM)	Family history Obesity Poor diet	Pancreas does not secrete enough insulin, or body does not use insulin properly. If dietary fat intake is excessive, pancreas may not be able to keep up with demand.	Diet modification and exercise may be enough. If not: oral antihyperglycemic agents. If these do not work: insulin.

When insulin is not available to remove accumulating glucose from the bloodstream, cells give up water to flush the vessels out and send the glucose to the kidneys. For that reason, signs and symptoms of hyperglycemia are increased urination (from flushing), increased thirst (the cells are dehydrated), and increased hunger (the body just flushed out its energy source). In the long run, body organs can become severely affected. Vision can worsen, wounds don't heal normally, fingers and feet can become numb, and kidney function can become impaired. When blood glucose is very high, the patient may become lethargic and exhibit fruity-smelling breath and ketoacidosis (inefficient burning of fat).

If the patient has low blood glucose, there is not sufficient energy to fuel the cells. Signs and symptoms of hypoglycemia are restlessness, shaky hands, lethargy, seizures, and coma (see Fast Tip 18.1).

CRITICAL THINKING

What would you do if a patient with diabetes mellitus came to your office and collapsed in the waiting room?

You must understand the types of insulin, its proper handling, and its proper injection to care for patients with diabetes mellitus safely.

Types of insulin

Insulin preparations are divided into three categories based on how quickly they start working and the length of action: short-acting, intermediate-acting, and long-acting (Table 18.3). When a patient's blood glucose is high, you may need to use a short-acting insulin to lower it. Short-acting insulin is

Fast Tip 18.1 Emergency Treatment of Hypoglycemia

If an insulin dose is too high and low blood glucose results, immediately give juice, honey, or hard candy if the patient is awake. A physician may also order dextrose IV or glucagon IM or IV to correct low blood glucose levels.

TABLE 18.3 Types of Insulin

TYPE	ACTION	ONSET OF ACTION (HOURS)	DURATION OF ACTION (HOURS)
Insulin Lispro	Short	0.25	2–5
Insulin Aspart	Short	0.25	3–5
Regular	Short	0.5–1	8–12
Semilente	Short	1–1.5	12–16
NPH	Intermediate	1–1.5	24
Lente	Intermediate	1–2.5	24
Insulin glargine	Long	1.1	24
Protamine zinc insulin	Long	4–8	36
Ultralente	Long	4–8	20–36

usually prescribed on a sliding scale, depending on the assessed blood glucose level. It may also be taken before meals; this way it starts to work as food is being digested. If a patient is npo for a test, insulin is not given because food is not given.

Intermediate-acting insulin is an insulin mixed with something that makes the body absorb the insulin more slowly. This type of insulin looks cloudy in the bottle and needs to be mixed before being injected.

Long-acting insulin can last an entire day. It is usually taken in the morning or at bedtime.

If a patient is fairly stable with the disease, short- and intermediate-acting insulin can be mixed to cover the next meal and a long time after the meal in one dose. The name of the insulin states the ratio of long-acting to short-acting insulin (e.g., 70/30). Here are examples of some combinations:

- Humalog   75/25
- Humulin   50/50
- Humulin   70/30
- Novolin   70/30

Handling insulin

Insulin should be refrigerated until use. After you have opened an insulin vial, gently roll it between your fingers (Fig. 18.2). Do not shake it. This insulin vial can be stored at room temperature if used within 1 month. Always label a container with the date opened and dispose of it 30 days after opening.

Injecting insulin

When injecting insulin, sites should be rotated on the patient's body so pockets of insulin do not accumulate. You may need to help the patient develop a chart of site rotation, such as that shown in Figure 18.3.

It saves discomfort and cost to the patient if you draw up regular- and longer-acting insulin into one syringe before injecting. Follow your office protocol, but usually you draw in the ordered amount of the clear, regular insulin and then draw in the cloudy, longer-acting insulin. Following these directions ensures that you do not inadvertently put some of the cloudy, longer-acting insulin into the clear, regular insulin vial.

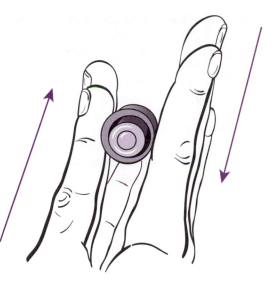

FIGURE 18.2. Proper insulin handling. Be sure to roll the insulin vial in your fingers before drawing up the injection; do not shake the vial.

Medications for Adrenal Disorders

The adrenal glands are located above the kidneys and secrete adrenocorticotropic hormone (ACTH). ACTH controls the fight or flight responses by simulating the release of cortisol and glucocorticoids. Through the negative feedback system, when the cortisol level increases, the hypothalamus tells the pituitary to shut off the release of ACTH. The adrenal gland secretes glucocorticoid hormones (hydrocortisone and cortisol) and the mineralocorticoid hormone aldosterone.

Corticosteroid and mineralocorticoid medications

Addison's disease occurs when the adrenal cortex undersecretes glucocorticoid hormones. The disease is treated with hydrocortisone tablets, a synthetic corticosteroid. If the level of aldosterone is also insufficient, it is replaced with oral doses of fludrocortisone acetate (Florinef).

Corticosteroid medications are also used to treat autoimmune diseases, inflammatory reactions, cerebral edema, dermatologic disorders, allergies, asthma, cancer, Crohn's disease, dermatitis, edema, rashes, rheumatoid arthritis, rhinitis, shock, transplant rejection, and ulcerative colitis.

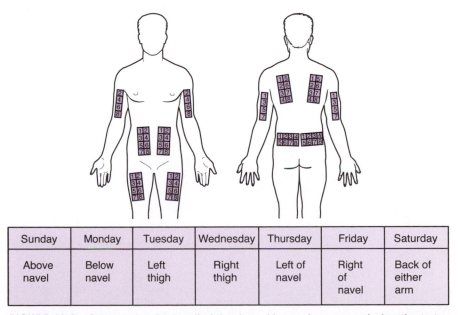

Sunday	Monday	Tuesday	Wednesday	Thursday	Friday	Saturday
Above navel	Below navel	Left thigh	Right thigh	Left of navel	Right of navel	Back of either arm

FIGURE 18.3. Site rotation for insulin injections. Use a chart to remind patients to rotate injection sites.

In Cushing's disease the adrenal cortex oversecretes the glucocorticoids mentioned above. Patients with Cushing's disease gain weight and have edema. Treatment is based on the cause of the excess production and may include surgery, irradiation, chemotherapy, and cortisol-inhibiting drugs.

Anabolic steroids

Anabolic steroids, which change the natural balance between tissue breakdown and building, are frequently abused by athletes trying to build muscle mass. For this reason, anabolic steroids are considered to be on Schedule III of controlled substances. They can be used to prevent muscle wasting in patients with acquired immunodeficiency syndrome (AIDS). Examples of anabolic steroids are oxandrolone and nandrolone decanoate. Side effects of these medications include aggressive behavior, atherosclerosis, and liver cancer.

SUMMARY

Most body functions are controlled by the endocrine system, so disorders affecting this system can have profound implications on the health of the patient. Having hormone levels that are extremely high or extremely low can cause various illnesses, so it is important to be aware of the various types of hormones. Patients may need to take hormone supplements to compensate for missing ones.

Activities

To make sure that you have learned the key points covered in this chapter, complete the following activities.

True or False
Write *true* if the statement is true. Beside the false statements, write *false* and correct the statement to make it true.

1. Hypoglycemia is low blood pressure. _____

2. Graves' disease is caused by too much thyroid hormone. _____

3. Lack of insulin causes hyperglycemia. _____

4. If a patient has taken too much insulin, give 4 oz of juice. _____

5. Melatonin is made in the pituitary gland. _____

6. Addison's disease is caused by low FSH. _____

7. Signs and symptoms of hypoglycemia are increased urination, increased thirst, and increased hunger. _____

8. NPH is used on a sliding scale. _____

9. Draw up regular insulin before NPH. _____

10. Cushing's disease is caused by too much ADH. _____

Multiple Choice
Choose the best answer for each question.

1. **Which of the following is a symptom/sign of hyperglycemia?**
   a. Tremor
   b. Dehydration
   c. Restlessness
   d. Seizures

2. **Which of the following is *not* a treatment for hypoglycemia?**
   a. Diet soda
   b. Candy
   c. Fruit juice
   d. Glucagon

3. **Which of the following is caused by hyperthyroidism?**
   a. Cushing's disease
   b. Addison's disease
   c. Graves' disease
   d. Myxedema

4. **Which hormone puts calcium from the bloodstream into the bones?**
   a. Parathormone
   b. Calcitonin
   c. T_3
   d. T_4

5. Which are controlled drugs?
   a. Diuretics
   b. Corticosteroids
   c. Anabolic steroids
   d. Contraceptives

Application Exercises

Respond to the following scenarios on a separate sheet.

1. Glucophage is ordered for Bilab Khatab, a newly diagnosed patient with diabetes. **Explain this medication's action to him.**
2. Steve Finch takes corticosteroids for a short time. **What are the side effects of this classification of medications in the short term and in the long term?**
3. David Paul Stavros has been recently diagnosed with Addison's disease. **Explain to him the side effects of his corticosteroid medications.**
4. Linda Ross has her thyroid removed because of thyroid cancer. **How will this affect her chance of getting osteoporosis? What might the prescriber prescribe for her?**
5. Lucinda Anderson has just been prescribed 75/25 insulin. In the past she has given herself two shots. **Explain what 75/25 insulin is and how it is used.**

Virtual Field Trips

Go to the following websites to find the information. If a website is not available, try to find the information through another source.

1. Go to your favorite drug website and find the classifications of these drugs.

   a. Levothyroid

   b. Humalog

   c. Clomid

   d. Prednisone

   e. Humulin

2. Visit http://www.bddiabetes.com and create a teaching tool for diabetics.

Essentials Review

For further study and practice with drug classifications learned in this chapter, complete the following table to the best of your ability. Use resources such as a PDR, the Internet, or printed drug guides for help.

CLASSIFICATION	PURPOSE	SIDE EFFECTS	CONTRAINDICATIONS/PRECAUTIONS/INTERACTIONS	PATIENT EDUCATION	EXAMPLES
Anabolic steroids					
Corticosteroids					
Insulin					
Oral antidiabetic agents					
Thyroid medications					

Reproductive and Urinary System Medications

*T*he reproductive system not only helps patients reproduce but also affects the way in which they perceive themselves. Reproductive disorders can cause pain and sometimes death if not treated. They can also affect the patient's ability to reproduce. The urinary system rids the body of harmful toxins while conserving precious electrolytes. Urinary system failure leads to death if not treated.

OBJECTIVES

At the end of this chapter, the student will be able to:

- Define all key terms.
- List actions of reproductive and urinary system hormones.
- Describe what happens to the body when a hormone is over- or underproduced.
- Discuss why hormones must be taken as directed.
- List the functions of the reproductive hormones.
- Describe how contraceptives work.
- Discuss how urinary system hormones affect bodily functions.
- List side effects of diuretics.
- Describe the effects of estrogens, progestins, androgens, ovulations stimulants, agents for cervical ripening, diuretics, oxytocin, tocolytics, and agents to treat erectile dysfunction.

KEY TERMS

Androgen	LH
BPH	Oxytocin
ERT	Progestin
Estrogen	Prolactin
FSH	Prostaglandin
HRT	STD
ICSH	Tocolytic

● REPRODUCTIVE SYSTEM MEDICATIONS

It makes sense to study reproductive disorder medications after studying the endocrine system because so many of these disorders are treated with hormones. (See the Master the Essentials table for descriptions of the most common reproductive system drugs.)

Master the Essentials: Reproductive and Urinary Medications

This table shows the various classes of reproductive and urinary medications and key side effects, contraindications and precautions, and interactions for each class.

CLASS	SIDE EFFECTS	CONTRAINDICATIONS/ PRECAUTIONS	INTERACTIONS
Androgens	Headache, increased or decreased libido, anxiety, depression, acne, hirsutism, nausea, gynecomastia; amenorrhea or virilization in women	Serious heart, kidney, or liver disease; hypersensitivity, pregnancy, male with breast or prostate cancer	Anticoagulants, insulin, propranolol, corticosteroids, cyclosporine
BPH medications	Decreased libido, mild impotence, palpitations, dizziness, somnolence, asthenia, nausea	Hypersensitivity, liver impairment	Alcohol, beta blockers, verapamil
Cervical ripening agent (dinoprostone)	Uterine hyperstimulation, GI effects, back pain, fetal bradycardia	Prior C-section, cephalopelvic disproportion, prior traumatic delivery, ruptured membranes, hypersensitivity, placenta previa	Oxytocics
Erectile dysfunction drugs	Fatal cardiovascular events, flushing, headache, abnormal vision, dyspepsia, back pain	Hypersensitivity, heart disease, kidney or liver impairment	Erythromycin, grapefruit, nitrates, alcohol, alpha blockers, amylodipine, angiotensin II receptor blockers, beta blockers, diuretics, enalapril, metoprolol, protease inhibitors

CLASS	SIDE EFFECTS	CONTRAINDICATIONS/ PRECAUTIONS	INTERACTIONS
Estrogens	Breast enlargement and tenderness, cardiovascular risk, decreased folic acid, edema, gallbladder disease, GI upset, headache, increased or decreased acne, increased triglycerides, irregular menstrual bleeding, visual disturbances, DVT, PE	Asthma, diabetes, heart problems, lactation, liver dysfunction, pregnancy, stroke, seizures, smoking, breast cancer, abnormal uterine bleeding, DVT, PE, MI, hypersensitivity	Anticoagulants, anti-infectives, corticosteroids, oral hypoglycemics, tricyclic antidepressants, thyroid hormones, hydantoins, topiramate
Loop diuretics	Increased blood glucose, fluid and electrolyte loss, GI problems, headache, hypotension, hearing loss	Children, cirrhosis, diabetes, kidney disease, lactation, pregnancy, anuria, hypersensitivity	Blood pressure medications, corticosteroids, lithium, digoxin, aminoglycosides, anticoagulants
Osmotic diuretics	CNS effects, fluid and electrolyte imbalances, increased or decreased blood pressure, rapid heart rate, swelling, headache, nausea, vomiting, diarrhea	Cardiovascular or kidney failure; pulmonary edema; active intracranial bleeding	Lithium
Ovulation stimulants	Ovarian hyperstimulation, headache, gynecomastia, injection site pain, vasomotor flushes	Liver disease, pregnancy, uncontrolled thyroid or adrenal disease, ovarian cysts, abnormal uterine bleeding, hypersensitivity	None reported
Oxytocin	Uterine rupture, embolism, fetal trauma and death, forceful contractions, hemorrhage, increased heart rate, nausea, vomiting	Cephalopelvic disproportion, fetal distress, placenta previa, scarred uterus, unfavorable fetal positions, prolonged use in severe toxemia, hypersensitivity	Cyclopropane anesthesia, sympathomimetics, vasoconstrictors
Potassium-sparing diuretics	GI distress, high blood potassium, low blood pressure, headache, drowsiness	Cirrhosis, lactation, pregnancy, renal impairment, hypersensitivity, serum potassium > 5.5 mEq/L	ACE inhibitors, lithium, NSAIDs, potassium supplements, digoxin
Progestins	Breast tenderness, decreased bone density, headache, irregular menses, swelling, insomnia, depression, nausea, weight changes	Cardiovascular disease, depression, edema, pregnancy, hypersensitivity, thrombophlebitis, thromboembolic disorder, breast cancer, undiagnosed vaginal bleeding, missed abortion	Aminoglutethimide, rifampin
Thiazide diuretics	High blood glucose; low chloride, potassium, and blood pressure	Anuria, hypersensitivity, renal decompensation, hepatic coma	Antidiabetic medications, corticosteroids, lithium, NSAIDs, digoxin, anesthetics, anticoagulants, antigout medications

Testosterone, estrogen, and progesterone are hormones that promote the health, growth, and functioning of the reproductive system. The testes in the male (testicles) produce testosterone. The ovaries in the female secrete female sex hormones (estrogen and progesterone) (Fig. 19.1).

Table 19.1 summarizes the reproductive hormones. As noted in Chapter 18, follicle-stimulating hormone (FSH) regulates sperm and egg production. Luteinizing hormone (LH) triggers release of the egg in women and promotes secretion of estrogen and progesterone. In men, LH is called interstitial cell-stimulating hormone (ICSH) and regulates testosterone production.

Medications for Disorders Related to Female Hormones

If the hormone levels are too high or too low in the female, fertility can be affected. Low hormone levels can lead to infertility; high hormone levels can lead to multiple births.

Contraceptive medications

Some of the most common drugs used for contraception are based on hormones that are naturally manufactured in the female reproductive system (Table 19.2). When administered in the form of a drug, they prevent pregnancy by overriding the body's own mechanism to make estrogens and progestins (the two main hormones secreted by the ovaries). The body, receiving hormones from an outside source regularly, simply stops manufacturing its own estrogens and progestins. The contraceptives are at such low doses of the hormones that it usually inhibits the body's ability to conceive—either by inhibiting ovulation (release of an egg from the ovary), inhibiting fertilization (joining of egg and sperm to form an embryo), preventing implantation (embedding of the embryo into the uterine wall), or preventing growth of the fetus.

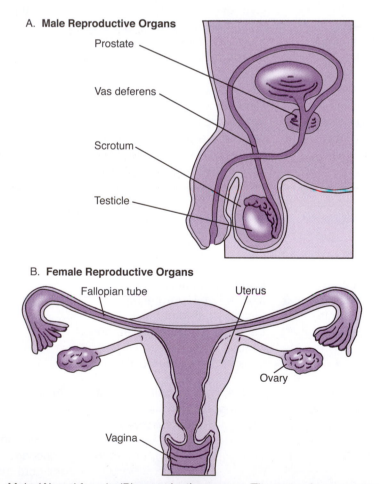

A. **Male Reproductive Organs**
- Prostate
- Vas deferens
- Scrotum
- Testicle

B. **Female Reproductive Organs**
- Fallopian tube
- Uterus
- Ovary
- Vagina

FIGURE 19.1. Male (A) and female (B) reproductive organs. The testes in a man secrete testosterone, and the ovaries in a woman secrete estrogen and progesterone.

TABLE 19.1 Reproductive Hormones

HORMONE	ACTION	TOO MUCH CAUSES...	TOO LITTLE CAUSES...
Prolactin	Stimulates milk production in the mammary gland	Overproduction of breast milk in women. Milk production in a non-nursing patient can be a sign of a pituitary tumor. Parlodel is used to suppress lactation in women who choose not to breastfeed, but a side effect is increased fertility.	Underproduction of milk in women; baby has difficulty nursing
Follicle-stimulating hormone (FSH)	Stimulates sperm production in men and egg production in women	Increased fertility	Men: sterility Women: irregular or absent menses
Luteinizing hormone (LH)	Stimulates release of the ripened egg in women (ovulation); also helps in the production of the female hormones (estrogens and progestins)	Multiple gestations (e.g., twins, triplets)	Infertility (woman cannot ovulate, so cannot conceive)
Interstitial cell-stimulating hormone (ICSH)	Stimulates production of androgens (male hormone testosterone)	Aggressiveness, excessive hair	Feminine attributes in men (e.g., high voice, small muscles)

TABLE 19.2 Examples of Contraceptive Medications

TYPE	ACTION
Monophasic tablets	Inhibit reproductive function
Biphasic tablets	Inhibit reproductive function
Triphasic tablets	Inhibit reproductive function
Implants (e.g., Norplant)	Inhibit pregnancy
Transdermals	Inhibit pregnancy
IUDs	Prevent implantation
Spermicides	Kill sperm
Barrier devices (e.g., diaphragm)	Prevent fertilization
Postcoital contraception	Prevents implantation
Abortifacient (e.g., RU-486)	Kills fetus within 49 days from period

Sometimes patients have symptoms of pregnancy while taking contraceptive pills or tablets. The reason for this is that the usual activity of the reproductive system is shut down, so it behaves as though it is pregnant (e.g., weight gain, mood swings, breast tenderness).

Hormone replacement therapy

Women going through menopause (permanent cessation of menses) may chose to take hormone replacement therapy (HRT) or estrogen replacement therapy (ERT). If a woman no longer has a uterus, ERT replaces her own estrogen, and there is no concern of building up the lining of the uterus. If the woman still has a uterus, estrogen is usually combined with a progestin in this therapy, so the endometrial lining is shed in the same way it would be in the presence of natural hormones. HRT has been shown to decrease bone loss and cardiovascular dysfunction. However, studies have shown an increased risk of breast cancer with its use.

If contraception fails or fails to be used properly, a woman can use postcoital high-dose estrogen to prevent pregnancy. In addition, ERT or HRT can be used to treat prostate cancer in men, because estrogen decreases testosterone levels.

Medications for abnormal uterine bleeding

Abnormal uterine bleeding is a condition in which vaginal bleeding occurs irregularly or too heavily. Correction of hormonal imbalance is usually indicated. Combination therapy of estrogen and progesterone, as oral contraceptives, can be given. Progestins (progesterone) alone can also be prescribed to regulate the rhythm and amount of menstruation.

Lupron (gonadotropin-releasing hormone) is frequently used to suppress creation of the endometrial lining in patients with endometriosis. It suppresses both ovarian and testicular function, and it can cause hot flashes, weight gain, and acne.

Medications for women in labor

Medications that women in labor may need include cervical ripening agents, oxytocin, and tocolytics.

Dinoprostone is a *prostaglandin* used for cervical ripening, or to prepare the cervix for labor. The gel form is inserted into the cervix; the vaginal insert is placed in the posterior fornix of the vagina. The cervix is then allowed time to gently soften. If oxytocin is to be used, 6–12 hours should pass before it is administered.

Oxytocin is the pituitary hormone that causes the uterus to contract. If labor fails to progress, synthetic oxytocin (Pitocin) can be given intravenously (IV) over time to gently encourage the uterus to contract. It is also given after the baby is born to contract the uterus and control postpartum bleeding.

Tocolytics have an effect opposite to that of oxytocin. They slow or stop uterine contractions and are indicated to prevent premature birth. Terbutaline, magnesium sulfate, calcium channel blockers, and nonsteroidal antiinflammatory drugs (NSAIDs) are agents used as tocolytics.

Infertility medications

Drugs are available to help women increase their fertility. Some cause the release of multiple eggs to increase the chance that one will be fertilized and grow into a fetus. These drugs are referred to as ovulation stimulants. Clomiphene (Clomid) is an example of a drug that increases FSH and LH. Menotropins (Pergonal) stimulates follicle ripening and release. Chorionic gonadotropin induces ovulation. The patient should be prepared for the possibility of not becoming pregnant or becoming pregnant with multiple fetuses.

Other disorders

Premenstrual dysphoric disorder (formerly premenstrual syndrome, or PMS) is frequently treated with selective serotonin reuptake inhibitors.

Women may also get infections in their reproductive system. Some are sexually transmitted diseases (STDs). Among the more popular drugs for vaginal infections are antibacterials such as metronidazole (MetroGel), antivirals such as acyclovir (Zovirax), and antifungals such as miconazole (Monistat).

Medications for Disorders Related to Male Hormones

Androgens are male sex hormones that promote maturation of the sexual organs and male sexual characteristics. Men who have low androgen levels may need testosterone to increase their masculine traits. Testosterone can also be used to lower estrogen in women with breast cancer, just as estrogen is used to lower testosterone in men with prostate cancer.

Medications to treat erectile dysfunction, decreased libido, and infertility

Erectile dysfunction, or impotence, is a fairly common disorder, frequently related to atherosclerosis, diabetes, stroke, and hypertension. It also can have psychological roots, such as guilt, fatigue, depression, and fear of failure to perform adequately.

Erectile dysfunction drugs such as phosphodiesterase type 5 inhibitors usually dilate the arteries leading to the penis and constrict the veins thus holding the blood in the penis and sustaining an erection. If erectile dysfunction is associated with physiological decline, it is vitally important that the patient give a complete history to the prescriber. A history of cardiovascular disease is a contraindication for use of several of these drugs.

 CRITICAL THINKING

> Why might erectile dysfunction drugs affect the entire cardiovascular system and not act just on the penis?

Reduced libido can be present in both men and women. Libido is affected not only by emotions but also by physiological changes in the body. For example, many medications decrease libido in men and women. Among them are Benadryl, Aldactone, Aldomet, Catapres, Chlor-Trimeton, Valium, alcohol, Zantac, Tagamet, Dopar, and Inderal. Amphetamines increase libido.

A variety of drugs can be used to treat male infertility, including human chorionic gonadotropin, a substance naturally present in pregnant women.

Medications used for benign prostatic hypertrophy

Many older men suffer from benign prostatic hypertrophy (BPH). This is a nonmalignant growth of the prostate gland that constricts the bladder, impeding outflow of urine (Fig. 19.2).

During its early stages, BPH can be treated with alpha-adrenergic blockers, such as terazosin or doxazosin. These drugs relax smooth muscle in the prostate gland and decrease the blockage.

● URINARY SYSTEM MEDICATIONS

The urinary system (Fig. 19.3) is closely linked with the reproductive system, especially in men. The most common medications used for this system are diuretics.

Diuretics

Diuretics increase excretion of body fluids from the kidneys. They are thus used to treat hypertension, heart failure, kidney failure, and liver failure. There are four categories of diuretic: loop, thiazide, potassium-sparing, and osmotic.

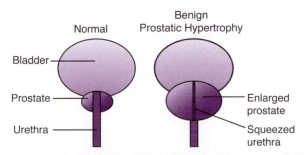

FIGURE 19.2. Benign prostatic hypertrophy (BPH). The prostate surrounds the male urethra. When the prostate becomes enlarged, it squeezes the urethra and limits the flow of urine.

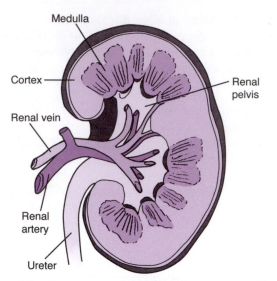

FIGURE 19.3. Urinary system. The kidneys are part of the urinary system. They act as the body's filtering system, retaining valuable electrolytes and fluids and getting rid of what is not needed. The fluid (urine) that is not needed travels through the ureters into the bladder and from there is excreted through the urethra.

A CLOSER LOOK: The Nephron

The kidneys regulate volume and content of urine. In doing so, they also affect blood pressure. The working unit of the kidney is the nephron. Each nephron determines which electrolytes are retained and which are disposed of outside the body. Thus, the kidneys have a large role in maintaining the acid-base balance in the body.

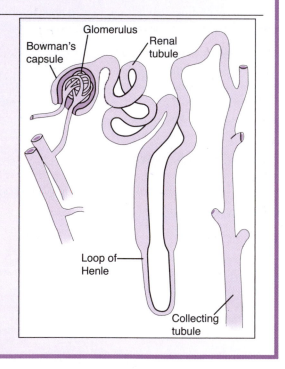

Loop diuretics
The most effective diuretics work in the loop of Henle, located in the nephron. Not surprisingly, they are called loop diuretics.

Thiazide diuretics
Thiazides block sodium reabsorption and increase water excretion. Where salt goes, water follows. These drugs are used to treat moderate high blood pressure and are less effective than loop diuretics.

Potassium-sparing diuretics

Although loop diuretics are highly effective, they rid the body of potassium, a valuable electrolyte. For that reason, potassium-sparing diuretics are frequently prescribed instead.

Osmotic diuretics

Osmotic diuretics such as mannitol are used to lower intraocular pressure and for renal failure.

Electrolyte imbalances and diuretics

Although diuretics may relieve congestion by getting fluid out of the body, they can have a devastating effect on the patient's electrolyte balance. The body needs electrolytes—sodium (Na), potassium (K), calcium (Ca), and magnesium (Mg). Intravenous (IV) infusion therapy may be needed to replenish lost electrolytes; alternatively, electrolytes can be taken orally to prevent imbalances.

Other Urinary Medications

Other common disorders of the urinary system include infection, gout, and urinary incontinence.

Urinary tract infections can cause frequency, urgency, pain, and blood in the urine. They are usually treated with broad-spectrum antibiotics, analgesics, antispasmodics, and muscle relaxants.

Gout, although it affects the musculoskeletal system, is caused by the inability of the kidneys to clear uric acid from the bloodstream. Antigout medications can cause rashes in hypersensitive individuals. (Information regarding antigout drugs can be found in Chapter 17.)

Certain muscle relaxants and antispasmodics can effectively treat urinary incontinence.

Enuresis (bed-wetting) can be treated effectively with DDAVP (nasally or orally) and oral imiprimine (Tofranil). You should also advise patients not to drink caffeinated drinks after 6 p.m. because they can irritate the bladder and cause enuresis.

Effects of Medications on Color of the Urine

One side effect of many medications is that they can change the color of urine. Usually this has no effect on the kidneys, but it may frighten the unprepared patient. Agents that change the color of urine include some anticoagulants, antidepressants, laxatives, barbiturates, and iron salts. Always check your drug handbook for information on urine color changes.

●●● SUMMARY

Many reproductive disorders are treated with hormones. The reproductive system does not just create babies, it has a profound effect on how we view ourselves. The urinary system eliminates wastes and regulates volume of body fluids. When it does not function well, toxic substances can build up in the body and lead to acute renal failure or even death.

Activities

To make sure that you have learned the key points covered in this chapter, complete the following activities.

True or False

Write *true* if the statement is true. Beside the false statements, write *false* and correct the statement to make it true.

1. High doses of estrogens and progestins act as contraceptives. _____

2. Erectile dysfunction is always fatal. _____

3. Androgens are used to treat breast cancer. _____

4. Tocolytics stimulate labor. _____

5. Testosterone is used to treat BPH. _____

Multiple Choice

Choose the best answer for each question.

1. Which of the following causes abortion?
   a. Norplant
   b. Triphasil
   c. Diaphragm
   d. RU-486

2. Which drug is used to treat vaginal fungi?
   a. Clomid
   b. Pitocin
   c. Metrogel
   d. Monistat

3. Which drug classification suppresses uterine contractions?
   a. Antispasmodics
   b. Thiazides
   c. Tocolytics
   d. SSRIs

4. Which hormone regulates sperm production?
   a. LH
   b. FSH
   c. Prolactin
   d. Oxytocin

5. Which is a sign of increased sodium retention?
   a. Increased edema
   b. Decreased temperature
   c. Decreased blood pressure
   d. Increased cramps

Application Exercises

Respond to the following scenarios on a separate sheet.

1. Michael Mullins comes to the office every week demanding Viagra. The physician refuses to order it for him because he has serious cardiovascular disease. **Explain to Mr. Mullins why he should not take Viagra for erectile dysfunction.**

2. Moriah Ryan is in labor with twins. Tocolytics have been prescribed to suppress the labor. **Explain the side effects to her.**

Virtual Field Trips

Go to the following websites to find the information. If a website is not available, try to find the information through another source.

1. Go to your favorite drug website and find the classifications of these drugs.
   a. Diuril
   b. Lasix
   c. Depo-Testosterone
   d. Vasopressin
   e. Detrol
   f. Pyridium
   g. Yutopar
   h. Premarin
   i. Viagra

2. Go to http://www.google.com or a similar search engine and research one drug from each category in the contraceptive table (monophasics through abortifacients). Create a poster to help teach teenagers about contraceptive options.

Essentials Review

For further study and practice with drug classifications learned in this chapter, complete the following table to the best of your ability. Use resources such as a PDR, the Internet, or printed drug guides for help.

CLASSIFICATION	PURPOSE	SIDE EFFECTS	CONTRAINDICATIONS/PRECAUTIONS/INTERACTIONS	EXAMPLES	PATIENT EDUCATION
BPH medications					
Erectile dysfunction drugs					
Estrogens					
Oxytocin					
Progestins					
Thiazide diuretics					

Eye and Ear Medications

*O*ur eyes and ears gather sensory data from the environment and send it to our brain. When these organs do not work properly, information may be blocked or distorted, leading to pain, anxiety, and the inability to react properly to the environment. For example, those with poor eyesight may fall because they cannot clearly see stairs. Fortunately, several medications are available for conditions of the eyes and ears. These medications must be carefully given to have optimal effect.

OBJECTIVES

At the end of this chapter, the student will be able to:

- Define all key terms.
- List the effects of medications on the eyes and ears.
- Describe the types of medications that are administered to treat eye disorders: miotics, prostaglandins, cyclopegic mydriatics, alpha blockers, beta blockers, carbonic anhydrase inhibitors, osmotic diuretics, ophthalmic nonsteroidal antiinflammatory drugs (NSAIDs), and ophthalmic antibiotics.
- Discuss how medications placed in the ear affect the ear and the body.
- Contrast the effects of systemic and topically applied medications.

KEY TERMS

Cerumen
IOP
Ototoxicity
Tinnitus
Tonometer
Vertigo

● EYE AND EAR MEDICATIONS

Various medications are used to treat conditions of the eyes and ears.

Medications for the Eye

Before examining drugs that affect the eye, it is important to review eye anatomy (Fig. 20.1). The eyes are protected by their placement in the orbits of the skull. Eyelids, eyelashes, and eyebrows protect the eye from irritants and infectious microbes. A hard sclera protects the outer eye, and the pupil regulates the amount of light that enters the eye. The outer eye is bathed with tears. The anterior chamber contains a watery aqueous humor (fluid). The dark cavern of the posterior chamber contains a viscous (thick) vitreous humor.

Images are projected through the pupil and lens onto the rods and cones of the retina. The inverted images are then sent to the brain via the optic nerve.

A CLOSER LOOK: Eye Health

Good eye health requires that patients have their eyes assessed annually. Even a family practitioner should be alert to the need to encourage every patient—particularly older ones—to see an ophthalmologist or optometrist annually. These specialists use a tonometer to measure pressure in the eye. If pressure builds in the eye, it is usually because the aqueous humor is not flowing out of the eye correctly. This causes intraocular pressure (IOP) to increase. Pressure on the optic nerve eventually can lead to blindness.

Several disorders that require medication treatment can occur in the eye, including glaucoma, irritation, and infection. Medications may also be used to make it easier to examine the eye. (See the Master the Essentials table for descriptions of the most common medications for disorders of the eye.)

Medications for glaucoma

Glaucoma is a leading cause of blindness. It can be caused by defective genes, injury, or disease. Some medications (e.g., glucocorticoids, antihypertensives, antihistamines, antidepressants) can predispose a patient to glaucoma. Glaucoma is more prevalent among patients with hypertension, migraine headache, nearsightedness, farsightedness, and older age.

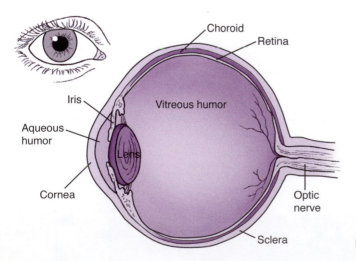

FIGURE 20.1. Anatomy of the eye.

Master the Essentials: Eye and Ear Medications

This table shows the various classes of eye and ear medications, the key side effects, contraindications, precautions, and interactions for each class.

CLASS	SIDE EFFECTS	CONTRAINDICATIONS/ PRECAUTIONS	INTERACTIONS
Ophthalmic alpha blockers	Hypertension, somnolence, oral dryness, ocular hyperemia, eye burning or stinging	Hypersensitivity	MAO inhibitors, TCAs, beta blockers, antihypertensives, digoxin
Antivertigo agents	Blurred vision, confusion, extrapyramidal symptoms, restlessness, sedation, hypotension, rash, dry mouth	Benign prostatic hypertrophy, children, glaucoma, hypertension, lactation, pregnancy, seizures, hypersensitivity	Alcohol, CNS depressants, muscle relaxants
Ophthalmic beta blockers	Headache, depression, arrhythmia, syncope, nausea, keratitis, visual disturbances, bronchospasm	Bronchial asthma, COPD, sinus bradycardia, AV block, heart failure, hypersensitivity	Oral beta blockers, calcium antagonists, digoxin, quinidine, phenothiazines
Carbonic anhydrase inhibitors	Ocular burning or stinging, blurred vision, bitter taste	Hypersensitivity	Salicylates
Cycloplegic mydriatics	Increased IOP, transient burning/stinging, dry mouth, dry skin	Primary glaucoma, hypersensitivity, children with history of reaction to atropine, pregnancy	None reported
Miotics	Corneal edema, clouding, stinging, burning, tearing, headache	Hypersensitivity, any condition where pupillary constriction is undesirable	Topical NSAIDs
Ophthalmic antibiotics	Burning sensation in the eyes, conjunctivitis, hypersensitivity reactions, rash, urticaria	Allergy, fungal or viral diseases in the eye	Corticosteroids
Ophthalmic local anesthetics	Stinging, burning	Hypersensitivity, prolonged use	None reported
Ophthalmic NSAIDs	Burning sensation in the eyes, decreased resistance to infection, increased IOP, slowed wound healing	Diabetes mellitus, infections, pregnancy, open-angle glaucoma, hypersensitivity	Acetylcholine chloride, carbachol

(table continued on page 324)

Master the Essentials: Eye and Ear Medications (continued)

CLASS	SIDE EFFECTS	CONTRAINDICATIONS/ PRECAUTIONS	INTERACTIONS
Osmotic diuretics	Dizziness, dry mouth, fluid and electrolyte imbalance, headache, tremors, nausea, vomiting, disorientation, confusion	Anuria, dehydration, pulmonary edema, hypersensitivity	None reported
Ophthalmic prostaglandins	Ocular hyperemia, decreased visual acuity, eye discomfort	Hypersensitivity, pregnancy	None reported

A CLOSER LOOK: Types of Glaucoma

Glaucoma occurs in two main types: open-angle glaucoma and closed-angle glaucoma (also called angle-closure glaucoma). Open-angle glaucoma is a chronic condition that develops over time. Frequent checkups and treatment can prevent open-angle glaucoma. Closed-angle glaucoma is an acute form that results from stress, injury, or certain medications. In this condition, the Schlemm canal (drainage tube for aqueous humor) becomes blocked. The patient may complain of blurred vision, extreme headache, difficulty concentrating, and bloodshot eyes. Acute glaucoma may require surgery to correct the position of the iris and to drain the aqueous humor. Drug treatments act by increasing the output of the aqueous humor at the Schlemm canal or decreasing the production of aqueous humor at the ciliary body.

Drugs used to treat glaucoma act by increasing the flow of aqueous humor; they include miotics and prostaglandins.

Drugs that increase the outflow of aqueous humor are called miotics. They also constrict the pupil. Some of these drugs activate cholinergic receptors, which decrease the IOP. They dilate the meshwork of the canals of Schlemm, allowing increased output of aqueous humor. As more aqueous humor is absorbed, the IOP decreases.

Prostaglandins do not affect pupil diameter but dilate the meshwork in the anterior chambers in the canals of Schlemm. However, one side effect of prostaglandins is that they change the pigmentation and thus the color of the iris.

Other medications decrease IOP by reducing the flow of aqueous humor. These agents include alpha and beta blockers, carbonic anhydrase inhibitors, and osmotic diuretics.

Alpha blockers dilate blood vessels in the eye and have a mild effect on the cardiovascular and respiratory systems. In low dosages, beta blockers affect the eye but do not have a systemic effect. If they do enter the cardiovascular system, they can cause constriction of the bronchi, slow the heart rate, and cause hypotension.

Carbonic anhydrase inhibitors decrease IOP. They can be administered topically or systemically and are especially good for open-angle glaucoma.

Osmotic diuretics are used for eye surgery to decrease the amount of aqueous humor rapidly.

Medications for eye irritation

For minor eye injury and irritation, local anesthetics, antimicrobials, nonsteroidal antiinflammatory drugs (NSAIDs), and glucocorticoids can be used. They can be administered as drops or salves or by injection. Some, such as eye lubricants, just soothe the outer eye. Others penetrate beyond the surface.

Ophthalmic NSAIDs should not be used for long-term treatment, because they can suppress the immune response.

Medications for eye infections

Antiinfectives are used for eye infections. Like infections elsewhere in the body, it is important to treat eye infections swiftly and completely. Eye infections can spread to other parts of the body—especially if patients rub their eyes with their fingers and then touch another part of the body. Meticulous hand washing is important, and patients should be advised to not rub the infected eye.

Medications for eye examinations

Some drugs are used to make it easier for a health care professional to examine the eyes. Cyclopegic mydriatics, for example, relax ciliary muscles and dilate the pupils so the examiner can peer into the eye.

Local ophthalmic anesthetic agents are used when removing foreign objects that get in the eye. The blink reflex is impaired, so tell the patient not to go out into sunlight without wearing darkened glasses.

Staining agents are nontoxic, water-soluble dyes used to diagnose corneal epithelial defects caused by infection or injury. They can also be used to find foreign bodies or contact lenses in the eye. The stain colors the object green.

Medications for the Ear

Otic, or ear, medications can be used to treat inflammation, wax buildup, or infections. To understand ear disorders, you must understand the anatomy of the ear, which is divided into the outer, middle, and inner ear (Fig. 20.2). Otic medications are usually deposited in the outer ear, or pinna, from where they flow through the auditory canal toward the eardrum. If the eardrum is intact, it provides a barrier to prevent infection from entering the inner ear.

Several types of medication are used to treat ear disorders. Antibiotics can be given directly into the ear to fight infection. Systemic antibiotics are needed for middle or inner ear infections.

Pain medications may also be prescribed for the pain that accompanies trauma or infection. Glucocorticoids are sometimes added to decrease the associated inflammation. (See the Master the Essentials table for descriptions of the most common medications for disorders of the ear.)

Medications for earwax

Mineral oil, earwax (*cerumen*) softeners (*cerumenolytics*), and hydrogen peroxide can be used to decrease the amount of earwax. Although earwax can protect the ear from infection, having too much of it can decrease hearing.

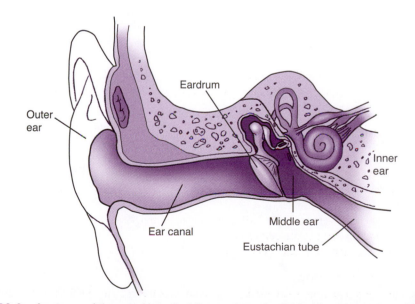

FIGURE 20.2. Anatomy of the ear. Note that the anatomy is divided into the outer, middle, and inner ear.

Medications for motion sickness and vertigo

In addition to hearing, the ear gives the brain information about balance. Motion sickness is caused by the ear's inability to determine the body's position relative to the motion. It can be treated with tablets or transdermal patches that are placed behind the ear. Medications should be taken 20–60 minutes before travel.

Drugs such as meclizine, which is an anticholinergic, are given for dizziness, or vertigo, and the nausea that sometimes accompanies it.

Medications and ototoxicity

It should be noted that many drugs can cause ototoxicity. Symptoms of ear damage include tinnitus (ringing in the ears), severe headache, ataxia, and balance disturbances.

SUMMARY

The eyes and ears gather crucial information for the brain. When they are diseased, there are systemic consequences. Good eye and ear health is fundamental to retaining our ability to see and hear. Patients should be encouraged to be alert to changes in their vision and hearing and to have a thorough assessment of these organs regularly.

Activities

To make sure that you have learned the key points covered in this chapter, complete the following activities.

True or False

Write *true* if the statement is true. Beside the false statements, write *false* and correct the statement to make it true.

1. Cerumen is earwax. _____

2. Ototoxicity occurs in the eyes. _____

3. Cyclopegic mydriatics relax ciliary muscles. _____

4. Drugs that decrease the outflow of aqueous fluid are miotics. _____

5. Anticholinergics decrease IOP. _____

Multiple Choice

Choose the best answer for each question.

1. Which is a physician specializing in the eye?
   a. Audiologist
   b. Ophthalmologist
   c. Optician
   d. Dermatologist

2. Which of the following are used to treat ear problems?
   a. Cerumenolytics
   b. Glucocorticoids
   c. Mydriatics
   d. Miotics

3. Which drugs dilate the pupils?
   a. Cerumenolytics
   b. Glucocorticoids
   c. Mydriatics
   d. Miotics

4. What class of diuretics is used to decrease IOP?
   a. Loop
   b. Osmotic
   c. Thiazide
   d. Potassium-sparing

5. Which type of drug is used to treat glaucoma?
   a. Cerumenolytics
   b. Miotics
   c. Cyclopegic mydriatics
   d. Glucocorticoids

Application Exercises

Respond to the following scenarios on a separate sheet.

1. Burns Ahrens has not had an eye checkup in years. You note that he has trouble reading the informed consent form. **What do you say?**

2. Adam Troy wants to join the military but is rejected after his physical examination because of earwax. He comes to your office to have his ears cleared. **What is likely to be prescribed?**

3. Bruce Scalise has glaucoma. He wants to smoke marijuana to decrease IOP. **What should you say to him?**

Virtual Field Trips

Go to the following websites to find the information. If a website is not available, try to find the information through another source.

1. Visit your favorite website and write the classification of each of the following.

    a. Timoptic

    b. Pilocarpine

    c. Visine

    d. Bonine

    e. Meclizine

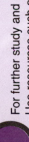

Essentials Review

For further study and practice with drug classifications learned in this chapter, complete the following table to the best of your ability. Use resources such as a PDR, the Internet, or printed drug guides for help.

CLASSIFICATION	PURPOSE	SIDE EFFECTS	CONTRAINDICATIONS/PRECAUTIONS/INTERACTIONS	EXAMPLES	PATIENT EDUCATION
Antivertigo agents					
Ophthalmic alpha blockers					
Ophthalmic beta blockers					
Miotics					
Osmotic diuretics					

329

Herbs, Vitamins, and Minerals

*T*his last chapter discusses herbs, vitamins, and minerals. Vitamins and minerals are vital to survival and good health, and herbal supplements have become popular treatments for many conditions. Remember, though, that the Food and Drug Administration (FDA) does not regulate herbal supplements. Vitamins and herbs are usually taken by mouth, but minerals can be given intravenously (IV), intramuscularly (IM), or orally.

OBJECTIVES

At the end of this chapter, the student will be able to:

● Define all key terms.
● Discuss the body's need for vitamins and minerals.
● List herbs that can be used to improve patient health.
● Discuss why some patients prefer herbs to prescription medications.
● Discuss why insurance companies do not usually pay for herbal remedies.

KEY TERMS

Aromatherapy
CAM
Homeopathy
Inorganic
Megadosage
Organic

HERBS, VITAMINS, MINERALS, AND MORE

This chapter primarily discusses herbs, vitamins, and minerals. Amino acids and lipids are included as well because, like vitamins and minerals, a proper diet helps maintain proper levels of these important nutrients. A wise allied health professional always asks patients if they are taking any supplements. Sometimes patients may not consider these agents to be medications, so ask about them specifically.

Herbal Medicines

Herbs have been used as medications for centuries. Many patients self-medicate with herbs. This practice may not always be harmful, but some herbs can be dangerous in the wrong quantities or when they interact with some medications. For example, St. John's wort can lower cyclosporine levels, which can ultimately cause rejection of a transplanted organ.

Herbs are a type of complementary and alternative medicine (CAM). CAM therapies include treatments and medications that are used as an adjunct to (complement) or instead of (alternative) conventional medical therapy. Sometimes the patient believes that conventional treatment did not eliminate the disease. Others may discount modern medical treatment as dangerous. Interestingly, most herbs have had less scientific testing than modern drugs.

Many CAM therapies emphasize an Eastern philosophy rather than a Western philosophy of healing (see Fast Tip 21.1). The Eastern philosophy stresses the body's ability to heal itself and uses herbs to promote self-healing. Disease is thought to be caused by imbalances in the body, and it is believed that health returns when balance is restored.

In the Western philosophy, the focus is on medications to target specific problems. It is believed that disease is caused by physiological disorders and that health is the absence of disease.

Recently, Eastern and Western philosophies are meeting halfway as integrative therapy, which combines conventional medical treatment with CAM therapies.

? CRITICAL THINKING

If a placebo (inactive medication) works almost 60% of the time, what does that tell you about the role of faith in healing?

If you visit any herbal store, you may be surprised to see the variety of products as well as the routes by which to administer them. Most are swallowed as tablets, but many are drunk as teas, chewed on as a root, or rubbed on the skin. Furthermore, some herbs (e.g., eucalyptus for asthma) are used as aromatherapy. They are burned and their aroma inhaled. Herbs are also just one type of plant substance used in homeopathy.

It is impossible to give a comprehensive list of herbs in this book, but you can learn about common ones in Table 21.1 and some helpful websites at the end of this chapter. Be careful about sources of information on herbs. Data about safety, efficacy, and dosing may not be available. Furthermore, because herbs are not regulated like most pharmaceutical preparations, there may be inconsistent amounts of an herb in different manufacturers' products.

○ *Fast Tip 21.1* Eastern and Western Healing Philosophies

You need to understand the different philosophies that patients and health care providers can have toward healing. If, for example, a patient who values the Eastern philosophy visits a provider who values Western philosophy, conflicts in the choice of treatment may result.

A CLOSER LOOK: Homeopathy

Homeopathy is a type of CAM based on the principle that "like cures like." This means that a patient takes a substance similar to the one that is harming the body, thereby training the body to fight the dangerous substance with a small amount of a similar substance.

A German physician, Samuel Hahnemann (1755–1843), developed these remedies. In those days, physicians cut people open and allowed them to bleed because they felt that it purged the body of evil disease. They also administered harsh enemas to force the body to purge itself. These measures did not seem to work and, in fact, killed many patients, so Dr. Hahnemann developed homeopathy.

Homeopathy is supposed to work according to three laws:

• A remedy starts healing from the top of the body and works downward.
• It starts from within the body, working outward, and from major to minor organs.
• Symptoms clear in reverse order to their manner of appearance.

There are more than 2000 homeopathic remedies available from animal, vegetable, and mineral sources. You can find them by doing an Internet search on homeopathy or visiting the National Homeopathy Center (http://www.homeopathic.org).

Homeopaths are people skilled in homeopathy who advise patients on the selection and dosing of homeopathic preparations. Homeopaths are usually not regulated by any medical board or governmental agency.

TABLE 21.1 Examples of Herbs and Possible Benefits

Aloe vera—cures acne, astringent, blood cleanser, cures burns, seals cuts, helps with shingles, tonic
Angelica—diaphoretic, tonic, antispasmodic, expectorant; induces fetal abortion
Barberry—respiratory aid, antiinfective
Camphor—bronchodilator
Caraway—antispasmodic
Cayenne pepper—decongestant, expectorant, emetic
Chamomile—calming, digestive aid, antiinfective, antiseptic, antispasmodic
Cedar—decreases oily skin, cures dandruff, tonic
Celery seed—expectorant, lithotrophic (expels stones)
Cumin—boosts immune system, sexual stimulant
Echinacea—boosts immune system
Evening primrose—decreases scaling and redness, prevents multiple sclerosis, decreases liver damage from alcohol, maintains hormonal balance, decreases inflammation, acts as an immunosuppressant
Feverfew—antispasmodic, decreases migraines
Garlic—stimulant, carminative, expectorant, fungicide, antibiotic, antispasmodic; decreases blood pressure and cholesterol
Ginger—digestive aid
Ginkgo biloba—increases blood flow, antiinfective
Ginseng—energizer, boosts immune system, increases concentration
Green tea—preventing cancer
Horehound—respiratory problems
Hyssop—antiretroviral
Kava kava—improves mood

(table continued on page 334)

TABLE 21.1 Examples of Herbs and Possible Benefits (continued)

Licorice—antiulcer, heals rashes, aids respiration
Melatonin—sleep
Mustard—digestive aid, antiinfective, emetic, laxative
Myrrh—analgesic, antispasmodic, antiinfective
Nutmeg—calming; hallucinogen in high doses
Onion—stimulant, expectorant, rejuvenates
Peppermint—digestive aid, stimulant, antispasmodic
Rosemary—improves hair, decreases muscle tension
Saffron—stimulant and expectorant
Saw palmetto—tonic, urinary antiseptic, increases sex drive
Senna—cathartic, antispasmodic, antiseptic
Skullcap—antianxiety, antispasmodic
St. John's wort—antidepressant, diuretic, antiviral, analgesic
Turmeric—digestive aid
Valerian—sedative
Witch hazel—astringent, antiinflammatory
Yams—antiinfective, antispasmodic
Yarrow—aids in blood clotting, diaphoretic, antiinflammatory, antiseptic, tonic, antispasmodic

Vitamins, Minerals, and More

Vitamins are organic nutrients with carbon that are essential to regulate the chemical processes in the body. These nutrients maintain strong bones, release energy from food, and control hormonal activity.

Minerals are inorganic (lack carbon) chemical elements that are necessary for the body's many processes.

Amino acids are compounds that contain an amino group and have an acidic function. There are eight "essential" amino acids: phenylalanine, valine, threonine, tryptophan, isoleucine, methionine, lysine, and leucine (Table 21.2). There are also 12 "nonessential" amino acids. They can usually be made from other substances in the body, if needed.

TABLE 21.2 Key Amino Acids

Phenylalanine—kills pain, acts as an antidepressant
Glycine—increases pituitary function, decreases spasms, increases blood glucose
Arginine—boosts immunity, decreases tremors, increases muscle tone, burns fat, promotes
   wound healing, protects the liver from toxins
Aspartic acid—disposes of ammonia, decreases fatigue, may improve stamina and endurance
Cysteine—protects against copper toxicity, decreases damage from free radicals (molecules that
   cause many kinds of chemical reactions in the body), may reverse damage done by smoking
   and alcohol abuse, protects against x-rays and radiation exposure damage
Glutamine—decreases craving for alcohol, heals peptic ulcers, acts as an antidepressant,
   energizes the brain, heals colitis
Histidine—increases suppressor T cells and decreases arthritis
Lysine—prevents or treats herpes, builds muscle mass, improves concentration, increases fertility
Methionine—eliminates fatty substances, decreases the risk of heart attack, regulates the
   nervous system, decreases tumors; is necessary for biosynthesis of taurine and cysteine
Phenylalanine—acts as an antidepressant, controls addictive behavior, increases alertness and
   sexual arousal, decreases hunger
Tryptophan—decreases pain sensitivity and craving for alcohol, acts as an antidepressant, acts
   as a sleep aid
Tyrosine—acts as an antidepressant, decreases stress and premenstrual syndrome, decreases
   addiction and withdrawal symptoms

TABLE 21.3 Examples of Lipid Supplements

Fish oils—reduce kidney disease, decrease cancer, stop arthritis progression; decrease blood pressure, cardiovascular effects, psoriasis

Inositol—dissolves fat, decreases anxiety, grows hair and nails, decreases cholesterol, improves sleep

Lecithin—decreases cardiovascular illness and memory loss, balances mood in bipolar disorder, acts as an antiviral, decreases gallstones, is palliative for viral hepatitis

---

Lipids (fats) are necessary for life and are available as supplements (Table 21.3). They are used to prevent wrinkles, unclog arteries, and decrease cholesterol and heart disease.

A healthy diet should provide a patient with sufficient vitamins, minerals, amino acids, and fats. If a patient does not maintain a healthy diet, supplements may be prescribed. They come in powders, capsules, liquids, and tablets.

Vitamins

The FDA has established recommended daily allowances for vitamins and minerals. Although deficiencies of vitamins and minerals can lead to illness, overdoses can also cause illness or death. Just because a small amount of a vitamin is good, it does not mean that megadosages (larger than the FDA recommendations) are better. The recommended daily allowance (RDA) for each vitamin varies for women, men, pregnant women, infants, and children.

Vitamins A, D, E, and K are stored in the liver. Vitamins B and C are not stored; they must be ingested daily, and excessive amounts are excreted through the kidneys.

CRITICAL THINKING

If an athlete takes excessive amounts of vitamins and complains that his urine has changed color and has a strong smell, what is the likely cause?

Essential vitamins

- *Vitamin A*—anticarcinogenic; heals skin disorders; improves vision; determines growth of bones, hair, teeth, skin, and gums. Deficiencies of vitamin A cause brittle nails, joint and muscle pain, jaundice, vertigo, irritability, headache, and coma if overdosed. Side effects of supplementation are prolonged infection, diabetes mellitus, hypothyroidism, and liver illness.
- *Vitamin B$_1$ (thiamine)*—protects against imbalances caused by alcohol consumption; decreases heart disease, neurological diseases, anemia, herpes, and other infections; treats diabetes mellitus; helps convert sugar into energy. Deficiencies of vitamin B$_1$ cause emaciation, constipation, anorexia, nausea, gastrointestinal (GI) upset, neuritis, pain, tingling in the extremities, loss of reflexes, muscle weakness, fatigue, ataxia, confusion, and memory loss.
- *Vitamin B$_2$ (riboflavin)*—works with enzymes to metabolize fats, proteins, and carbohydrates; aids vision; improves growth and reproductive system; helps skin, hair, and nails grow; can improve athletic performance; decreases cancer; improves anemias. Deficiencies of vitamin B$_2$ cause glossitis, cheilosis, and dermatitis.
- *Vitamin B$_3$ (niacin)*—prevents and treats schizophrenia; aids in cell respiration; decreases cholesterol; cures migraines; decreases blood pressure; alleviates arthritis, acts as an antioxidant; produces energy from food; improves skin, nerves, and tongue. Deficiencies of nicotinic acids can cause peripheral vascular damage, dermatitis, and diarrhea. Side effects of niacin include headache, flushing, burning sensation, postural hypotension, and jaundice.
- *Vitamin B$_5$ (pathothenic acid)*—encourages wound healing; produces energy; decreases stress on the body; improves metabolism; decreases fatigue; boosts the immune system.
- *Vitamin B$_6$ (pyridoxine)*—boosts the immune system; decreases diabetes mellitus; assimilates proteins and fats; decreases skin and nervous system disorders; improves nausea; decreases

PMS and menopausal symptoms; stops muscle cramps and spasms; decreases cancer; acts as a natural diuretic.

- *Vitamin B$_9$ (folic acid)*—improves lactation; decreases cancer; improves skin and appetite; acts as an analgesic; decreases infection; metabolizes RNA and DNA; forms blood; decreases spina bifida in fetuses. Deficiencies of folic acid cause anorexia, diarrhea, decreased weight, weakness, sore mouth, and irritability. Overdoses can cause allergic reactions.
- *Vitamin B$_{12}$ (cobalamin)*—improves memory and concentration; utilizes food for energy; increases growth; decreases cancer; acts as an antiallergen. Deficiencies of cobalamin cause anemia, ataxia, numbness, and irritability. Side effects are numbness, decreased muscle coordination, irritability, and confusion.
- *Vitamin C (ascorbic acid)*—increases wound healing; decreases cholesterol and heart disease; boosts the immune system; makes healthy bones and teeth; nourishes the sex organs; alleviates male infertility; decreases cancer; improves vision; acts as an antihistamine and antioxidant. Deficiencies of ascorbic acid cause fragility of capillaries, poor wound healing, and degenerative bone disease. Side effects are muscle weakness, cramping, sore and bleeding gums and mouth.
- *Vitamin D*—prevents osteoporosis; treats psoriasis; boosts immune system; decreases cancer; makes strong bones and teeth. Deficiencies of vitamin D cause tooth and bone deformation and fractures, osteomalacia, osteoporosis, and tetany. Side effects of vitamin D given in excess include nausea, vomiting, diarrhea, kidney stones, dizziness, redness of skin, muscle and bone pain, cardiac arrhythmias, vertigo, and tinnitus.
- *Vitamin E*—acts as an antioxidant and diuretic; decreases PMS and miscarriage; increases immunity; decreases fatigue; treats skin problems and baldness; heals burns and wounds; improves neurological functioning. Side effects are muscle weakness and abnormal red blood cell counts. In large dosages, vitamin E significantly decreases clotting time.
- *Vitamin H (biotin)*—decreases hair turning gray, eases muscular aches and pains, cures eczema and dermatitis, decreases baldness.
- *Vitamin K*—clots blood. Deficiencies of vitamin K cause increased clotting time, blood in urine, petechiae, bruising, and blood in stool. Overdose can cause a hypersensitivity reaction.

Minerals

Minerals are necessary for the body to function properly, but they do not contain carbon as vitamins do.

- *Calcium*—decreases osteoporosis and cancer as well as heart disease and high blood pressure; alleviates arthritis; keeps skin healthy; decreases leg cramps; encourages healthy heart rhythms; helps metabolize iron; decreases insomnia. Deficiencies can cause bone deformities and fractures, leg cramps, tetany, and heart dysrhythmias. Side effects are constipation and irritation of tissue if an IV infusion infiltrates.
- *Chromium*—improves the production of insulin; metabolizes carbohydrates and fats; improves the cholesterol level; improves synthesis of proteins in the body, increasing resistance to infection and decreasing hunger. Deficiencies can cause diabetes mellitus.
- *Cobalt*—decreases pernicious anemia, increases the production of red blood cells, helps the synthesis of DNA and choline, decreases blood pressure; aids the nervous system and the formation of myelin. Deficiencies of cobalt cause blood abnormalities and neurological disorders.
- *Copper*—decreases cancer and cardiovascular (CV) disorders; improves arthritis; boosts the immune system; acts as an antioxidant. Deficiencies can cause infection and CV disease.
- *Fluoride*—decreases dental caries and osteoporosis; improves heart functioning; decreases calcium buildup in organs. Deficiencies cause tooth cavities and kidney stones.
- *Iron (ferrous)*—increases energy and physical performance; decreases cancer and learning disabilities; boosts the immune system; decreases iron-deficiency anemia; encourages sleep. Deficiencies cause fatigue, anemia, pallor, pica (craving to eat nonfoods such as clay and laundry starch), lethargy, weakness, vertigo, air hunger, confusion, irregular heartbeat, learning disabilities in children, and insomnia. Too much iron can cause constipation.
- *Germanium*—maintains homeostasis; decreases blood pressure and cholesterol; boosts the immune system; acts as an analgesic and antiinfective; helps patients with chronic Epstein-Barr virus syndrome and acquired immunodeficiency syndrome (AIDS)-related diseases.

- *Iodine*—aids metabolism; reduces fibrocystic disease in breasts; protects against toxic effects of exposure to radioactive materials; prevents goiter and thyroid disorders; loosens mucus in the respiratory tract; acts as an antiseptic. Deficiencies produce goiters and thyroid disease.
- *Magnesium*—produces energy; replicates cell materials; transmits nerve impulses; prevents kidney stones and gallstones; repairs body cells; is required for hormonal activity. Deficiencies produce kidney stones and gallstones, endocrine disorders, and nerve numbness.
- *Manganese*—aids the nervous system; necessary for synthesis of structural proteins and normal bone structure; helps with female sex hormones; metabolizes glucose; is needed for formation of thyroxine in the thyroid gland; improves brain function; decreases nervous disorders. Deficiencies affect the endocrine and nervous systems.
- *Molybdenum*—necessary for the utilization of iron, carbohydrates, and fats; excretes uric acid; decreases impotence and cancer; prevents dental caries; alleviates anemia. Deficiencies cause cavities, anemia, impotence, gout, and malabsorption.
- *Phosphorus*—forms bones and teeth, cofactor for many enzymes; activates B-complex vitamins; produces energy; increases endurance; fights fatigue; forms RNA and DNA. Deficiencies cause malformed bones and teeth, poor growth and healing, fatigue, and malabsorption.
- *Potassium*—stabilizes the internal structure of cells; activates enzymes that control energy production; decreases blood pressure and stroke; improves athletic performance; acts with sodium to conduct nerve impulses. Deficiencies cause confusion, muscular weakness, paralysis, arrhythmias, lethargy, and fatigue. Side effects include decreased blood pressure, listlessness, paralysis, and confusion.
- *Selenium*—improves vision, skin, and hair; boosts the immune system; decreases cancer; improves liver function; decreases CV disease; detoxifies alcohol and other drugs; increases male potency and sex drive; decreases hot flashes and menopausal symptoms; alleviates dandruff. Deficiencies cause immune, CV, liver, and sexual disorders.
- *Silicon*—decreases CV disease and osteoporosis; prevents hair from falling out; helps bones, skin, and fingernails grow. Deficiencies can cause hair, skin, CV, and bone disorders.
- *Sodium and chloride*—found in every cell. If the body is deficient in sodium chloride, body fluid replacement is needed. Deficiencies usually result from dehydration or blood/fluid loss. Symptoms are thirst and hunger for salty foods.
- *Vanadium*—decreases dental caries and blood glucose; produces red blood cells and tissue growth; metabolizes fat; decreases cholesterol; diminishes heart disease. Deficiencies can cause cavities and diabetes mellitus as well as CV and GI disorders.
- *Zinc*—boosts the immune system; prevents cancer; improves senses of sight, taste, and smell; decreases hair loss and acne; alleviates rheumatoid arthritis. Deficiencies can cause alcohol tolerance, anemia, poor wound healing, decreased taste, hair loss, and dermatitis. Toxic amounts can cause nausea and vomiting.

Wrap Up

There are comprehensive lists of herbs, vitamins, minerals, amino acids, and lipids according to the systems they affect in Appendix G.

 SUMMARY

This chapter closes the book by stressing that what you put in your mouth is important for the body to function correctly. Not only should food be tasty, it must contain the necessary vitamins, minerals, amino acids, and lipids. Excessive quantities of food can lead to obesity, and too small quantities can lead to malnutrition. Herbs and vitamin supplements are not regulated by the government, although they can have a powerful effect on our bodies. You should be familiar with complementary and alternative treatments and medications your patient may be using.

Activities

To make sure that you have learned the key points covered in this chapter, complete the following activities.

True or False

Write *true* if the statement is true. Beside the false statements, write *false* and correct the statement to make it true.

1. Vitamin B is necessary for good vision. _____

2. Vitamin C is stored in the liver. _____

3. Ginger helps with digestion. _____

4. Saw palmetto helps the urinary tract function correctly. _____

5. Potassium is a form of vitamin B. _____

Multiple Choice

Choose the best answer for each question.

1. Which of the following vitamins is *not* stored in the liver?
   a. A
   b. B
   c. D
   d. K

2. Which is *not* a principle of homeopathy?
   a. Symptoms clear up in reverse order from the order of appearance.
   b. Healing starts from within the body.
   c. Homeopathy is regulated by the FDA.
   d. Healing starts from the top down.

3. Which herb is used for nausea?
   a. Ginger
   b. Ginkgo
   c. Ginseng
   d. Garlic

Application Exercises

Respond to the following scenarios on a separate sheet.

1. Pu Beiji asks why there is so little research on CAM. **What do you reply?**
2. Rita Chabelewski is taking megadosages of vitamins. **Is that good? Why or why not?**

Virtual Field Trips

Go to the following websites to find the information. If a website is not available, try to find the information through another source.

1. Visit http://www.drweil.com and research one form of alternative therapy.
2. Go to http://www.safemedication.com and download information on the safety of herbal medications.

Essentials Review

For further study and practice with vitamins and minerals learned in this chapter, complete the following table to the best of your ability. Use resources such as a PDR, the Internet, or printed drug guides for help.

CLASSIFICATION	PURPOSE	SIDE EFFECTS	CONTRAINDICATIONS/PRECAUTIONS/INTERACTIONS	PATIENT EDUCATION
Vitamin A				
Vitamin B B_1 B_2 B_3 B_5 B_6 B_9 B_{12}				
Vitamin C				
Vitamin D				
Vitamin E				
Vitamin H				
Vitamin K				
Calcium				
Chromium				
Cobalt				
Copper				

(box continued on page 340)

CLASSIFICATION	PURPOSE	SIDE EFFECTS	CONTRAINDICATIONS/PRECAUTIONS/INTERACTIONS	PATIENT EDUCATION
Fluoride				
Iron				
Germanium				
Iodine				
Magnesium				
Manganese				
Molybdenum				
Phosphorus				
Potassium				
Selenium				
Silicon				
Sodium chloride				
Vanadium				
Zinc				

Drug Classifications

Drugs are classified according to what they do in the body. They may be used to treat specific illnesses or unpleasant symptoms and to diagnose diseases. It is important to understand the general effects of classifications. You can then learn about drugs more easily because those in the same classification share many of the same purposes and effects.

A

Analgesics—reduce pain. Non-narcotic analgesics are used for mild pain. Narcotic analgesics are used to treat moderate to severe pain.

Anti-Alzheimer agents—work to manage the dementia that occurs with Alzheimer's disease. They are not curative.

Antianemics—prevent and treat anemias, which are usually caused by low iron levels in the blood.

Antianginals—treat and prevent angina, or chest pain.

Antianxiety medications—used to treat anxiety, such as generalized anxiety disorder (GAD) or post-traumatic stress disorder (PTSD).

Antiarrhythmics—suppress cardiac arrhythmias, or irregular heart beats.

Antiasthmatics—manage both acute and chronic attacks of bronchospasm or asthma.

Anticholinergics—have many uses, including slowing a fast heart rate and relieving spasms of the respiratory system and nasal discharge. They may also be used to treat nausea and vomiting, motion sickness, and dizziness; some decrease gastric secretions and increase esophageal sphincter muscle tone. Finally, anticholinergics can be used for treating eye and urinary tract disorders as well as neurological disorders.

Anticoagulants—prevent blood from clotting. They can cause a prolonged bleeding time (a laboratory test).

Anticonvulsants—decrease the incidence and severity of seizures. Sometimes they are used for immediate relief of symptoms (usually given intramuscularly for this purpose) and at other times for chronic suppression of seizures (usually given orally for this purpose). Blood levels may be measured to evaluate the effectiveness of the therapy.

Antidepressants—treat depression and elevate mood, usually in conjunction with psychotherapy. They are also used to treat anxiety, bed-wetting, and chronic pain syndromes; for smoking cessation and eating disorders; and for obsessive-compulsive and generalized anxiety disorders.

Antidiabetics—manage diabetes mellitus. In some cases injecting or inhaling insulin is necessary. In others, tablets can be given to stimulate the body to release its own insulin.

Antidiarrheals—control and give symptomatic relief for both acute and chronic diarrhea.

Antiemetics—manage nausea, vomiting, and motion sickness.

Antifungal agents—treat fungal infections. Usually they are rubbed on the skin or mucosa. Severe cases may require systemic treatment with an oral form.

Antihistamines—relieve symptoms associated with allergies, including nose inflammation, itching, and vessel swelling. They are used to treat anaphylaxis.

Antihypertensives—decrease blood pressure. They are usually taken orally to reduce chronic hypertension, although some may be given intravenously in an emergency.

Antiinfectives—treat bacterial infections. They may be used for a current infection or to prevent infection (prophylaxis). For example, frequently antiinfectives can be given before surgery to prevent infections that might result from opening the patient's body during surgery.

Antiinflammatories—decrease inflammation and swelling.

Antineoplastics—fight new growths caused by cancer. They are also used against other autoimmune diseases, such as rheumatoid arthritis.

Antiparkinsonian agents—treat Parkinson's disease, a neurological disorder caused by low levels of dopamine, a chemical substance that transmits nerve impulses in the body.

Antiplatelet agents—prevent thromboembolic (clots that move) events, such as a stroke (cerebrovascular accident, or CVA) or heart attack. They are frequently used after cardiac surgery and can be combined with anticoagulants and thrombolytic (clot-busting) drugs.

Antipsychotic drugs—treat both acute and chronic psychoses, such as schizophrenia. They are also used to suppress tics that originate in the brain, such as with Tourette's syndrome.

Antipyretics—lower fevers due to infection, inflammation, or cancer.

Antiretrovirals—manage human immunodeficiency virus (HIV) infections. They increase the CD4 cell count and decrease the viral load.

Antirheumatics—manage symptoms of rheumatoid arthritis (pain and swelling), slow joint destruction, and preserve joint function.

Antituberculars—prevent and treat tuberculosis. They are also used to prevent meningitis and influenza.

Antiulcer agents—prevent or treat stomach ulcers. They are also used in the management of gastroesophageal reflux disease (GERD).

Antiviral medications—manage viral inflections, such as herpes, chickenpox, influenza A, and cytomegalovirus (CMV) infection.

B

Beta blockers—help to manage blood pressure, chest pain, fast heart rates, vessel narrowing, migraine headaches, glaucoma (eye), and heart failure. They can also prevent heart attacks and manage symptoms of low thyroid function.

Bone resorption inhibitors—primarily used to treat and prevent osteoporosis in postmenopausal women. They are also used to manage high blood calcium and Paget's disease of bone.

Bronchodilators—treat reversible airway obstruction due to asthma or chronic obstructive pulmonary disease (COPD).

C

Calcium channel blockers—treat high blood pressure, chest pain, and coronary artery spasm. They act to control the rhythm of the heart and to prevent neurological damage.

Central nervous system stimulants—treat narcolepsy, attention deficit disorder (ADD), and attention deficit with hyperactivity disorder (ADHD).

Corticosteroids—correct adrenocortical insufficiency. In large dosages, corticosteroids are used for antiinflammatory, immunosuppressive, and antineoplastic activity. They can be used to reduce blood calcium and to treat autoimmune diseases. Topically, they are used to decrease inflammation and allergic conditions. Inhaled corticosteroids are used for asthma and vasoconstriction. They are also used for eye disorders.

D

Diuretics—used alone or in combination to reduce high blood pressure and swelling due to congestive heart failure (CHF) and other disorders. Potassium-sparing diuretics conserve potassium while decreasing fluid.

H

Headache suppressants—change vascular tension to decrease pain.

Hormones—treat deficiencies in diabetes mellitus (insulin), diabetes insipidus (desmopressin), thyroid function (thyroid hormones), and menopause (hormone replacement therapy with estrogens and progestins). They can also be used to treat hormone-sensitive tumors and as contraceptives.

I

Immunosuppressants—prevent transplant rejection. However, they also suppress the body's own immune system.

L

Laxatives—treat and prevent constipation. They are also used to clean the bowel in preparation for radiologic or endoscopic procedures.

Lipid-lowering agents—part of a total plan to reduce fats in blood, including diet and exercise.

M

Minerals/electrolytes/pH modifiers—treat deficiencies or excesses of electrolytes to maintain correct acid/base balance.

N

Natural/herbal products—used for a wide variety of disorders. As discussed earlier in the book, the Food and Drug Administration (FDA) does not regulate herbal remedies, so the quality and effectiveness of herbal remedies can vary. Herbs are used extensively to treat menopausal symptoms, improve mood, reduce nausea, prevent motion sickness, boost the immune system, strengthen muscles, and improve gastric and urinary functioning.

Nonsteroidal antiinflammatory drugs (NSAIDs)—control mild to moderate pain, fever, and inflammatory conditions such as rheumatoid arthritis and osteoarthritis. Ophthalmic NSAIDs decrease inflammation after eye surgery.

S

Sedative-hypnotics—provide sedation. They are frequently given before procedures or to induce sleep.

Skeletal muscle relaxants—reduce spasticity associated with neurological disorders or for symptomatic relief of musculoskeletal conditions.

T

Thrombolytic agents—dissolve clots and prevent heart attacks. As their name suggests, they are "clot-busters."

V

Vaccines/immunizing agents—prevent infectious diseases by promoting the body's own production of antibodies against diseases.

Vitamins—prevent and treat vitamin deficiencies. They are also used as supplements in metabolic disorders.

W

Weight control agents—used in the management of obesity. This therapy should be combined with a reduced-calorie diet and exercise.

Drug Classification Index by Generic Name

GENERIC NAME	TRADE NAME	CLASSIFICATION
acetaminophen	Acephen, Aceta, Aminofen, Apacet, APAP, Aspirin Free Anacin, Aspirin Free Pain Relief, Children's Pain Reliever, Dapacin, Feverall, Extra Strength Dynafed (Billups, P.J.), Extra Strength Dynafed E.X., Genapap, Genebs, Halenol, Infant's Pain Reliever, Liquiprin, Mapap, Maranox, Meda, Neopap, Oraphen-PD, Panadol, paracetamol, Redutemp, Ridenol, Silapap, Tapanol, Tempra, Tylenol, Uni-Ace	antipyretics, nonopioid analgesics
acyclovir	Zovirax	antivirals
adenosine	Adenocard, Adenoscan	antiarrhythmics
albuterol	AccuNeb, Airet, Proventil, Proventil HFA, salbutamol, Ventodisk, Ventolin, Ventolin HFA, Volmax, VoSpira ER	bronchodilators
alendronate	Fosamax	bone resorption inhibitors
allopurinol	Alloprim, Lopurin, Zyloprim	antigout agents, antihyperuricemics
alprazolam	Niravam, Xanax, Xanax XR	antianxiety agents
alteplase	Activase, Cathflo Activase, tissue plasminogen activator, t-PA	thrombolytics
aminocaproic acid	Amicar, epsilon-aminocaproic acid	hemostatic agents
amiodarone	Cordarone, Pacerone	antiarrhythmics (class III)
amitriptyline	Elavil, Endep	antidepressants
amlodipine	Norvasc	antihypertensives
amoxicillin	Amoxil, DisperMox, Trimox, Wymox	antiinfectives, antiulcer agents
amoxicillin/clavulanate	Augmentin, Augmentin ES, Augmentin XR	antiinfectives
amphetamine mixtures	Adderall, Adderall XR, Amphetamine Salt	central nervous system stimulants
amphotericin B liposome	AmBisome	antifungals
ampicillin	Marcillin, Omnipen, Penbritin, Polycillin, Principen, Totacillin	antiinfectives

GENERIC NAME	TRADE NAME	CLASSIFICATION
atenolol	Tenormin	antianginals, antihypertensives
atorvastatin	Lipitor	lipid-lowering agents
atropine	Atro-Pen	antiarrhythmics
azathioprine	Azasan, Imuran	immunosuppressants
azithromycin	Zithromax, Zmax	agents for atypical mycobacteria, antiinfectives
baclofen	Kemstro, Lioresal	antispasticity agents, skeletal muscle relaxants (centrally acting)
beclomethasone (nasal)	Beconase AQ	antiinflammatories (steroidal)
benazepril	Lotensin	antihypertensives
benzonatate	Tessalon	allergy, cold, and cough remedies, antitussives (local anesthetic)
benztropine	Cogentin	antiparkinsonian agents
bethanechol	Duvoid, Urabeth, Urecholine	urinary tract stimulants
bicalutamide	Casodex	antineoplastics
bisoprolol	Monocor, Zebeta	antihypertensives
bumetanide	Bumex	diuretics
bupropion	Wellbutrin, Wellbutrin SR, Wellbutrin XL, Zyban	antidepressants, smoking deterrents
buspirone	BuSpar	antianxiety agents
butalbital, acetaminophen	Bucet, Phrenilin, Phrenilin Forte, Tencon	nonopioid analgesics (combination with barbiturate)
butalbital, acetaminophen, and caffeine	Esgic-Plus, Fioricet	nonopioid analgesics (combination with barbiturate)
butalbital, aspirin, and caffeine	Fiorinal	nonopioid analgesics (combination with barbiturate)
candesartan	Atacand	antihypertensives
captopril	Capoten	antihypertensives
carbamazepine	Atretol, Carbatrol, Epitol, Equetro, Tegretol, Tegretol-XR, Teril	anticonvulsants, mood stabilizers
carbidopa/levodopa	Parcopa, Sinemet, Sinemet CR	antiparkinsonian agents
carboplatin	Paraplatin	antineoplastics
carisoprodol	Soma, Vanadom	skeletal muscle relaxants (centrally acting)
carvedilol	Coreg	antihypertensives
cefdinir	Omnicef	antiinfectives
cefprozil	Cefzil	antiinfectives
cefuroxime	Ceftin, Zinacef	antiinfectives
celecoxib	Celebrex	antirheumatics, nonsteroidal antiinflammatory agents
cephalexin	Keflex	antiinfectives
cetirizine	Zyrtec	allergy, cold, and cough remedies; antihistamines
chlordiazepoxide	Libritabs, Librium	antianxiety agents, sedative-hypnotics

GENERIC NAME	TRADE NAME	CLASSIFICATION
chlorpheniramine	Aller-Chlor, Allergy, Chlo-Amine, Chlorate, Chlor-Trimeton, Chlor-Trimeton Allergy 4 Hour, Chlor-Trimeton Allergy 8 Hour, Chlor-Trimeton Allergy 12 Hour, PediaCare Allergy Formula, Phenetron, Telechlor, Teldrin	allergy, cold, and cough remedies; antihistamines
cidofovir	Vistide	antivirals
cimetidine	Tagamet, Tagamet HB	antiulcer agents
ciprofloxacin	Cipro, Cipro XR, Proquin XR	antiinfectives
citalopram	Celexa	antidepressants
clarithromycin	Biaxin, Biaxin XL	agents for atypical mycobacteria, antiinfectives, antiulcer agents
clindamycin	Cleocin, Cleocin T, Clinda-Derm, Clindagel, ClindaMax, Clindesse, Clindets, C/T/S, Evoclin	antiinfectives
clonazepam	Klonopin	anticonvulsants
clonidine	Catapres, Catapres-TTS, Duraclon	antihypertensives
clopidogrel	Plavix	antiplatelet agents
clorazepate	Gen-XENE, Tranxene, Tranxene-SD	anticonvulsants, sedative-hypnotics
clozapine	Clozaril, FazaClo	antipsychotics
codeine	None given	allergy, cold, and cough remedies; antitussives; opioid analgesics
colchicine	None given	antigout agents
cyclobenzaprine	Flexeril	skeletal muscle relaxants (centrally acting)
cyclosporine	Gengraf, Neoral, Sandimmune	immunosuppressants, antirheumatics (DMARDs)
cyproheptadine	Periactin, PMS-Cyproheptadine	allergy, cold, and cough remedies; antihistamines
darbepoetin	Aranesp	antianemics
desloratadine	Clarinex	allergy, cold, and cough remedies; antihistamines
desmopressin	DDAVP, DDAVP Rhinal Tube, DDAVP Rhinyle Drops, Octostim, Stimate	hormones
diazepam	Diastat, D-Val, Valium	antianxiety agents, anticonvulsants, sedative-hypnotics, skeletal muscle relaxants (centrally acting)
dicyclomine	Bentyl	antispasmodics
digoxin	Digitek, Lanoxicaps, Lanoxin	antiarrhythmics, inotropics
diltiazem	Cardizem, Cardizem LA, CartiaXT, Dilacor XR, Diltia XT, Nu-Diltiaz, Tiamate, Tiazac	antianginals, anti-arrhythmics (class IV), antihypertensives
dinoprostone	Cervidil Vaginal Insert, Prepidil Endocervical Gel, Prostin E Vaginal Suppository	cervical ripening agent

GENERIC NAME	TRADE NAME	CLASSIFICATION
diphenhydramine (oral, parenteral)	Allergy Medication, AllerMax, Banophen, Benadryl, Benadryl Allergy, Benadryl Dye-Free Allergy, Compoz, Compoz Nighttime Sleep Aid, Diphen AF, Diphen Cough, Diphenhist, Dormin, Genahist, 40 Winks, Hyrexin-50, Maximum Strength Nytol, Maximum Strength Sleepinal, Midol PM, Miles Nervine, Nighttime Sleep Aid, Nytol, Scot-Tussin Allergy DM, Siladril, Silphen, Sleep-Eze 3, Sleepwell 2-night, Snooze Fast, Sominex, Tusstat, Twilite, Unisom Nighttime Sleep-Aid	allergy, cold, and cough remedies; antihistamines; antitussives
dipyridamole	Dipridacot, Persantine, Persantine IV	antiplatelet agents, diagnostic agents (coronary vasodilators)
dobutamine	Dobutrex	inotropics
docetaxel	Taxotere	antineoplastics
dolasetron	Anzemet	antiemetics
donepezil	Aricept, Aricept ODT	anti-Alzheimer's agents
dopamine	Intropin	inotropics, vasopressors
doxazosin	Cardura	antihypertensives
doxepin	Sinequan, Zonalon	antianxiety agents, antidepressants, antihistamines (topical)
doxorubicin hydrochloride	Adriamycin PFS, Adriamycin RDF, Rubex	antineoplastics
enalapril, enalaprilat	Vasotec, Vasotec IV	antihypertensives
enoxaparin	Lovenox	anticoagulants
epinephrine	Adrenalin, Ana-Guard, AsthmaHaler Mist, AsthmaNefrin (racepinephrine), EpiPen, microNefrin, Nephron, Primatene, S-2, Sus-Phrine	antiasthmatics, bronchodilators, vasopressors
epoetin	EPO, Epogen, erythropoietin, Procrit	antianemics
eprosartan	Teveten	antihypertensives
eptifibatide	Integrilin	antiplatelet agents
erythromycin (topical)	Akne-Mycin, A/T/S, Del-Mycin, E/Gel, Erycette, Erygel, EryMax, Erysol, Staticin, Theramycin Z, T-Stat	antiinfectives
esmolol	Brevibloc	antiarrhythmics (class II)
esomeprazole	Nexium	antiulcer agents
estropipate	Ogen, Ortho-Est, piperazine estrone sulfate	hormones
etodolac	Lodine, Lodine XL	antirheumatics, nonopioid analgesics
famotidine	Mylanta AR, Pepcid, Pepcid AC Maximum Strength, Pepcid RPD	antiulcer agents
felodipine	Plendil	antianginals, antihypertensives
fenofibrate	Antara, Lofibra, Tricor, Triglide	lipid-lowering agents

GENERIC NAME	TRADE NAME	CLASSIFICATION
fentanyl (parenteral)	Sublimaze	opioid analgesics
fentanyl (transdermal)	Duragesic	opioid analgesics, analgesic adjuncts
fexofenadine	Allegra	allergy, cold, and cough remedies; antihistamines
filgrastim	G-CSF, granulocyte colony-stimulating factor, Neupogen	colony-stimulating factors
finasteride	Propecia, Proscar	hair regrowth stimulants
fluconazole	Diflucan	antifungals (systemic)
flumazenil	Romazicon	antidotes (for sedative-hypnotics)
fluoxetine	Prozac, Prozac Weekly, Sarafem	antidepressants
flurazepam	Dalmane	sedative-hypnotics
fluticasone (nasal)	Flonase	antiinflammatories (steroidal)
fluvastatin	Lescol, Lescol XL	lipid-lowering agents
folic acid	folate, Folvite, vitamin B	antianemics, vitamins
fosinopril	Monopril	antihypertensives
furosemide	Lasix	diuretics
gabapentin	Gabarone, Neurontin	analgesic adjuncts, therapeutic; anticonvulsants; mood stabilizers
gatifloxacin	Tequin	antiinfectives
gemfibrozil	Lopid	lipid-lowering agents
gemifloxacin	Factive	antiinfectives
gentamicin	Garamycin, G-Mycin, Jenamicin	antiinfectives
glimepiride	Amaryl	antidiabetics
glipizide	Glucotrol, Glucotrol XL	antidiabetics
glucagon	GlucaGen	hormones
glyburide	DiaBeta, Glynase PresTab, Micronase	antidiabetics
glycopyrrolate	Robinul, Robinul-Forte	antispasmodics
granisetron	Kytril	antiemetics
guaifenesin	Alfen Jr, Altarussin, Breonesin, Diabetic Tussin, Ganidin NR, Guiatuss, Hytuss, Hytuss-2X, Mucinex, Naldecon Senior EX, Organidin NR, Robitussin, Scottussin Expectorant, Siltussin DAS, Siltussin SA	allergy, cold, and cough remedies; expectorant
haloperidol	Haldol, Haldol Decanoate	antipsychotics
heparin	Hep-Lock, Hep-Lock U/P	anticoagulants
hydralazine	Apresoline	antihypertensives
hydrocodone	Hycodan, Tussigon (U.S. antitussive formulations contain homatropine)	allergy, cold, and cough remedies (antitussive); nonopioid analgesics; opioid analgesics
hydromorphone	Dilaudid, Dilaudid-HP, Hydrostat IR, PMS Hydromorphone	allergy, cold, and cough remedies (antitussives); opioid analgesics
hydroxychloroquine	Plaquenil	antimalarials, antirheumatics (DMARDs)
hydroxyzine	Atarax, Hyzine-50, Vistaril	antianxiety agents, antihistamines, sedative-hypnotics

GENERIC NAME	TRADE NAME	CLASSIFICATION
hyoscyamine	Anaspaz, A-Spas S/L, Cystospaz, Cystospaz-M, Donnamar, ED-SPAZ, Gastrosed, Levbid, Levsin, Levsinex, L-hyoscyamine, NuLev	antispasmodics
ibuprofen, oral	Advil, Advil Migraine Liqui-Gels, Children's Advil, Children's Motrin, Excedrin IB, Genpril, Haltran, Junior Strength Advil, Medipren, Menadol, Midil Maximum Strength Cramp Formula, Motrin, Motrin Drops, Motrin IB, Motrin Junior Strength, Motrin Migraine Pain, Nu-Ibuprofen, Nuprin, PediaCare Children's Fever	antipyretics, antirheumatics, nonopioid analgesics, nonsteroidal antiinflammatory agents
ibutilide	Corvert	antiarrhythmics (class III)
imipenem/cilastatin	Primaxin	antiinfectives
imipramine	Norfranil, Tipramine, Tofranil, Tofranil PM	antidepressants
indapamide	Lozol	antihypertensives, diuretics
indomethacin	Indochron E-R, Indocin, Indocin I.V., Indocin SR	antirheumatics, ductus arteriosus patency adjuncts (IV only), nonsteroidal antiinflammatory agents
insulin, regular (injection, concentrated)	Humulin R, Humulin R Regular U-500 (Concentrated), Iletin II Regular, Novolin R, Velosulin BR	antidiabetics, hormones
ipratropium	Atrovent HFA	allergy, cold, and cough remedies; bronchodilators
irbesartan	Avapro	antihypertensives
ketoconazole (systemic)	Nizoral	antifungals (systemic)
ketorolac	Toradol	nonsteroidal antiinflammatory agents, nonopioid analgesics
labetalol	Normodyne, Trandate	antianginals, antihypertensives
lactulose	Cephulac, Cholac, Chronulac, Constilac, Constulose, Duphalac, Enulose, Evalose, Heptalac, Kritalose, Lactulose PSE, Portalac	laxatives
lamotrigine	Lamictal	anticonvulsants
lansoprazole	Prevacid	antiulcer agents
leuprolide	Eligard, Lupron, Lupron Depot, Lupron Depot-PED, Lupron Depot-3 Month, Viadur	antineoplastics
levalbuterol	Xopenex	bronchodilators
levofloxacin	Levaquin	antiinfectives
levothyroxine	Levo-T, Levothroid, Levoxyl, Novothyrox, Synthroid, T_4, Unithroid	hormones
linezolid	Zyvox	antiinfectives
lisinopril	Prinivil, Zestril	antihypertensives
lithium	Eskalith, Eskalith-CR, Lithobid, Lithonate, Lithotabs	antimanic, mood stabilizers

GENERIC NAME	TRADE NAME	CLASSIFICATION
lomefloxacin	Maxaquin	antiinfectives
loperamide	Diar-aid Caplets, Imodium, Imodium A-D, Kaopectate II Caplets, Maalox Antidiarrheal Caplets, Neo-Diaral, Pepto Diarrhea Control	antidiarrheals
loratadine	Alavert, Children's Loratidine, Claritin Hives Relief, Claritin Reditabs, Claritin, Claritin 24-Hour Allergy, Clear-Atadine, Dimetapp Children's ND Non-Drowsy Allergy, Non-Drowsy Allergy Relief for Kids, Tavist ND	antihistamines
lorazepam	Ativan	analgesic adjuncts, antianxiety agents, sedative-hypnotics
losartan	Cozaar	antihypertensives
lovastatin	Mevacor	lipid-lowering agents
magnesium sulfate (IV) (9.9% Mg; 8.1 mEq/L)	None given	mineral and electrolyte replacements/supplements
mannitol	Osmitrol, Resectisol	diuretics
meclizine	Antivert, Antrizine, Bonine, Dramamine Less Drowsy Formula, Meni-D, Vergon	antiemetics, antihistamines
medroxyprogesterone	Amen, Curretab, Cycrin, Depo-Provera, Depo-Sub Q Provera 104, Provera	antineoplastics, contraceptive hormones
megestrol	Megace	antineoplastics, hormones
meloxicam	Mobic	nonsteroidal antiinflammatory agents
meperidine	Demerol, pethidine	opioid analgesics
mesalamine	Asacol, Canasa, Pentasa, Rowasa	gastrointestinal antiinflammatories—therapeutic
metaxalone	Skelaxin	skeletal muscle relaxants (centrally acting)
metformin	Fortamet, Glucophage, Glucophage XR, Riomet	antidiabetics
methadone	Methadose	opioid analgesics
methocarbamol	Carbacot, Robaxin	skeletal muscle relaxants (centrally acting)
methotrexate	amethopterin, Folex, Folex PFS, Rheumatrex, Trexall	antineoplastics, antirheumatics (DMARDs), immunosuppressants
methylphenidate	Concerta, Metadate CD, Metadate ER, Methylin, Methylin SR, Ritalin, Ritalin LA, Ritalin-SR	central nervous system stimulants
metoclopramide	Clopra, Octamide, Octamide-PFS, Reclomide, Reglan	antiemetics
metolazone	Mykrox, Zaroxolyn	antihypertensives, diuretics
metoprolol	Lopressor, Toprol-XL	antianginals, antihypertensives
metronidazole	Flagyl, Flagyl ER, Metric 21, MetroCream, MetroGel, MetroGel-Vaginal, Metro IV, MetroLotion, Metryl, Noritate, Protostat	antiinfectives, antiprotozoals, antiulcer agents

GENERIC NAME	TRADE NAME	CLASSIFICATION
midazolam	Versed	antianxiety agents, sedative-hypnotics
mirtazapine	Remeron, Remeron Soltabs	antidepressants
misoprostol	Cytotec	antiulcer agents, cytoprotective agents
moexipril	Univasc	antihypertensives
mometasone (nasal)	Nasonex	antiinflammatories (steroidal)
montelukast	Singulair	allergy, cold, and cough remedies; bronchodilators
morphine	Astramorph, Astramorph PF, Avinza, DepoDur, Duramorph, Infumorph, Kadian, MS, MS Contin, MSIR, MSO$_4$, OMS Concentrate, Oramorph SR, RMS, Roxanol, Roxanol Rescudose, Roxanol-T	opioid analgesics
moxifloxacin	Avelox	antiinfectives
mupirocin	Bactroban, Bactroban Nasal	antiinfectives
nabumetone	Relafen	antirheumatics, nonsteroidal antiinflammatory agents
nadolol	Corgard	antianginals, antihypertensives
naloxone	Narcan	antidotes (for opioids)
naproxen	Aleve, Anaprox, Anaprox DS, Apo-Napro-Na DS, EC-Naprosyn, Naprelan, Napron X, Naprosyn	nonopioid analgesics, nonsteroidal antiinflammatory agents, antipyretics
naratriptan	Amerge	vascular headache suppressants
nefazodone	Serzone	antidepressants
neostigmine	Prostigmin	antimyasthenics
niacin		vitamins
niacinamide	Edur-Acin, Nia-Bid, Niac, Niacels, Niacor, Niaspan, Nicobid, Nico-400, Nicolar, nicotinamide, Nicotinex, nicotinic acid, Slo-Niacin, vitamin B	lipid-lowering agents, vitamins
nicardipine	Cardene, Cardene IV, Cardene SR	antianginals, antihypertensives
nifedipine	Adalat, Adalat CC, Nifedical XL, Procardia, Procardia XL	antianginals, antihypertensives
nimodipine	Nimotop	subarachnoid hemorrhage therapy agents
nitrofurantoin	Furadantin, Macrobid, Macrodantin	antiinfectives
nitroglycerin	Deponit, Minitran, Nitrek, Nitro-Bid, Nitro-Bid IV, Nitrocot, Nitrodisc, Nitro-Dur, Nitrogard, Nitroglyn E-R, Nitrol, Nitrolingual, Nitrong, Nitro-par, NitroQuick, Nitrostat, Nitro-Time, Transderm-Nitro, Tridil	antianginals
nizatidine	Axid, Axid AR	antiulcer agents
norfloxacin	Noroxin	antiinfectives
nortriptyline	Aventyl, Pamelor	antidepressants
NPH insulin (isophane insulin suspension)	Humulin N, Novolin N, NPH Iletin II	antidiabetics, hormones
nystatin	Mycostatin, Nilstat, Nystex	antifungals (topical/local)
octreotide	Sandostatin, Sandostatin LAR	antidiarrheals, hormones
ofloxacin	Floxin	antiinfectives

GENERIC NAME	TRADE NAME	CLASSIFICATION
olanzapine	Zyprexa, Zyprexa Zydis	antipsychotics, mood stabilizers
olmesartan	Benicar	antihypertensives
omeprazole	Prilosec, Prilosec OTC, Zegerid	antiulcer agents
ondansetron	Zofran	antiemetics
orphenadrine	Antiflex, Banflex, Flexoject, Flexon, Mio-Rel, Myolin, Myotrol, Norflex, Orfro, Orphenate	skeletal muscle relaxants (centrally acting)
oxazepam	Serax	antianxiety agents, sedative-hypnotics
oxcarbazepine	Trileptal	anticonvulsants
oxybutynin (oral)	Ditropan	urinary tract antispasmodics
oxybutynin (transdermal)	Oxytrol	urinary tract antispasmodics
pamidronate	Aredia	bone resorption inhibitors
pancrelipase	Cotazym, Cotazym E.C.S. 8, Cotazym E.C.S. 20, Cotazym-S, Creon 10, Creon 25, Enzymase-16, Ilozyme, Ku-Zyme HP, Lipram-CR20, Lipram-PN10, Lipram-PN16, Lipram-UL12, Lipram-UL18, Lipram-UL20, Pancoate, Pancrease, Pancrease MT 4, Pancrease MT 10, Pancrease MT 16, Pancrease MT 20, Pancrebarb MS-8, Protilase, Ultrase MT 12, Ultrase MT 20, Viokase, Zymase	digestive agent
pantoprazole	Protonix, Protonix I.V.	antiulcer agents
pentamidine	NebuPent, Pentam 300	antiprotozoals
pentoxifylline	Trental	blood viscosity reducing agent
perindopril	Aceon	antihypertensives
phenazopyridine	Azo-Standard, Baridium, Geridium, Prodium, Pyridiate, Pyridium, Pyridium Plus, Urodine, Urogesic, UTI Relief	nonopioid analgesics
phenobarbital	Luminal, Solfoton	anticonvulsants, sedative-hypnotics
phentolamine	Regitine	agents for pheochromo-cytoma
phytonadione	AquaMEPHYTON, Mephyton, vitamin K	antidotes, vitamins
pioglitazone	Actos	antidiabetics (oral)
piroxicam	Feldene	antirheumatics, nonsteroidal antiinflammatory agents
polyethylene glycol	MiraLax	laxatives
potassium chloride	Cena-K, Gen-K, K+ Care, K+ 10, Kaochlor, Kaochlor S-F, Kaon-Cl, Kay Ciel, KCl, K-Dur, K-Lease, K-Lor, Klor-Con, Klorvess Liquid, Klotrix, K-Lyte/Cl Powder, K-Med, K-Norm, K-Sol, K-Tab, Micro-K, Micro-K ExtenCaps, Micro-LS, Potasalan, Roychlor, Rum-K, Slow-K, Ten-K	mineral and electrolyte replacements/supplements

GENERIC NAME	TRADE NAME	CLASSIFICATION
pramipexole	Mirapex	antiparkinsonian agents
pravastatin	Pravachol	lipid-lowering agents
prazosin	Minipress	antihypertensives
prednisone	Deltasone, Meticorten, Prednicen-M, Sterapred, Winpred	corticosteroids (intermediate acting), immune modifiers
procainamide	Procanbid, Promine, Pronestyl, Pronestyl-SR	antiarrhythmics (class IA)
prochlorperazine	Compazine, Ultrazine	antiemetics, antipsychotics
progesterone	Crinone, Prochieve, Prometrium	hormones
promethazine	Antinaus, Pentazine, Phenadoz, Phenergan, Promacot, Promet, Prorex	antiemetics, antihistamines, sedative-hypnotics
propafenone	Rythmol	antiarrhythmics (class IC)
propofol	Diprivan, Disoprofol	general anesthetics
propoxyphene napsylate	Darvon N	opioid analgesics
propranolol	Inderal, Inderal LA, InnoPran XL	antianginals, antiarrhythmics (Class II), antihypertensives, vascular headache suppressants
protamine sulfate	None given	antidotes (heparin)
pseudoephedrine	Congestaid, Decofed, Dimetapp Decongestant Pediatric, Dimetapp Maximum Strength 12-Hour Non-Drowsy Extentabs, Drixoral 12 Hour Non-Drowsy Formula, Efidac 24, Genafed, Halofed, Kid Kare, Medi-First Sinus Decongestant, PediaCare Infants' Decongestant Drops, Pediatric Nasal Decongestant, Silfedrine, Simply Stuffy, Sinustop, Sudafed, Sudafed Childrens's Non-Drowsy, Sudafed Non-Drowsy Maximum Strength, Sudafed 12 Hour, Sudodrin, Triaminic Allergy Congestion Softchews, Unified	allergy, cold, and cough remedies; nasal drying agents/decongestants
pyridoxine	Beesix, Doxine, Nestrex, Pyri, Rodex, Vitabee 6, vitamin B_6	vitamins
quetiapine	Seroquel	antipsychotics, mood stabilizers
quinapril	Accupril	antihypertensives
quinine	None given	antimalarials
rabeprazole	Aciphex	antiulcer agents
raloxifene	Evista	bone resorption inhibitors
ramipril	Altace	antihypertensives
ranitidine	Apo-Ranitidine, Zantac, Zantac 75	antiulcer agents
repaglinide	Gluconorm, Prandin	antidiabetics
rifampin	Rifadin, Rimactane	antituberculars
risedronate	Actonel	bone resorption inhibitors
risperidone	Risperdal, Risperdal Consta, Risperdal M-TAB	antipsychotics, mood stabilizers
rizatriptan	Maxalt, Maxalt-MLT	vascular headache suppressants
rosiglitazone	Avandia	antidiabetics
salmeterol	Serevent	bronchodilators

GENERIC NAME	TRADE NAME	CLASSIFICATION
sargramostim	Leukine, rHu GM-CSF (recombinant human granulocyte/macrophage colony-stimulating factor)	colony-stimulating factors
scopolamine	Isopto Hyoscine, Transderm Scōp	antiemetics
sertraline	Zoloft	antidepressants
sildenafil	Revatio, Viagra	antiimpotence agents
simvastatin	Zocor	lipid-lowering agents
sirolimus	Rapamune	immunosuppressants
sodium bicarbonate	Baking soda, Bell-Ans, Citrocarbonate, Neut, Soda Mint	antiulcer agents
sodium chloride (IV/oral)	Slo-Salt	mineral and electrolyte replacements/supplements
sodium citrate and citric acid	Bicitra, Oracit, Shohl's Solution modified	antiurolithics, mineral and electrolyte replacements/ supplements
sotalol	Betapace, Betapace AF	antiarrhythmics (classes II and III)
stavudine	d4T, Zerit, Zerit XR	antiretrovirals
sumatriptan	Imitrex	vascular headache suppressants
tacrine	Cognex	anti-Alzheimer's agents
tamoxifen	Nolvadex	antineoplastics
tamsulosin	Flomax	none assigned
telmisartan	Micardis	antihypertensives
temazepam	Restoril	sedative-hypnotics
terazosin	Hytrin	antihypertensives
terbinafine	Lamisil	antifungals (systemic)
terbutaline	Brethaire, Bricanyl	bronchodilators
theophylline	Elixophyllin, Quibron-T, Theochron, Theo-24, Uniphyl	bronchodilators
thiamine	Biamine, vitamin B_1	vitamins
thyroid	Armour thyroid, Thyrar, Thyroid Strong, Westhroid	hormones
ticlopidine	Ticlid	antiplatelet agents
timolol	Blocadren	antihypertensives, vascular headache suppressants
tirofiban	Aggrastat	antiplatelet agents
tizanidine	Zanaflex	antispasticity agents (centrally acting)
tolterodine	Detrol, Detrol LA	urinary tract antispasmodics
topiramate	Topamax	anticonvulsants, mood stabilizers
torsemide	Demadex	antihypertensives
tramadol	Ultram	analgesics (centrally acting)
trandolapril	Mavik	antihypertensives
trazodone	Desyrel, Trialodine, Trazon	antidepressants
triazolam	Halcion	sedative-hypnotics
trimethoprim/ sulfamethoxazole	Bactrim, Bactrim DS, Cofatrim, Cotrim, Cotrim DS, Septra, Septra DS, SMZ/TMP, Sulfatrim, Sulfatrim DS, TMP/SMX, TMP/SMZ	antiinfectives, antiprotozoals
valacyclovir	Valtrex	antivirals
valsartan	Diovan	antihypertensives
vancomycin	Lyphocin, Vancocin, Vancoled	antiinfectives
venlafaxine	Effexor, Effexor XR	antidepressants, antianxiety agents

GENERIC NAME	TRADE NAME	CLASSIFICATION
verapamil	Apo-Verap, Calan, Calan SR, Covera-HS, Isoptin, Isoptin SR, Verelan, Verelan PM	antianginals, antiarrhythmics (class IV), antihypertensives, vascular headache suppressants
warfarin	Coumadin	anticoagulants
zaleplon	Sonata	sedative-hypnotics
zidovudine	azidothymidine, AZT, Retrovir	antiretrovirals
zolpidem	Ambien, Ambien CR	sedative-hypnotics

Pregnancy Drug Categories and Controlled Substances Schedules

PREGNANCY DRUG CATEGORIES

Category A
Adequate, well-controlled studies in pregnant women have not shown an increased risk of fetal abnormalities.

Category B
Animal studies have revealed no evidence of harm to the fetus; however, there are no adequate and well-controlled studies in pregnant women. *or* Animal studies have shown an adverse effect, but adequate and well-controlled studies in pregnant women have failed to demonstrate a risk to the fetus.

Category C
Animal studies have shown an adverse effect, and there are no adequate and well-controlled studies in pregnant women. *or* No animal studies have been conducted, and there are no adequate and well-controlled studies in pregnant women.

Category D
Studies—adequate and well-controlled or observational—in pregnant women have demonstrated a risk to the fetus. However, the benefits of therapy may outweigh the potential risk.

Category X
Studies—adequate and well-controlled or observational—in animals or pregnant women have demonstrated positive evidence of fetal abnormalities. Use of the product is contraindicated in women who are or may become pregnant.

CONTROLLED SUBSTANCES SCHEDULES

Classes or schedules are determined by the Drug Enforcement Agency (DEA), an arm of the United States Department of Justice, and are based on the potential for abuse and dependence liability (physical and psychological) of the medication. Some states have stricter prescription regulations. Physicians, dentists, podiatrists, and veterinarians may prescribe controlled substances. Nurse practitioners and physician's assistants may prescribe controlled substances with certain limitations.

Schedule I (C-I)
Potential for abuse is so high as to be unacceptable. May be used for research with appropriate limitations. Examples are LSD and heroin.

Schedule II (C-II)
High potential for abuse and extreme liability for physical and psychological dependence (amphetamines, opioid analgesics, dronabinol, certain barbiturates). Outpatient prescriptions must be in writing.

Source: Deglin J. and Vallerand AH. (2006). Davis's Drug Guide for Nurses, 10th edition. Philadelphia: F.A. Davis.

In emergencies, telephone orders may be acceptable if a written prescription is provided within 72-hours. No refills are allowed.

Examples of Schedule II drugs included in *Davis's Drug Guide for Nurses*:

Amphetamine
Codeine (single entity; solid dosage form or injectable)
Fentanyl
Hydromorphone
Methylphenidate
Morphine

Schedule III (C-III)

Intermediate potential for abuse (less than C-II) and intermediate liability for physical and psychological dependence (certain nonbarbiturate sedatives, certain nonamphetamine CNS stimulants, limited dosages of certain opioid analgesics). Outpatient prescriptions can be refilled five times within 6 months from date of issue if authorized by prescriber. Telephone orders are acceptable.

Examples of Schedule III drugs included in *Davis's Drug Guide for Nurses*:

Codeine (in combination with nonopioid analgesics; solid oral dosage forms)
Hydrocodone (in combination with nonopioid analgesics)
Nandrolone decanoate

Schedule IV (C-IV)

Less abuse potential than Schedule III with minimal liability for physical or psychological dependence (certain sedative-hypnotics, certain antianxiety agents, some barbiturates, benzodiazepines, chloral hydrate, pentazocine, propoxyphene). Outpatient prescriptions can be refilled six times within 6 months from date of issue if authorized by prescriber. Telephone orders are acceptable.

Schedule IV drugs included in *Davis's Drug Guide for Nurses*:

Alprazolam
Codeine (elixir or oral suspension with acetaminophen)
Diazepam
Pentazocine
Phenobarbital
Zolpidem

Schedule V (C-V)

Minimal abuse potential. Number of outpatient refills determined by prescriber. Some products (cough suppressants with small amounts of codeine, antidiarrheals containing paregoric) may be available without prescription to patients >18 years of age.

Schedule V drugs included in *Davis's Drug Guide for Nurses*:

Buprenorphine
Diphenoxylate/atropine

Routine Pediatric and Adult Immunizations

Immunization recommendations change frequently: For the latest recommendations see http://www.cdc.gov/nip.

Routine Pediatric Immunizations (0–18 years)

GENERIC NAME (BRAND NAMES)	ROUTE/DOSAGE	CONTRAINDICATIONS/ PRECAUTIONS	ADVERSE REACTIONS/ SIDE EFFECTS	NOTES
DTaP: diphtheria toxoid, tetanus toxoid, and acellular pertussis vaccine (Daptacel, Infanrix, Tripedia)	0.5 mL IM at 2, 4, 6, and 15–18 mo; booster at 4–6 yr (4th dose in series may be given at 12 mo)	Acute infection, immunosuppressive therapy, previous CNS damage, or convulsions	Redness, tenderness, induction at site; fever, malaise; myalgia; urticaria; hypotension; neurological reactions; allergic reactions (all less than with DTwP)	Individual components may be given as separate injections if unusual reactions occur
Tetanus toxoid, reduced diphtheria toxoid and acellular pertussis vaccine absorbed (Tdap, Adacell, Boostrix)	0.5 mL IM to replace one dose of DTaP at from age 10 to 18 (Boostrix) or 11 to 18 (Adacel)	Previous reactions to DTaP, one progressive neurological disease, or recent (within 7 days) CNS pathology	Fatigue, headache, gastrointestinal symptoms, pain at injection site	Pertussis protection in addition to diphtheria and tetanus designed to protect against older children becoming ill with pertussus and passing it on to very young unprotected children in whom the disease has heightened morbidity
Polio vaccine, inactivated (IPV, IPOI, Poliovax)	0.5 mL subcut at 2, 4, and 6–18 mo with a booster at 4–6 yr	Hypersensitivity to neomycin, streptomycin, or polymyxin B; acute febrile illness	Erythema, induration, pain at injection site; fever	Oral polio vaccine (OPV) is no longer recommended for use in the United States
Measles, mumps, and rubella vaccines (M-M-R II)	Single dose 0.5 mL subcut at 12–15 mo with a booster at 4–6 yr or 11–12 yr	Allergy to egg, gelatin, or neomycin, active infection; immunosuppression	Burning, stinging, pain at injection site; arthritis/arthralgia (40%); fever, encephalitis; allergic reactions	If unusual reactions occur, individual components may be given as separate injections
Haemophilus b conjugate vaccine (PedvaxHIB, ActHIB, HibTITER)*	0.5 mL IM at 2, 4, and 6 mo (6-mo dose not needed for PedvaxHIB, with a booster at 12–15 mo	If co-administered with other immunizations, consider contraindications of all products	Induration, erythema, tenderness at injection site, fever	

*Available in varying concenrations.

GENERIC NAME (BRAND NAMES)	ROUTE/DOSAGE	CONTRAINDICATIONS/ PRECAUTIONS	ADVERSE REACTIONS/ SIDE EFFECTS	NOTES
Hepatitis B vaccine (Engerix-B, Recombivax HB)	10 mcg IM Engerix-B or 5 mcg IM Recombivax HB; 1st dose at 0–2 mo, 2nd dose at 1–4 mo, and 3rd dose at 6–18 mo (1st and 2nd dose about 1 mo apart). Dose is same for patients up to 20 yr old *Infants born to HBsAg-positive mothers:* Administer 0.5 mL of hepatitis B immune globulin within 12 hr of birth and 1st dose of 5 mcg Recombivax or 10 mcg of Engerix B IM and 2nd dose at 1–2 mo, 3rd dose at 6 mo *Children up to 10 yr:* 2.5 mcg Recombivax HB or 10 mcg Engerix-B IM as 3-dose series; 2nd dose 1 mo after 1st dose, 3rd dose 4 mo after 1st dose, and 2 mo after 2nd dose *Children up to 11–19 yr:* 5 mcg Recombivax HB or 10 mcg Engerix-B as 3-dose series; 2nd dose 1 mo after 1st dose, 3rd dose 4 mo after 1st dose, and 2 mo after 2nd dose. *Children 11–15 yr:* may also be given as two doses of 10 mcg/mL (Recombivax HB) 4–6 mo apart	Hypersensitivity to yeast	Local soreness	Children who have not been vaccinated as infants should complete the series by 12 yr

(table continued on page 362)

Routine Pediatric Immunizations (0–18 years) (continued)

GENERIC NAME (BRAND NAMES)	ROUTE/DOSAGE	CONTRAINDICATIONS/PRECAUTIONS	ADVERSE REACTIONS/SIDE EFFECTS	NOTES
Meningococcal polysaccharide, diphtheria toxoid conjugate vaccine (Menactra)	0.5 mL IM single dose at 11–12 yr or before entry to high school (15 yr)	Hypersensitivity to any components	Fatigue, malaise, anorexia, pain at injection site	Goal is to decrease invasive meningococcal disease. Routine vaccination with meningococcal vaccine also is recommended for college freshmen living in dormitories and other high-risk populations (military recruits, travelers to areas in which meningococcal disease is prevalent); other high-risk patients may elect to receive vaccine
Varicella vaccine (Varivax)	0.5 mL IM single dose at 12–18 mo; those without a history of chickenpox should be vaccinated by the 11–12 yr visit; children around age 13 yr should receive two doses 1 mo apart	Allergy to gelatin or neomycin; active infection; immunosuppression, including HIV	Local soreness, fever	Given to children who have not been vaccinated or have not had chickenpox. Salicylates should be avoided for 6 wk following vaccination
Hepatitis A vaccine (Havrix, Vaqta)	Children 2–18 yr: 0.5 mL IM (pediatric formulation), repeated 6–12 mo later (pediatric dose form)	Acute febrile illness	Local reactions, headache	Recommended for children in areas with high rates of hepatitis A and other high-risk groups
Pneumococcal 7-valent conjugate vaccine (Prevnar)	Infants: 0.5 mL IM for four doses at 2, 4, 6, and 12–15 mo	Hypersensitivity to all components including diphtheria toxoid; moderate to severe febrile illness; thrombocytopenia or coagulation disorder. Use cautiously in patients receiving anticoagulants; safe use in children < 6 wk not established	Erythema induration, tenderness, nodule formation at injection site, fever	Antineoplastics, corticosteroids, radiation therapy, and immunosuppressants decrease antibody response; product is a suspension—shake before use

GENERIC NAME (BRAND NAMES)	ROUTE/DOSAGE	CONTRAINDICATIONS/ PRECAUTIONS	ADVERSE REACTIONS/ SIDE EFFECTS	NOTES
Influenza vaccine Injection: Fluarix, Fluvirin, Fluzone Intranasal: FluMist	*Older infants and children starting at 7–11 mo of age:* Three doses of 0.5 mL IM, two doses at least 4 wk apart, 3rd dose after 1 yr birthday *Starting at 12–23 mo of age:* two doses of 0.5 mL IM at least 2 mo apart *Starting 2–6 yr:* single dose 0.5 mL IM *Injection Children 6–35 mo:* 0.25 mL IM one or two doses (two doses at least 1 mo apart for initial season) followed by single dose annually. *Children 3–8 yr:* 0.5 mL IM one or two doses (two doses at least 1 mo apart for initial season) followed by single dose annually. *Children ≥ 9 yr:* 0.5 mL IM single dose annually *Nasal Children 5–8 yr:* If not previously immunized with FluMist—two doses of 0.5 mL intranasally (given as one 0.25-mL dose in each nostril) at least 2 mo apart, then one dose annually. If previously immunized with FluMist, one dose of 0.5 mL intranasally (given as one 0.25-mL dose in each nostril) annually. *Children ≥ 9 yr:* one dose of 0.5 mL intranasally (given as one 0.25-mL dose in each nostril) annually	Hypersensitivity to eggs/egg products. Hypersensitivity to thimerosal (injection only). Fluvirin should be used in children > 4 yr only. Avoid use in patients with acute neurological compromise. FluMist should be avoided in patients receiving salicylates or who are immunocompromised	*Injection:* local soreness, fever myalgia, possible neurological toxicity *Intranasal:* upper respiratory congestion, malaise	Immunosuppression may decrease antibody response to injection and increase the risk of viral transmission with intranasal route
Human papilloma virus	Series of three intramuscular injections over a 6-month period. The second and third dosages should be given 2 and 6 months after the first dose	Hypersensitivity to yeast or any vaccine component. Not recommended for use in pregnancy	Heart problems, blood clotting, neurological toxicity	Recommended for 11–12 yr old girls before sexual activity begins. Does not protect against all cervical cancers or HPV types

NURSING IMPLICATIONS

ASSESSMENT

Assess previous immunization history and history of hypersensitivity.

Assess patient for history of asthma or reactive airway disease. Patients with positive history should not receive FluMist.

Assess for history of latex allergy. Some prefilled syringes may use latex components and should be avoided in those with hypersensitivity.

POTENTIAL NURSING DIAGNOSES

Infection, risk for (indications).

Knowledge, deficient, related to medication regimen (patient/family teaching).

IMPLEMENTATION

Measles, mumps, and rubella vaccine; trivalent oral poliovirus vaccine; and diphtheria toxoid, tetanus toxoid, and pertussis vaccine may be given concomitantly.

Do not administer FluMist concurrently with other vaccines or in patients who have received a live virus vaccine within 1 mo or an inactivated vaccine within 2 wk of vaccination.

Administer each immunization by appropriate route:

   PO: polio (Orimune)

   Subcut: measles, mumps, rubella, polio (IPOL, Poliovax)

   IM: diphtheria, tetanus toxoid, pertussis

   Intranasal: FluMist

PATIENT/FAMILY TEACHING

Inform parent of potential and reportable side effects of immunization. Physician should be notified if patient develops fever higher than 39.4°C (103°F); difficulty breathing; hives; itching; swelling of eyes, face, or inside of nose; sudden, severe tiredness or weakness; convulsions.

Review next scheduled immunization with parent.

EVALUATION

Effectiveness of therapy can be demonstrated by prevention of diseases through active immunity.

Routine Adult Immunizations

GENERIC NAME (BRAND NAMES)	INDICATIONS	DOSAGE/ROUTE	CONTRAINDICATIONS	ADVERSE REACTIONS/SIDE EFFECTS
Hepatitis A vaccine (Havrix, Vaqta)†	High-risk patients, some health care workers, food handlers, clotting disorders, travel to endemic areas, chronic liver disease	1 mL IM, followed by 1 mL IM 6–18 mo later (adult dose form)	Hypersensitivity to alum or 2-phenoxyethanol	Local soreness, headache
Hepatitis B vaccine (Engerix-B, Recombivax HB)	High-risk patients, health care workers, all unvaccinated adolescents	Three doses of 1 mL IM, given at 0, 1–2, and 4–6 mo	Anaphylactic allergy to yeast.	Local soreness
Influenza vaccine *Injection* (Fluzone, Fluvirin); *nasal:* (FluMist)	All adults	*Injection:* 0.5 mL IM annually; *intranasal for adults < 50:* Single 0.5-mL dose given as 0.25 mL in each nostril annually	Hypersensitivity to eggs/egg products; thimerosal (injection only). Avoid use in patients with acute neurological compromise. FluMist should be avoided in patients receiving salicylates or who are immunocompromised	*Injections:* local soreness, fever, myalgia, possible neurological toxicity *Intranasal:* upper respiratory congestion, malaise Immunosuppression may decrease antibody response to injection and increase the risk of viral transmission with intranasal route
Measles, mumps, and rubella vaccines (M-M-R II)	Adults with unreliable history of MMR illness or immunization, occupational exposure	0.5 mL subcut, single dose in those with unreliable history, two doses 1 mo apart for those with occupational exposure	Allergy to egg, gelatin, or neomycin; active infection; immunosuppression; pregnancy; also avoid becoming pregnant for 4 wk after immunization	Burning, stinging, pain at injection site; arthritis/arthralgia; fever; encephalitis; allergic reactions

(table continued on page 366)

†Less commonly used vaccines are not included.

Routine Adult Immunizations (continued)

GENERIC NAME (BRAND NAMES)	INDICATIONS	DOSAGE/ROUTE	CONTRAINDICATIONS	ADVERSE REACTIONS/SIDE EFFECTS
Meningococcal polysaccharide, diphtheria toxoid conjugate vaccine (Menactra)	Recommended for college freshmen living in dormitories and other high-risk populations (military recruits, travelers to areas in which meningococcal disease is prevalent); other high-risk patients may elect to receive vaccine	0.5 mL IM single dose at 11–12 yr or before entry to high school (15 yr)	Hypersensitivity to any components	Fatigue, malaise, anorexia, pain at injection site
Pneumococcal vaccine, polyvalent (Pneumovax 23, Pnu-Imune 23)	Everyone > 65 yr, high-risk patients with chronic illnesses including HIV, and other high-risk patients	0.5 mL IM; high-risk patients (asplenics) should have a booster after 6 yr	Safety during first trimester of pregnancy not established	Local soreness
Tetanus toxoid, reduced diphtheria toxoid, and acellular pertussis; vaccine absorbed (Tdap, Adacell)	Pertussis protection in addition to diphtheria and tetanus designed to protect against those becoming ill with pertussis passing it on to very young unprotected children in whom the disease has heightened morbidity	0.5 mL IM to replace one dose of DTaP	Previous reactions to DTaP, progressive neurological disease or recent (within 7 days) CNS pathology	Fatigue, headache, gastrointestinal symptoms, pain at injection site
Tetanus-diphtheria (Adult Td)	All adults	*Unimmunized:* two doses 0.5 mL IM 1–2 mo apart, then a 3rd dose 6–12 mo later *Immunized:* booster every 10 yr	Neurological or severe hypersensitivity reaction to prior dose	Local pain and swelling
Varicella vaccine (Varivax)	Any adult without a history of chickenpox or herpes zoster	0.5 mL subcut; repeated 4–8 wk later	Allergy to gelatin or neomycin; active infection; immunosuppression, including HIV; pregnancy; family history of immunodeficiency; blood/blood product in past 5 mo	Salicylates should be avoided for 6 wk following vaccination

Source: Adapted from the recommendations of the National Immunization Program: http://www.cdc.gov/nip. In: Deglin J. and Vallerand AH. (2006). *Davis's Drug Guide for Nurses.* 10th edition. Philadelphia: FA Davis.

E

Administering Medications to Children

GENERAL GUIDELINES

Medication administration to a pediatric patient can be challenging. Prescribers should order dosage forms that are age-appropriate for their patients. If a child is unable to take a particular dosage form, ask the pharmacist if another form is available or for other options.

ORAL LIQUIDS

Pediatric liquid medicines may be given with plastic medicine cups, oral syringes, oral droppers, or cylindrical dosing spoons. Parents should be taught to use these calibrated devices rather than using household utensils. If a medicine comes with a particular measuring device, do not use the device with another product. For young children, it is best to squirt a little of the dose at a time into the side of the cheek away from the bitter taste buds at the back of the tongue.

EYEDROPS/OINTMENTS

Tilt the child's head back and gently press the skin under the lower eyelid and pull the lower lid away slightly until a small pouch is visible. Insert the ointment or drop (one drop at a time) and close the eye for a few minutes to keep the medicine in the eye.

EARDROPS

Shake otic suspensions well before administration. For children < 3 years of age, pull the outer ear outward and downward before instilling drops. For children ≥ 3 years, pull the outer ear outward and upward. Keep the child on his or her side for 2 minutes and place a cotton plug in ear.

NOSE DROPS

Clear nose of secretions prior to use. A nasal aspirator (bulb syringe) or a cotton swab may be used in infants and young children. Ask older children to blow their nose. Tilt child's head back over a pillow and squeeze the dropper without touching the nostril. Keep child's head back for 2 minutes.

SUPPOSITORIES

Keep refrigerated for easier administration. Wearing gloves, moisten the rounded end with water or petroleum jelly prior to insertion. Using your pinky finger for children < 3 years of age and your index finger for those ≥ 3 years, insert the suppository into the rectum about $1/_2$ to 1 inch beyond the sphincter. If the suppository slides out, insert it a little farther than before. Hold the buttocks together for a few minutes and have the child hold the position for about 20 minutes, if possible.

TOPICALS

Clean affected area and dry well prior to application. Apply a thin layer to the skin and rub in gently. Do not apply a covering over the area unless instructed to do so by the prescriber.

METERED-DOSE INHALERS

Generally the same principles apply to children as to adults, except the use of spacers is recommended for young children.

Source: Deglin J. and Vallerand AH. (2006). Davis's Drug Guide for Nurses, 10th edition. Philadelphia: FA Davis.

Pediatric Dosage Calculations

Most drugs in children are dosed according to body weight (mg/kg) or body surface area (BSA) (mg/m^2). Care must be taken to convert body weight from pounds to kilograms (1 kg = 2.2 lb) before calculating doses based on body weight. Doses are often expressed as mg/kg/day or mg/kg/dose; therefore, orders written "mg/kg/d" which is confusing, *require clarification from the prescriber*.

Chemotherapeutic drugs are commonly dosed according to the BSA, which requires an extra verification step (BSA calculation) prior to dosing. Medications are available in multiple concentrations; therefore, *orders written in "mL" rather than "mg" are not acceptable and require clarification*.

Dosing also varies by indication; therefore, diagnostic information is helpful when calculating doses. The following examples are typically encountered when dosing medication in children.

Example 1. Calculate the dose of amoxicillin suspension in milliliters for otitis media for a 1-year-old child weighing 22 lb. The dose required is 40 mg/kg/day divided b.i.d., and the suspension comes in a concentration of 400 mg/5 mL.

Step 1. Convert pounds to kilograms:	22 lb × 1 kg/2.2 lb = 10 kg
Step 2. Calculate the dose in milligrams:	10 kg × 40 mg/kg/day = 400 mg/day
Step 3. Divide the dose by the frequency:	400 mg/day ÷ 2 (b.i.d.) = 200 mg/dose b.i.d.
Step 4. Convert the milligrams dose to milliliters:	200 mg/dose ÷ 400 mg/5 mL = 2.5 mL b.i.d.

Example 2. Calculate the dose of ceftriaxone in milliliters for meningitis for a 5-year-old weighing 18 kg. The dose required is 100 mg/kg/day given IV once daily, and the drug comes prediluted in a concentration of 40 mg/mL.

Step 1. Calculate the dose in milligrams:	18 kg × 100 mg/kg/day = 1800 mg/day
Step 2. Divide the dose by the frequency:	1800 mg/day ÷ 1 (daily) = 1800 mg/dose
Step 3. Convert the milligrams dose to milliliters:	1800 mg/dose ÷ 40 mg/mL = 45 mL once daily

Example 3. Calculate the dose of vincristine in milliliters for a 4-year-old with leukemia who weighs 37 lb and is 97 cm tall. The dose required is 2 mg/m^2, and the drug comes in 1 mg/mL concentration.

Step 1. Convert pounds to kilograms:	37 lb × 1 kg/2.2 lb = 16.8 kg
Step 2. Calculate the BSA:	✓16.8 kg × 97 cm/3600 = 0.45 m^2
Step 3. Calculate the dose in milligrams:	2 mg/m^2 × 0.67 m^2 = 1.34 mg
Step 4. Calculate the dose in milliliters:	1.34 mg ÷ 1 mg/mL = 1.34 mg

Source: Deglin J. and Vallerand AH. (2006). *Davis's Drug Guide for Nurses,* 10th edition. Philadelphia: FA Davis.

Examples of Herbs, Vitamins, Minerals, Amino Acids, and Lipids Used in Illness by System

NEUROLOGICAL

Illness	Product that may help
Addictions	Oats; vitamin B
Anxiety	Lady's slipper, lime blossom, oats, skullcap; vitamin B
Depression	Balm, oats, rosemary, vervain; vitamins B_6, B_{12}, C
Encephalitis	Catnip, chamomile, echinacea, garlic, skullcap; vitamin C; zinc
Epilepsy	Valerian, vervain; vitamins B_5, B_6, D; taurine
Guillain-Barré syndrome	Echinacea, ginseng, oats, skullcap, valerian root, vervain; vitamins B, E; calcium, magnesium, manganese, zinc
Insomnia	Catnip, calcium, chamomile, lavender, lime flowers; vitamins B, C, folic acid; zinc
Memory loss	Ginseng, rosemary; vitamin B; lecithin
Migraines	Balm, feverfew, rosemary, skullcap; vitamins B_5, C, E
Multiple sclerosis	Vitamins B_3, B_6, B_{12}, C, E, folic acid; magnesium, zinc
Neuralgia	Chamomile, peppermint; vitamins B_1, B_2; chromium
Obsessions/compulsions	Valerian, hops, chamomile, passiflora
Parkinson's disease	Angelica; vitamins B, C
Phobias	Valerian; vitamins B, C
Shingles	Oats, skullcap, St. John's wort; vitamins C, E
Stress	Balm, chamomile, ginseng, lavender, oats, passiflora; vitamins B, C; L-tyrosine
Stroke	Ginkgo biloba, rosemary, yarrow; vitamin E; fish oil
Syncope (fainting)	Ginger, peppermint, rosemary

INTEGUMENTARY

Illness	Product that may help
Abscess	Echinacea, red clover, thyme
Alopecia (hair loss)	Ginger, nettles, rosemary; inositol, vitamin B; calcium, magnesium; choline
Athlete's foot	Echinacea; vitamin C
Boils	Echinacea, thyme
Cold sores	St. John's wort; vitamin C; zinc
Corns and calluses	Garlic, lemon juice; vitamins A, E
Dandruff	Lavender, rosemary; vitamins B, C, E; zinc
Dermatitis	Thyme, verbena
Diaper rash	Golden seal, marigold; zinc
Eczema	Aloe vera, chamomile, chickweed, marigold, oats; vitamins A, B, C

Edema	Dandelion, yarrow
Perspiration	Lavender, marigold
Prickly heat	Sandlewood; vitamin C
Psoriasis	Nettles, yarrow; vitamins A, B, C, E
Seborrhea	Burdock, butternut, meadowsweet
Sunburn	Aloe vera; vitamin E
Urticaria	Balm, chamomile, chickweed
Warts	Dandelion

CARDIOVASCULAR

Illness	Product that may help
Anemia	Alfalfa, angelica, dandelion, nettles, watercress; vitamins B, B_{12}, C; calcium, copper, iron
Aneurysm	Garlic; vitamins C, E
Angina	Garlic, hawthorne, motherwort, dietary fiber; fish oil
Atherosclerosis	Lavender, hawthorne, rosemary, dietary fiber
Bruising	Witch hazel; vitamin C; zinc
High blood pressure	Cramp bark, hawthorn, limeflowers, dietary fiber; calcium, magnesium, potassium
Low blood pressure	Broom, ginger, rosemary
Palpitations	Broom, mistletoe, motherwort; vitamin E
Raynaud's disease	Cayenne, ginger; vitamin C
Varicose veins	Marigold; vitamins C, E

IMMUNE

Illness	Product that may help
AIDS	Echincacea, garlic, ginseng, hyssop, licorice; vitamin C; zinc
Allergies	Angelica, chamomile, echinacea, elderflower, garlic, ginseng, red clover, wild yam; vitamins B, C
Cancer	Green tea
Chickenpox	Burdock, comfrey, peppermint
Enlarged spleen	Echinacea, garlic, ginseng, licorice
Measles	Elderflower, garlic; vitamins C, E
Pertussis (whooping cough)	Comfrey, hyssop, lemon
Rubella	Elderflower, peppermint, yarrow; vitamin E
Worms	Cayenne pepper, wormwood tea

RESPIRATORY

Illness	Product that may help
Asthma	Hyssop, motherwort, tumeric; vitamin B_6
Bronchitis	Anise, garlic, ginseng, peppermint; vitamins A, B, C
Cold	Echinacea, ginger, ginseng, peppermint; vitamin C; zinc
Cough	Aniseed, goldenseal, licorice, mustard, thyme
Emphysema	Peppermint, slippery elm bark
Epistaxis (nosebleed)	Lavender
Flu (influenza)	Fenugreek, ginseng, licorice; vitamin C
Hayfever	Chamomile, eucalyptus, lavender; vitamin C
Hyperventilation	Lady's slipper, skullcap; vitamin B
Pleurisy	Sage, comfrey root
Pneumonia	Garlic, ginseng; vitamin C
Sinusitis	Elderflower, goldenseal
Tracheitis	Comfrey root; vitamin C
Tuberculosis	Echinacea, garlic, ginseng, licorice

GASTROINTESTINAL

Illness	Product that may help
Anal fissure	Butternut, cascara, dandelion, licorice, yellow duck
Cirrhosis	Chamomile, grapefruit, juniper, lemon, orange
Constipation	Licorice, rhubarb, senna, dietary fiber; vitamin B
Crohn's disease	Hops, peppermint; vitamins A, B, D
Diarrhea	Myrrh; vitamins B_1, B_3, K
Flatulence	Dill
Gallstones	Dandelion leaves
Gastroenteritis	Comfrey root
Gingivitis	Comfrey, goldenseal, myrrh; vitamin C
Grinding teeth	Angelica, ginseng
Halitosis	Mint, parsley, rosemary, tarragon, thyme, watercress
Hemorrhoids	Bayberry, dandelion, witch hazel
Hepatitis	Barberry, dandelion, goldenseal, verbena, wild yam; vitamin C
Indigestion	Dandelion, dill, peppermint
Irritable bowel syndrome	Balm, chamomile, ginger, peppermint, slippery elm; vitamins A, B_6
Jaundice	Barberry, dandelion, goldenseal, verbena, yams
Laryngitis	Echinacea, sage; vitamin C
Motion sickness	Angelica, chamomile, fennel, ginger, peppermint
Mouth ulcers	Myrrh; vitamins A, B_2, E
Nausea	Ginger; vitamin B_6
Pancreatitis	Licorice, yellow dock
Peptic ulcers	Comfrey, licorice, slippery elm
Sore throat	Garlic, goldenseal; vitamin C; zinc
Thrush	Aloe vera, barberry
Tonsilitis	Chamomile, echinacea, elderberry, garlic, myrrh, safe, wild indigo, yarrow; vitamin C; fish oil
Tooth abscess	Comfrey, olive oil, garlic, myrrh
Toothache	Cayenne

MUSCULOSKELETAL

Illness	Product that may help
Arthritis	Bladderwrack, dandelion, feverfew, white willow; vitamins A, C, E; copper; fish oil
Bunion	Comfrey, marshmallow, slippery elm
Bursitis	Ginseng, slippery elm
Fractures	Comfrey, horsetail; calcium, magnesium, phosphorus
Gout	Nettles
Osteoporosis	Comfrey, dandelion, horsetail, nettles, white willow, wild yams; calcium, fluoride
Restless leg syndrome	Chamomile, valerian; vitamin E; zinc
Rheumatoid arthritis	Feverfew, slippery elm, white willow
Sciatica	Elderberry, juniper
Sprains and strains	Burdock, chamomile, ginger; vitamin C, beta-carotene; selenium, zinc

ENDOCRINE

Illness	Product that may help
Diabetes mellitus	Alfalfa, fenugreek, garlic, onions
Insomnia	Melatonin
Obesity	Bladderwrack, nettles; chromium
Thyroid disease	Angelica, bugleweed, bladderwrack, onions, garlic; iodine, zinc

REPRODUCTIVE

Illness	Product that may help
Breastfeeding problems	Caraway, dill, fennel, slippery elm, St. John's wort; vitamin E
Breast problems	Golden seal, marigold, nettles, yellowduck; vitamins A, E
Infertility	Agnus castus, balm, false unicorn root, passiflora, skullcap; vitamins B_6, E; zinc
Menopause	Black cohosh, dandelion, dong quai, ginseng, gingko biloba, licorice, milk thistle, valerian; vitamins A, B, C, E; magnesium, zinc
Menstrual problems	Angelica, catnip, peppermint, thyme, yarrow; vitamins A, B_6; iron, zinc
PMS	Chamomile, false unicorn, skullcap, yellowduck; vitamins A, B_6, C, E; chromium, iron, magnesium, zinc

URINARY

Illness	Product that may help
Bladder and kidney stones	Yarrow; vitamins B_6, C, D
Cystitis	Buchu, cornsilk, coughgrass, yarrow; vitamin C
Ejaculation	Lady's slipper, skullcap; vitamin B
Enuresis	St. John's wort
Erection	Anise, damiana, peppermint, saw palmetto; zinc, L-tryptophan
Incontinence	Horsetail, ginkgo biloba
Male problems	Damiana, saw palmetto; vitamins B_6, E; zinc; fish oil
Priapism	Broom, ginger, lavender; vitamins C, E
Urethritis	Buchu, cornsilk, coughgrass, yarrow; vitamin C

EYES

Illness	Product that may help
Cataract	Vitamins A, C, E
Conjunctivitis	Chamomile, echinacea, goldenseal
Eyelid twitching	Chamomile, lavender, vervain
Eyestrain	Chickweed, marigold; vitamins A, B_{12}
Glaucoma	Vitamins A, B_1, B_{12}, C
Stye	Chamomile, echinacea, marigold

EARS

Illness	Product that may help
Earache	St. John's wort, olive oil
Ear wax	Chamomile, elderflower, marigold
Otitis externa (outer)	Chamomile, elderflower, goldenseal, mullein oil, St. John's wort
Otitis intima (inner)	Angelica, ginger root, licorice
Otitis media (middle)	Chamomile, echinacea, goldenrod, goldenseal
Tinnitus	Black cohosh, feverfew; vitamins A, C; magnesium, manganese, potassium

Glossary

A

Absorption—passage of a substance through some surface of the body into body fluids and tissues

a.c.—before meals

ACE inhibitors—drugs that inhibit angiotension-converting enzyme from working

Acne—inflammatory disease of the sebaceous glands of the skin

Acromegaly—chronic syndrome of growth hormone excess, most often caused by a pituitary macroadenoma; characterized by gradual coarsening and enlargement of bones and facial features

ACTH—adrenocorticotropic hormone

a.d.—right ear

Addicting—a substance that encourages dependence on it

Addison's disease—gradual, progressive failure of the adrenal glands and insufficient production of steroid hormones

Addition—to combine two or more numbers together

Additive—effect that one drug or substance contributes to the action of another drug or substance

ADH—antidiuretic hormone

ADI—American Drug Index

Adrenergic—relating to nerve fibers that release norepinephrine or epinephrine at the synapses

Adverse effects—undesired side effects or toxicity caused by a treatment

Aerobic—taking place in the presence of oxygen

Agonist—drug that binds to the receptor and stimulates the receptor's function

Alopecia—absence or loss of hair

Alveoli—plural of alveolus; an air sac in the lungs

Ampule—a small glass container that can be sealed and its contents sterilized

Anaerobic—taking place in the absence of oxygen

Anaphylaxis—hypersensitivity reaction between an allergenic antigen and immunoglobulin E bound to mast cells; stimulates the sudden release of immunologic mediators locally or throughout the body

Androgens—substances producing or stimulating the development of male characteristics, such as the hormones testosterone and androsterone

Angina pectoris—oppressive pain or pressure in the chest caused by inadequate blood flow and oxygenation to heart muscle

Anoxia—absence of oxygen

Antagonist—that which counteracts the action of something else, such as a muscle or drug

Antihistamines—a drug that opposes the action of histamine

Antiinfluenza agents—drugs used to combat the influenza virus

Antispasmodics—drugs that prevent or relieve spasm

Antitussives—drugs that prevent or relieve coughing

Apothecary—druggist or pharmacist

Aromatherapy—use of fragrant oils in baths, as inhalants, or during massage to relieve stress and to treat skin conditions

a.s.—left eye

Atherosclerosis—the most common form of arteriosclerosis, marked by cholesterol-lipid-calcium deposits in the walls of the arteries

Attenuate—to render thin or make less virulent

a.u.—both ears

Aura—a subjective, but recognizable sensation that precedes and signals the onset of a convulsion or migraine headache

Automatic stop order—an order that discontinues a medication at a certain time

Autonomic—self-controlling, functioning independently

Avoirdupois—a system of weighing or measuring articles in which 7000 grains equal 1 pound

B

Bactericidal—capable of killing bacteria

Bacteriostatic—inhibits the growth of bacteria

Barrel—part of the syringe through which the plunger passes

Benign—not recurrent or progressive, not malignant

Beta-adrenergic agent—a synthetic or natural drug that stimulates beta-receptors

b.i.d.—two times per day

Biotransformation—chemical alteration that a substance undergoes in the body

Bisphosphonates—any of a class of medications that inhibit the resorption of bones by osteoclasts

Blister pack—method of delivering medications; usually contains one dose in each small sac

Blood-borne pathogens—microorganisms capable of producing disease, transmitted by body fluids

Booster—additional dose of an immunizing agent to increase the protection afforded by the original series of injections

BPH—benign prostatic hypertrophy

Brand name—drug name given by the drug manufacturer

BSA—body surface area (computed using height and weight)

Buffered—treated in such a way to offset the reaction of an agent administered in conjunction with it

Bulk—mass

BUN—blood urea nitrogen

C

c̄—with

C & S—culture and sensitivity

Calcitonin—hormone produced by the human thyroid gland that is important for maintaining a dense, strong bone matrix and regulating the blood calcium level

Calibrated—determined as accurate

CAM—complementary and alternative medicine

Cannula—tube used to deliver oxygen or through which a trocar is withdrawn after insertion

Cap.—abbreviation for capsule

Caplets—delivery mode for medication that is similar to both capsules and tablets

Capsules—delivery mode for medication that holds a measured drug inside a substance that dissolves

Carcinogen—any substance or agent that produces cancer or increases the risk of developing cancer in humans or animals

Centi—prefix used in the metric system to denote one-hundredth (1/100)

Cerumen—earwax; secreted by the glands at the outer third of the ear canal

Chemical name—drug name that reflects the chemical makeup of the drug

CHF—congestive heart failure

Cholinergic—agent that produces the effect of acetylcholine

Clinical trials—scientific tests that research the efficacy and safety of a medication

CO_2—carbon dioxide

Comedos—a small skin lesion of acne vulgaris and seborrheic dermatitis

Compendium of Drug Therapy—several volumes published yearly by Biomedical Information Corporation and distributed to prescribers—*Compendium of Patient Information* and *Compendium of Drug Therapy*; they include photographs of some drugs and phone numbers of poison control centers and pharmaceutical companies

Compound—mix

Condyloma—a wart, found on the genitals or near the anus, with a textured surface that may resemble coral, cauliflower, or cobblestone

Contractility—having the ability to contract or shorten

Contraindications—symptoms or circumstances that make treatment with a drug or device unsafe or inappropriate

Control group—group of people in clinical trials who receive the placebo or usual treatment, in contrast to the group given the treatment or medication being studied

Controlled substances—substances monitored under the Comprehensive Drug Abuse Prevention and Control Act, a law enacted in 1971 to control the distribution and use of all depressant and stimulant drugs and other drugs of abuse or potential abuse as may be designated by the Drug Enforcement Administration of the Department of Justice

Conversion factor—numbers used to change a mathematical number from one condition to another

COPD—chronic obstructive pulmonary disease

CPAP—continuous positive air pressure

CrCl—creatinine clearance

Cream—semi-solid delivery system for medications

Cretinism—congenital condition caused by a lack of thyroid hormones, characterized by arrested physical and mental development, myxedema, dystrophy of the bones and soft tissues, and lowered basal metabolism

Crystalloid—substance capable of crystallization, which in solution can be diffused through animal membranes; the opposite of colloid

CSF—cerebrospinal fluid

Cumulation—increasing in effect by successive additions

Curative—having healing or remedial properties

Cushing's disease—caused by excessive production of adrenocoticotropic hormone (ACTH) in the body

CVA—cerebrovascular accident

Cyanosis—blue, gray, slate, or dark purple discoloration of the skin or mucous membranes caused by deoxygenated or reduced hemoglobin in the blood

D

d/c—discontinue(d)

DEA—Drug Enforcement Agency, of the Department of Justice

Débride—to perform the action of débridement, the removal of foreign material and dead or damaged tissue, especially in a wound

Deci—prefix used in the metric system to denote one-tenth (1/10)

Decimal—numeric system using numbers from 0 to 9

Decongestants—agent that reduces congestion, especially nasal

Delayed action—action occurring a considerable time after a stimulus

Deltoid—triangular muscle on the upper arm

Delusion—false belief brought about without appropriate external stimulation and inconsistent with the individual's own knowledge and experience

Dementia—a progressive, irreversible decline in mental function, marked by memory impairment and, often, deficits in reasoning, judgment, abstract thought, registration, comprehension, learning, task execution, and use of language

Denominator—number on lower part of a fraction; used to divide into the numerator

Dependent—supported, nurtured, or relying on another person or variable

Depression—mood disorder marked by loss of interest or pleasure in living

Desired dose—dose of medication ordered by the prescriber

Destructive—causing injury or death

Dextrose—glucose, sugar

Diabetes insipidus—excessive urination caused by inadequate amounts of antidiuretic hormone (ADH) in the body or by failure of the kidney to respond to ADH

Diabetes mellitus—chronic metabolic disorder marked by hyperglycemia

Diagnostic—pertaining to the disease or syndrome a person has or is believed to have

Dialysis—passage of a solute through a membrane

Dimensional analysis—calculating dosages using the measurement, such as milligrams or milliliters, to set up the calculation

Distribution—dividing and spreading of a medication to a target organ

Dividend—number being divided in a division problem

Division—to separate into smaller parts

Divisor—number doing the division in a division problem

DMARD—disease-modifying antirheumatic drug

Dorsogluteal—injection site in the gluteus maximus on the dorsal (back) side

Double-blind—neither the patient nor the researcher in the clinical trial knows who has the placebo and who has the drug being tested

Drip chamber—part of an intravenous line where the medication drips into the chamber at a regulated rate

Drug Facts and Comparisons—is updated monthly; compares and evaluates medications, so it is frequently used by pharmacists to compare drugs; drugs are grouped by their classification, so similar drugs are indexed together

Drug Information—of the American Health-System Formulary Service; a volume published annually for the Health-System Pharmacists in Bethesda, MD; concise and more general that the PDR but contains no photographs

Drug Topics Red Book—book that contains both over-the-counter (OTC) and prescription drugs and their prices

DVT—deep vein thrombosis

Dwarfism—condition of being abnormally small

Dyspnea—difficult breathing

Dysrhythmias—abnormal heart rhythms

Dystonia—prolonged involuntary muscular contractions that may cause twisting of body parts, repetitive movements, and increased muscular tone

E

Eczema—general term for an itchy red rash that initially weeps or oozes serum and may become crusted, thickened, and scaly

EEG—electroencephalogram

Effervescent—bubbling, rising in little bubbles of gas

Efficacy—ability to produce a desired effect

Electrolytes—substances that, in solution, conduct an electric current and are decomposed by its passage

Elix.—abbreviation for elixir

Elixirs—sweetened, aromatic, hydroalcoholic liquids used when compounding oral medication

Embolus—mass of undissolved matter present in a blood or lymphatic vessel and brought there by the blood or lymph

Emulsions—mixtures of two liquids not mutually soluble

Endogenous—produced or originating from within a cell or organism

Enema—introduction of a solution into the rectum and colon to stimulate bowel activity and cause emptying of the lower intestine for feeding or therapeutic purposes; sometimes used to give anesthesia or to aid in radiographic studies

Enteric-coated—coated with a substance so the drug is dissolved and absorbed only in the small intestine

Equivalent—equal in power or force or value

ERT—estrogen replacement therapy

Estrogens—any natural or artificial substance that induces estrus and the development of female sex characteristics; more specifically, estrogenic hormones produced by the ovaries

ETOH—ethyl alcohol

Excretion—elimination of waste products from the body

Expectorants—agents, such as guaifenesin, that promote clearance of mucus from the respiratory tract

Expiration—death or end of usefulness

Extremes—numbers on the far ends (front and back) of a ratio and proportion problem

F

FDA—Food and Drug Administration

Filter—to pass a liquid through any porous substance that prevents particles larger than a certain size from passing through

Flow regulator—piece of equipment on the intravenous line that regulates the rate of passage of fluid; can be used to stop or start the flow

Formula—rule prescribing how to calculate a dosage; for example, $D/H \times Q$ = answer

Fraction—ratio of a numerator to a denominator

FSH—follicle-stimulating hormone

G

GABA—gamma-aminobutyric acid

Gauge—a device for measuring the size, capacity, amount, or power of an object or substance

Gel—semi-solid condition of a precipitated or coagulated colloid, jelly, or jelly-like colloid

Generic name—official name of the drug; nonproprietary

Geriatric—branch of health care concerned with care of the aged

GH—growth hormone

Gigantism—excessive development of a body or body part

Glucocorticoids—general classification of adrenal cortical hormones primarily active in protecting against stress and affecting protein and carbohydrate metabolism

gm—abbreviation for gram

Gout—form of arthritis marked by the deposition of monosodium urate crystals in joints and other tissues

gr—abbreviation for grain

Graves' disease—a distinct type of hyperthyroidism caused by an autoimmune attack on the thyroid gland

gtt—abbreviation for drop

H

Habituated—process of becoming accustomed to a stimulus

Half-life—time required for half the nuclei of a radioactive substance to lose their activity by undergoing radioactive decay

Hallucination—false perception having no relation to reality and not accounted for by any exterior stimulus

HDL—high-density lipid

Hemostasis—arrest of bleeding or of circulation

HIPAA—Health Insurance Portability and Accountability Act

HMO—health maintenance organization

Homeopathy—school of American healing, founded by Dr. Samuel Hahnemann; based on the idea that very dilute doses of medicines that produce symptoms of a disease in healthy people can cure that disease in affected patients

Household—measuring system used by lay persons, not apothecaries, in their homes

HPV—human papillomavirus

HRT—hormone replacement therapy

HTN—hypertension

Hub—central structure into which other structures are anchored, attached, or stabilized

Hydantoins—colorless bases; glycolyl urea; derived from urea and allantoin

Hyperglycemia—abnormally high blood sugar levels, as are found in people with diabetes mellitus or people treated with some drugs

Hyperlipidemia—abnormally high lipids in the blood

Hypocalcemia—abnormally low calcium in the blood

Hypodermic—under or inserted under the skin

Hypoglycemia—abnormally low glucose in the blood

Hypoxia—oxygen deficiency in body tissues

I

ICSH—interstitial cell-stimulating hormone

ID—intradermal

IDDM—insulin-dependent diabetes mellitus

Idiosyncratic—relating to idiosyncracy; how a person differs from another

IM—intramuscular

Impaired provider—professional caregiver who is under the influence of a drug or disease and thus not as competent

Implanted device—object inserted into the body

Improper—referring to a fraction, one in which the numerator is larger than the denominator

IND—investigational new drug

Induration—area of hardened tissue

Inert—having little or no tendency or ability to react with other chemicals, not active

Infarction—area of tissue in an organ or part that undergoes necrosis following cessation of blood supply

Infiltration—deposition and accumulation of an external substance in a cell, tissue, or organ, such as fat deposition in a damaged liver

Infusion—any liquid substance (other than blood) introduced into the body for therapeutic purposes

Inhalation—introduction of dry or moist air or vapor into the lungs for therapeutic purposes, such as by metered-dose bronchodilators in the treatment of asthma

Inhaler—device for administering medications by inhalation

Inorganic—not containing carbon; not derived from animal or vegetable matter

Inscription—body of the prescription, which gives the names of the drug prescribed and the dosage

Inserts—implanting something inside something else

Inspiration—inhalation, breathing in

Intradermal—within the dermis, intracutaneous

Intramuscular—within a muscle

Invert—to turn inside out or upside down

IOP—intraocular pressure

Ischemia—temporary deficiency of blood flow to an organ or tissue

IUD—intrauterine device, usually for contraception

IV—intravenous

IV push—inject quickly, not drip, a small amount of medication into an intravenous line

J

Jellies—thick, semi-solid, gelatinous masses

K

Keratization—process of keratin formation that takes place in keratocytes as they progress upward through the layers of the epidermis of skin to the stratum corneum

Kilo—prefix used in the metric system to denote 1000

L

Lactated Ringer's—intravenous medication containing fluid, dextrose, and electrolytes in a healthy combination, developed by Sydney Ringer

LDL—low-density lipid

LH—lutineizing hormone

Liniments—liquid vehicle (usually water, oil, or alcohol) containing a medication to be rubbed on or applied to the skin

Lipids—fats

Lotion—liquid medicinal preparation for local application to, or bathing, a part

Lowest common denominator—number on the bottom of a fraction that is common to the multiples of another number but is the least denominator those numbers have in common

Lozenge—small, dry, medicinal solid to be held in the mouth until it dissolves

Lumen—space within a tube

Lymphatic—pertaining to the lymph system

M

Magma—mass left after extraction of principal; salve or paste; suspension of finely divided material in a small amount of water

Malignant—growing worse; resisting treatment; said of cancerous growth; tending or threatening to produce death; harmful

Mania—mental disorder characterized by excessive excitement

MAO inhibitors—medication that affects the action of monoamine oxidase at the synapse; used to treat depression and Parkinson's disease

Mast cell stabilizer—stabilizes large tissue cells; resembles a basophil; essential for inflammatory reactions; does not circulate in the blood

mcg—microgram; one millionth part of a gram

Means—numbers in the center of a ratio and proportion problem, not those at the ends

Megadosages—overly large dosages

Melanocytes—cells that form melanin; found in the lower epidermis of the skin

Melatonin—peptide hormone produced by the pineal gland; influences sleep-wake cycles and other circadian rhythms

Meniscus—curved upper surface of a liquid in a container

mEq—milliequivalent; one thousandth of a chemical equivalent

Metabolism—breaking down into its constituents

Metastasis—change in location of a disease

Metric—measurement system based on grams for weight, liters for liquid, and meters for distance

mg—milligram, one-thousandth of a gram

MI—myocardial infarction, heart attack

Micro—small

Migraine headache—familiar disorder marked by periodic, usually unilateral, pulsatile headaches that begin during childhood or early adult life and tend to recur with diminishing frequency in later life

Milli—prefix used in the metric system to denote one-thousandth (1/1000)

Mixed—when referring to numbers, a fraction that contains a whole number and a fractional part

mL—milliliter, one-thousandth of a liter

Mortar—vessel with a smooth interior in which crude drugs are crushed or ground with a pestle

Mucolytic—medication that breaks down mucus, improving breathing

Multiplication—adding repetitively

Myxedema—clinical and metabolic manifestations of hypothyroidism in adults, adolescents, and children

N

NDA—new drug application

Nebulizer—apparatus for producing a fine spray or mist

Negative feedback system—result of a process that reverses or shuts off a stimulus

Neurotransmitter—substance released when the axon terminal of a presynaptic neuron is excited and acts by inhibiting or exciting a target cell

Nevus (nevi)—congenital discoloration of a circumscribed area of the skin due to pigmentation; a mole

NIDDM—non-insulin-dependent diabetes mellitus

Nit—egg of a louse or any other parasitic insect

Nodule—a small node or cluster of cells

npo—nothing by mouth

NSS—normal saline solution; isotonic solution

Numerator—number on the top of a fraction

O

O_2—oxygen

o.d.—right eye

Ointment—viscous, semi-solid vehicle to apply medication to the skin

Ophthalmic—pertaining to the eye

Oral—concerning the mouth; taking medications by mouth

Ordered dose—dose ordered by the prescriber

Organic—containing carbon; composed of animal or vegetable matter

o.s.—left eye

OSHA—Occupational Safety and Health Administration

Osmosis—passage of a solvent through a semi-permeable membrane that separates solutions of different concentrations

Osteoarthritis—inflammation of bone and joints

Osteomalacia—softening of bone

Osteoporosis—loss of bone mass that occurs throughout the skeleton, predisposing patients to fractures

OTC—over-the-counter

Otic—pertaining to the ear

Ototoxicity—having a detrimental effect on the eighth nerve or organs of hearing

o.u.—both eyes

Oxytocin—pituitary hormone that stimulates the uterus to contract, thus inducing parturition

oz—ounce

P

Packed cells—red blood cells that have been separated from plasma; used in treating conditions that require red blood cells but not liquid components of whole blood

Palliative—relieving or alleviating without curing

Papules—small lump or pimple—typically larger than a grain of salt but smaller than a peppercorn—that rises above the surface of the neighboring skin

Paranoia—condition in which patients show persistent persecutory delusions or delusional jealousy

Parasympathetic—of or pertaining to the craniosacral division of the autonomic nervous system

Parathormone—hormone produced by the parathyroid; increases blood calcium

Parenteral—denoting any medication route other than the alimentary canal, such as intravenous, subcutaneous, intramuscular, or mucosal

Particulate—made up of particles

Patch—drug delivery system that enhances uptake of a medicine through the skin

p.c.—after meals, on a full stomach

PCA—patient-controlled analgesia; delivery of pain medication that is controlled by the patient

PDR—Physician's Desk Reference

Pediatric—concerning the treatment of children

Percent—number divided by 100

Peripheral—located at, or pertaining to, the periphery; occurring away from the center

Pernicious anemia—chronic, macrocytic anemia; an autoimmune disease marked by a reduction in the mass of circulating red blood cells

Pestle—device for macerating drugs in a mortar

Pharmacodynamics—study of drugs and their actions in living organisms

Pharmacokinetics—study of metabolism and action of drugs with particular emphasis on the time required for absorption, duration of action, distribution in the body, and method of excretion

Pharmacology—study of drugs and their origin, nature, properties, and effects on living organisms

Phlebitis—inflammation of the vein

Piggyback—when medication is hung above another IV line and delivered before the main line is allowed to drip in

Placebo—inactive substance given to satisfy a patient's demand for medicine; a drug or treatment used as a nonspecific or inactive control in a test of a therapy that is suspected of being useful for a particular disease or condition

Plasma—liquid part of blood or lymph

Plaster—topical preparation in which the constituents are formed into a tenacious mass of substance harder than an ointment and spread on muslin, linen, skin, or paper

Platelet—round or oval disk found in the blood of vertebrates; fragments of megakaryocytes that contribute to forming a clot

Plunger—part of a syringe that pushes the medication through the needle

PO—by mouth

Polymerized hemoglobin—hemoglobin that has been chemically changed; when added to solutions, polymerized hemoglobin gives concentrated hemoglobin; used only when other blood products are not available

Polypharmacy—concurrent use of a large number of drugs, a condition that increases the likelihood of unwanted side effects and adverse drug-drug interactions

Port—doorway, opening

Potency—power

Powder—an aggregation of fine particles of one or more substances that may be passed through fine meshes; a dose of such a powder, contained in a paper

PPD—purified protein derivative; substance used in an intradermal test for tuberculosis

Prime—a number that cannot be divided evenly, except by the number 1

Priming—removing air from an intravenous line by allowing fluid to flow through it

Progestin—corpus luteum hormone that prepares the endometrium for implantation of the fertilized ovum; a term used to cover a large group of synthetic drugs that have a progesterone-like effect on the uterus

Prolactin—hormone produced by the anterior pituitary gland; in humans, in association with estrogen and progesterone, stimulates breast development and the formation of milk during pregnancy

Proper—in mathematics, a fraction in which the numerator is smaller than the denominator

Prophylactic—pertaining to prevention

Proportion—in mathematics, a comparison or relationship of numbers

Proprietary name—name given to a medication by the pharmaceutical company that developed it; trade name

Prostaglandins—any of a large group of biologically active, carbon-20, unsaturated fatty acids produced by the metabolism of arachidonic acid through the cyclooxygenase pathway

Protective cap—a top devised to maintain sterility or to prevent access by children

Psoriasis—chronic skin disorder in which red, scaly plaques with sharply defined borders appear on the body surface

Psychotropic—affecting the mind, emotions, or behaviors

Q

q.i.d.—four times per day

Quotient—answer in a division problem

R

Random—in research, a method used to assign subjects to experimental groups without introducing bias into a study

Ratio—relation in degree or number between two things

Reconstitute—return a substance previously altered for preservation or storage to its original state

Releasing factor—relieves restraint

Replacement—restoration of something depleted or missing

Respiration—interchange of gases

Rheumatoid arthritis—acute and chronic conditions marked by inflammation, muscle soreness and stiffness, and pain in joints and associated structures

Rickets—disease of bone formation in children, most commonly the result of vitamin D deficiency; marked by inadequate mineralization of developing cartilage and newly formed bone; causes abnormalities in the shape, structure, and strength of the skeleton

Rosacea—chronic eruption, usually localized in the middle of the face, in which papules and pustules appear on a flushed or red background

Rx—means take; prescription; therapy

S

s̄—without

Saline—salty solution

Salves—ointments; viscous, semi-solid vehicles to apply medications to the skin

SC—under the skin, subcutaneous

Scored—marked with a line to facilitate taking a half of a tablet

Seborrhea—disease of the sebaceous glands marked by an increase in the amount; often an alteration of the quality of the fats secreted by the sebaceous glands

Shock—clinical syndrome marked by inadequate perfusion and oxygenation of cells, tissues, and organs; usually a result of marginal or markedly lowered blood pressure

SIADH—syndrome of inappropriate antidiuretic hormone

Signature—part of the prescription; giving instructions to the patient

Smoking cessation—stopping smoking

Solutions—liquids containing dissolved substances

Somatic—pertaining to the body

Somatotropin—human growth hormone

Spacers—attachments to inhalers that promote easier hand-holding; save the medication in a chamber for entry during the next inhalation

Spastic—afflicted with spasms

Spike—in relation to IV therapy, opening an IV bag with a sharp device to allow fluid to flow out of the bag

ss—half

SSRIs—selective serotonin reuptake inhibitors; drugs used to treat depression related to low amounts of the neurotransmitter serotonin

Standing orders—orders that a prescriber leaves to administer certain medications automatically, usually in the prescriber's absence

Stat orders—orders to be executed immediately

Status asthmaticus—persistent and intractable asthma

Status epilepticus—continuous seizure activity without a pause

STD—sexually transmitted disease

Street name—slang name for a drug; drug name used on the "street"

Subcutaneous—under the skin

Sublingual—under the tongue

Subscription—the part of the prescription that contains directions for compounding ingredients

Substance abuse—misuse or improper use of medications

Subtraction—removing one amount from another

Succinimides—class of antiseizure drugs that delay calcium moving over the neurons

Sum—answer to an addition problem

Superinfection—new infection caused by an organism different from that which caused the initial infection

Superscription—beginning of the prescription, denoted by the symbol R_x, meaning take

Suppository—semi-solid substance for introduction into the rectum, vagina, or urethra, where it dissolves

Suspension—state of a solid when its particles are mixed with, but not dissolved in, a fluid or another solid

Sympathetic—division of the autonomic nervous system that produces a general rather than a specific effect and prepares the body to cope with stressful circumstances

Synapse—space between the junction of two neurons

Synergism—action of two or more agents or organs working with each other

Synthetic—related to or made by synthesis; artificially prepared

Syrup—concentrated solution of sugar in water to which specific medicinal substances are usually added

Systemic—concerning a system or organized according to a system, pertaining to the whole body rather than one of its parts

T

t—teaspoon

T—tablespoon

T$_3$—triiodothyronine, a thyroid hormone

T$_4$—thyroxine, a thyroid hormone

Tab.—abbreviation for tablet

Tablets—a small, disk-like mass of medicinal powder

Telephone orders—orders received from a prescriber over the telephone

Tension headache—head pain that feels like pressure on the skull

Teratogenic—literally, creating a monster; anything that adversely affects normal cellular development in the embryo or fetus

Therapeutic dose—dose that causes the medication to promote wellness

Thrombus—blood clot that adheres to the wall of a blood vessel or organ

t.i.d.—three times daily

Timed-release—medication that is released over a period of time to allow continuous treatment

Tinnitus—subjective ringing, buzzing, tinkling, or hissing sound in the ear

Tip—part of the syringe where the needle is attached

Titer—standard of strength per volume of a volumetric test solution

TNF—tumor necrosis factor

Tocolytic—capable of relieving uterine contraction by reducing the excitability of myometrial muscle

Tolerance—capability to endure a large amount of a substance without an adverse effect and show decreased sensitivity to subsequent doses of the same substance

Tonometer—instrument for measuring tension or pressure

Topical—pertaining to a definite surface area; local

Toxic—pertaining to, resembling, or caused by poison

Toxin—poisonous substance

TPN—total parenteral nutrition; the patient would get nutrition only through this parenteral route

Trade name—name given to a drug by the pharmaceutical company that developed it; brand name

Transdermal—method of delivering medicine by placing it in a special gel-like matrix that is applied to the skin

Troches—solid, discoid, or cylindrical masses consisting of chiefly medicinal powder, sugar, and mucilage

TSH—thyroid-stimulating hormone

Tuberculin—a solution of purified protein derivative of tuberculosis that is injected intradermally to determine the presence of a tuberculosis infection

U

Units—a determined amount; insulin is usually measured in units

Urticaria—multiple swollen raised areas on the skin that are intensely itchy and last up to 24 hours

USP/DI—published by the United States Pharmacopeial Convention, Inc., in Rockville, MD. The first of this two-volume set is *Drug Information for Health Providers* and is written primarily for prescribers. The other volume, *Advice for the Patient*, is written in language that is easy for patients to understand. It gives tips for proper use of drugs and includes a pronunciation key

USP/NF—United States Pharmacopeia/National Formulary

V

Vasopressin—causes contraction of smooth muscle, including blood vessels

Vastus lateralis—muscle on the side of the thigh; usual site for injecting medication in infants

Ventrogluteal—site for injecting medication, wherein patient is lying on the side and the gluteus maximus muscle is accessed

Verbal orders—orders given by a prescriber that are not written

Verruca(e)—wart(s)

Vertigo—sensation of moving around in space or having objects move about the person

Vial—small bottle for medicine or chemicals

Viscous—sticky, gummy, gelatinous

Vitamins—an accessory, but vital, nutrient that serves as a coenzyme or cofactor in an essential metabolic process

VLDL—very low density lipid

W

Wheal—more or less round, temporary elevation of the skin, white in the center with a pale red periphery, accompanied by itching

Whole blood—all blood components, including plasma

Whole numbers—numbers that have no fractional component, except to be placed over 1

Withdrawal—cessation of administration of a drug, especially a narcotic; cessation of ingesting alcohol to which the individual has become either physiologically or psychologically addicted

Z

Z-track—intramuscular injection route that displaces the skin before entry in order to decrease skin staining

Index

Note: Page numbers followed by f refer to figures; page numbers followed by t refer to tables; page numbers followed by b refer to boxes.